THE PATIENT'S GUIDE TO SURGERY

THE PATIENT'S GUIDE TO SURGERY

How to Make the Best of Your Operation

by

Lawrence Galton

With an introduction by

Walter L. Mersheimer, M.D., F.A.C.S.
Professor and Chairman,
Department of Surgery, New York Medical College
Director of Surgery,
Flower-Fifth Avenue, Metropolitan, and Bird S.
Coler Hospitals, New York, N.Y.

HEARST BOOKS • NEW YORK

Copyright © 1976 by Lawrence Galton.
Published by arrangement with the author.

Manufactured in the United States of America.

All rights reserved.

ISBN 0-87851-400-7

Library of Congress Catalog Number 76-2339

Contents

PART ONE

v

PART TWO

Foreword

"How much should the patient be told?" is a question physicians are constantly confronted with. One old practitioner's answer was: "The patient has no more right to all the knowledge in my head than he has to all the medicine in my saddlebags." The doctor prescribed the dose of information as well as the dose of therapeutics. As dogmatic as that attitude seems today, at least it recognizes the important difference between knowing something and understanding it. What a patient knows without understanding may do more harm than good. Too little information breeds uncertainty and often needless fear. Too much irrelevant information, or worse, misinformation, can be equally disturbing and even dangerous to the patient.

New findings in medicine are now so widely published that physicians are sometimes challenged by patients with newspaper clippings about new treatments and procedures that are still under experimentation and far from ready for general use. Drugs, too, are now so easily available that self-medication is a common danger. Some conditions respond to medical treatment; others require the skill of surgeons to correct.

Today, the best answer to "How much should the patient be told?" is "As much as he can absorb." Such instruction, however, may require more time than the doctor can well afford, or be expressed in such technical terminology that it is of little practical help. Too often, the brevity of the dialogue results in a hiatus between doctor and patient rather than a closer bond.

In THE PATIENTS GUIDE TO SURGERY Lawrence

Galton has taken a giant step toward improving the physician/patient relationship. An experienced medical writer broadly knowledgeable in many areas of medicine, he bridges the information and understanding gap.

To an individual and his family, an operation may appear to be a severe crisis, if not a catastrophe. It signals, first of all, a condition that will not improve without surgery. Second, it involves an undeniable risk, though not nearly as great a risk as many imagine. Third, it usually creates a financial strain, both in the cost of the operation and hospitalization, and in time lost from work. At the very least, it is an alien and unpleasant experience that no one can meet with complete equanimity.

All this Mr. Galton looks at with the patient, helping him to know the worst and thereby to endure it, and to know the best and to gain confidence from that knowledge. With specific chapters on common operations in all areas of the body, he helps the patient prepare for almost any operation he may undergo. It is not the author's purpose to include every operation, nor all the possible variations of the over 150 operations that he does discuss. He does aim to provide the information essential to understanding for those many millions of individuals who for themselves or through those close to them will be facing surgery some time during their lives. He includes enough detail to give an accurate picture of the specific ailment, medical and surgical treatment, postoperative care and convalescence, and avoids the clinical detail that may confuse the layman. The compendium is laudably complete.

If this were the entire value of the book, it would be well worthwhile. But the aim is not only to present useful information clearly. Armed with knowledge, the patient is easier in mind and thus can contribute to his own rapid recovery. To make the patient an intelligent participant in the entire process is fundamental to the author's purpose. Offering him counsel in the selection of a surgeon in the first place, Mr. Galton points out that an operation need not be accepted merely because a physician recommends it. The decision is up to the patient, who may do well to seek more than one professional opinion. The patient has a right to ask questions, both about the operation and about its costs and consequences, and the good physician welcomes such questions. The recently published Patient's Bill of Rights is quoted in full.

Equally valuable are the sections that prepare the patient for the operation, telling him just what he can expect to encounter in the unfamiliar world of the hospital. He is frankly told to expect some pain, fatigue, and depression, and neither to fear them unduly nor to suffer stoically without reporting anything that seems to be wrong. Do not judge the seriousness of the operation by its length, Mr. Galton wisely warns, and the same is true of the period of convalescence.

Parents will be grateful for the chapter on "Helping a Child Through Surgery," which reviews methods now in use for preparing the child mentally and suggests how parents may use similar methods.

In many ways, this book fills a long-felt need. It belongs in family as well as school and municipal libraries, where it will be available with information to allay the fear that springs from ignorance.

RICHARD O. BULLIS, M.D., F.A.C.S.

FRANCIS E. BROWNE, M.D., F.A.C.S.

Introcuction

This is a book for the concerned and deeply curious. And anyone facing surgery is that.

Succinctly and clearly, it provides information that patients and their families need, want, and do best to have, but that is not always available when needed. Not that most doctors do not wish to provide it, but their opportunities for doing so most effectively are often limited. It isn't only that there are limits on time with patients. All of us can absorb only so much at one sitting about something that is strange and alien. And much about surgery—the operating room, surgical procedures, the hospital, even the body itself in any meaningful detail—is, for most of us, unfamiliar ground.

Patients and their families have many questions. They may ask some of the surgeon and receive answers. But many others occur to them—after the consultation and in the hours or days before the operation and afterward as well. What exactly *will* happen? What *has* happened? What *is* happening now, why, and is it normal . . . to be expected . . . no cause for worry?

This book does a great service by answering such questions and anticipating many others.

It does another service by providing background about tools, techniques, and practices of surgery that also help to illuminate the immediate operation and what is to be expected.

And it does further service by discussing when surgery is needed and when it may not be, and by providing suggestions that can help patients reassure themselves.

A patient who is informed, prepared, and understanding is better able to cope with the prospect of surgery and to cooperate before and after it. As a result, he or she has a greatly increased likelihood of coming through it more smoothly, experiencing less mental anguish, recovering more rapidly, and obtaining greater total benefit. To all of this, this book can contribute. And I am very pleased that it is now available.

WALTER L. MERSHEIMER

Professor and Chairman,
Department of Surgery, New York Medical College
Director of Surgery,
Flower-Fifth Avenue, Metropolitan, and Bird
S. Coler Hospitals, New York, N. Y.

Author's Preface

If this book serves its purpose well, it will be because of the help I have had from many scores of distinguished physicians and surgeons—far too many to list here—who over the years have taken the time to discuss with me at length the medical and surgical aspects of our most common health problems. I owe gratitude, too, to many of those surgeons for allowing me to watch them at work and for explaining in detail everything they did and why, and very special thanks to Drs. Francis E. and Lawrence Browne for their intensive help and advice.

I am indebted, too, to many hundreds of others with whom I have not had the opportunity to talk personally but of whose research and clinical reports in the latest medical and surgical literature I have made extensive use.

The Library of the New York Academy of Medicine has been most helpful in providing access to scores of medical and surgical journals in which the latest research and clinical reports are published.

Additionally, I have had the use of many varied bulletins, reports, and other publications of many private and public agencies—most notably among them, the American Cancer Society, American College of Surgeons, American Heart Association, American Geriatrics Society, American Medical Association, National Foundation, and National Institutes of Health.

Not least of all, I am indebted to the many patients, not limited to family and friends, who have talked to me about their doubts and anxieties, questions they have had about their operations which were left unanswered and sometimes even unasked, and what, looking back, they feel it would have been most helpful for them to know.

Making the Best of Your Operation

How to Use This Book

You've just been told that you or someone close to you will need an operation. Or perhaps you suspect that one may be necessary for yourself or a loved one.

Your first interest is likely to be: What is this operation? What does the surgeon actually do? What happens before, during, and after? Is the procedure painful? Is it crippling in any way? What may it "take out" of one in addition to any tissue that may be removed, repaired, or replaced?

You want information about the specific operation of immediate interest to *you* rather than generalizations about surgery.

And this is what comes very early in this book. Unless yours is a very rare operation, you will find facts about it in Part One: about the procedure itself, type of anesthesia, special preoperative care (if any) needed, postoperative care and recovery, success rate, limitations (if any) afterward. If more than one type of operative procedure is available, the alternatives are discussed.

You will also find in the discussion information about the nature of your problem, how it could have developed, what its causes (if known) may be, and what medical treatment may be helpful and may be tried before surgery is considered. You will gain insights into what determines when surgery is clearly necessary or advisable. And to reassure yourself, you may wish to discuss the necessity or advisability with your surgeon. You have the right to such a discussion.

1

In fact, you have many rights and needs. What can be called, without exaggeration, *near-miracles* are accomplished daily in operating rooms today. The technical prowess—based on increases in fundamental knowledge about the body, advances in surgical tools and methods, more and more intensive training of surgeons—is great. But if a combination of expert surgeon, competent supporting personnel, and first-rate hospital facilities is essential for the best outcome, so, to a great extent, is an informed, knowledgeable and psychologically prepared patient.

In addition to knowing about your own operation, you can benefit from an understanding of surgery, including its origins, development, and latest advances; from pertinent background material about hospital procedures, organization, and hierarchy; from guidelines that can help you make an intelligent choice of surgeon and hospital; from information about fees; and from knowing about rights you have and can exercise in the hospital.

And so this book, after discussing specific operations, goes on to cover these other aspects of surgery in Part Two. There, too, once you have done what is natural—which is, first of all, to look up the operation of immediate concern to you—you will find additional information on pre- and postoperative care, anesthesia, radiology, laboratory tests, and other related matters.

Preparing and Helping Yourself Psychologically

You probably realized it long ago: Almost any professional encounter with a physician may involve some degree of emotional stress. Even the healthiest person undergoing a routine checkup may experience apprehension until the examination is over and all is found to be well.

Certainly, when you are to undergo surgery, some degree of apprehension is to be expected. While each of us may react in his own way to an impending operation, we all experience some anxiety and fear—of the unknown, of possible dire consequences, of possible disability, of the future. Even aside from the operation itself, the hospital world is an alien one about which most of us know very little. All of us need reassurance. And much reassurance can come from understanding. The more you know about your operation, its nature, the necessity for it, the outlook for its success, and about other pertinent matters you will find in Parts One and Two of this book, the less the emotional stress is likely to be.

Hopefully, the information you find in this book can make a contribution. But it is not likely that any book can be all-sufficient. If you need further information and help, you can obtain them.

Do avoid certain common errors. One is heroic pretension. You gain nothing by acting as though your operation is too trivial to take notice of and by trying to pretend that when you wake up afterward all will be fine. All *is* likely to be fine—but not necessarily immediately. Unless you are realistically prepared for some degree of temporary discomfort and perhaps for some temporary adjustments you must make, you may find these unnecessarily stressful.

Another common error is to be unduly frightened and to *stay* unduly frightened. There is no shame in having fears, but it is a shame to let them continue and to be stressed by them when they can be greatly ameliorated or even eliminated.

Nor should you rely on having well-meaning friends "fill you in" on the "facts" even if they may have had similar operations. Their recitals, although not necessarily meant to be, tend to be too dramatic and to lack accuracy.

Help from your surgeon

However apocryphal the story may seem, it is a true one: An educated, sophisticated man was told by a surgeon that he would need a herniorrhaphy—just that, and no more. He delayed for weeks before seeking advice from his internist because he felt "unable to accept the loss of my testes." Such fear is common among men scheduled for herniorrhaphy because examination for the condition involves palpation of the scrotal area. When he was reassured by the internist that removal of the testes was not part of the operation, which would be devoted solely to repairing the hernia, he was able to return to the surgeon and undergo uneventful surgery.

The case illustrates two problems. The first is that surgeons, like other doctors, sometimes take too much for granted, and may assume that patients understand at least some technical terms or even that they have no specific worries. As a result, they may fail to provide adequate explanations unless asked for them.

The second problem is that many patients hesitate to ask, and may even avoid asking, for explanations, especially from a doctor they may not have known for a long time, which is likely to be the case with a surgeon. They may hesitate to ask out of awe or embarrassment, feeling—wrongly—that asking would indicate undue ignorance.

As a surgical patient, you are a consumer of surgical service. As a consumer of any service, you have a right to ask questions that seem important to you. You would probably not hesitate at all to ask any questions that occur to you when you call in a repairman to fix a TV set. "Fixing" you is even more vital to you, and your reasonable questions are expected by surgeons as part of their professional business. More and more surgeons encourage and try to anticipate them as much as possible.

Not that, with the best will, they always succeed. For physician and patient, concepts of illness and treatment differ. The physician is accustomed to dealing with bodily functions in anatomic and other scientific terms; the patient, of course, is not. Yet there is a natural tendency for the doctor to assume that patients share his information—particularly intelligent, educated patients. .

The assumption often extends to all aspects of surgery and is the reason for the "beautiful incision" reaction, for example. The surgeon remarks approvingly how good a healing surgical wound looks—but the patient, viewing his cut skin, which may still be full of thread and strange-looking drains, may have an eerie feeling of unreality and is unable to reconcile what he sees and what the surgeon says because the surgeon's experience provides different information from his.

Similarly, as technological developments add more and more complex equipment around hospital beds, the hospital staff comes to look upon the equipment as a natural part of the sickroom, which needs no explanation, but the patient doesn't see it that way and may find it frightening. Quite likely, in your own work, you routinely use some procedures and equipment that may seem mysterious to others—and, unless reminded, you may assume that what you use is obvious enough.

Don't hesitate, as a surgical patient, to ask questions that seem important to you if surgeon and hospital staff fail to anticipate them. The chances are the failing is human —forgetful, not deliberate.

Beliefs and fantasies

Patients often bring to surgery feelings and beliefs that can be stressful—and if you can identify any that you have, you'll benefit by discussing them with your surgeon.

Perhaps, for example, like many patients, you have established in your own mind a hierarchy of importance for various body organs. In a nonsense verse, Gelett Burgess wrote:

I'd rather have Fingers than Toes,
I'd rather have Eyes than a Nose;
And as for my Hair
I'm glad it's all there,
I'll be awfully sad when it goes.

For most people, according to the studies of Dr. Richard S. Blacher of Mount Sinai Hospital and School of Medicine, New York City, the kidneys rank higher in the organ hierarchy than does the pancreas, yet the pancreas is a vital organ. An adult man undergoing circumcision may, because of the body part involved, suffer greater anguish than if he were undergoing removal of the spleen, although the spleen operation is a more major one.

Sometimes individual background determines the anxiety with which an operation is viewed. Among patients studied by Dr. Blacher, for example, was a young woman with a long history of a duodenal ulcer for whom surgery was recommended finally. But at the last moment, she became panicky and refused the operation. It was only when it was discovered that her father had died after surgery for stomach cancer that she could be reassured about the vast difference between her condition and her father's, and she then agreed to the necessary operation. The fact was that the young woman had originally given the cause of her father's death not as stomach cancer but leukemia, in an unsuccessful effort to dissociate her own illness from his. Not until she let the real reason for her panic be known could she be helped.

Some patients come to surgery anxious because they see illness as a punishment for sins. Usually, this is obscured although there is a hint of it in such expressions as "What have I done to deserve this?"

As a result of his findings, Dr. Blacher has urged doctors to give careful consideration to surgery from the patient's viewpoint. "The physician," he points out, "because he is reality-oriented, may lose sight of the fact that the person who is ill views his body and his illness as fantasy." If the patient cannot bridge the gap, "the physician must be aware that what he says and does may not be quite understood: and he must be alert to possible breakdowns in communication, since these may hinder an otherwise successful procedure. . . . Especially important for the physician to keep in mind is the fact that his natural habitat is not that of the patient. The patient comes into the physician's bailiwick as an alien into a threatening land, and he is frightened by the landmarks that the physician barely notices. The physician's awareness of this anxiety will go far toward making the patient's sojourn an easier one." If you have what you think may be irrational fears, don't hesitate to discuss them. It has become apparent that they are to be found among surgical patients of all educational, social, and economic backgrounds and are, if anything, more prevalent among the educated than the uneducated.

Added help

Apart from concerns about your condition and the outcome of your surgery, why shouldn't you experience anxiety when, as a surgical patient, you must relinquish for a time your usual social role, tolerate some separation from family and friends, accept a relatively passive-dependent position and place a high level of trust in others, many of whom are strangers; and, to boot, must experience the petty annoyances of hospital routines and regulations!

If you seem to be free from all anxiety, you may only be using denial. It's best to drop the denial, face your anxiety, and talk it out. And if the surgeon cannot help by providing information, clarification and reassurance, psychiatric counseling may be of great value. It need not be extended counseling; even a single session may work wonders. Some hospitals maintain liaison psychiatric services for this purpose and the surgeon may call upon such a service to supplement his efforts. If such a service is not available, he may suggest a visit or two for private psychiatric counseling. This is not often necessary, but when it is, it can contribute greatly to smoother surgery and convalescence.

A healthy attitude of mind is important. Even if you thought, rightly, when you entered the hospital that yours was a good attitude, it is possible for some weakening to occur. If that happens, by all means face the fact and realize there is nothing shameful about it. Discuss your feelings with your doctor and, if it seems advisable, with a psychiatrist.

Helping a Child Through Surgery

There is much you can do as a parent to prepare your child for surgery and to ease his way through it.

Avoiding some errors

A child can't be expected to understand automatically the need for hospitalization. If he is inadequately prepared for the hospital experience, he can't understand the need for injections and for diagnostic and other procedures, all of which are alien to him and may cause some degree of discomfort. If inadequately prepared, his tendency may be to think he is being punished by being sent to a hospital.

Some parents make the mistake of being afraid to tell their children the truth about their hospitalization for fear that they will become unmanageable or will "go to pieces." And some, not clear themselves about what is going to happen, try to avoid explanations or make incorrect ones.

Explaining

The child's surgeon may provide an explanation for the child about why the operation is to be performed, how it will help to make him feel better, what will happen before, during, and after the operation.

You can cooperate closely with the surgeon. Note carefully what he tells the child. You may need to repeat his explanation later, perhaps several times. You can learn the facts about the operation and the preoperative and postoperative measures that may be used, and the course of recovery generally to be expected.

There is no need to go into great detail with a child. Do try to answer his questions truthfully. If you don't know the answer to a question, don't hesitate to say that you don't know rather than risk shattering the child's faith by fibbing. If the question seems important to the child, the surgeon may think it wise to give you the answer to pass on to the child.

While you cannot expect to erase completely a child's fears, by giving him truthful answers and a representative overall picture, you can reduce those fears and help him face them.

Another thing: the chances are very good that the child's morale will be higher the more gentle, loving, and sympathetic you are without being tearful and despondent— and to avoid being tearful and despondent, you yourself need to find out as much as possible about the operation and its likelihood of success.

A positive attitude on your part can do much to help the child. Children are often highly sensitive to suggestion. One indication of this is the fact that many anesthesiologists have found it helpful to give beneficial suggestions to a child just before putting him to sleep. The anesthesiologist may tell a child: "You will have some discomfort but not real pain when you wake up." The quiet remark seems to carry over when the child wakes up, and there is often a marked reduction in the number and amount of sedatives and pain-relievers the child needs postoperatively.

Keep any promise you make to the child. If you promise that you will be in his room when he returns from the operation, do be there. He may feel let down and even frightened if you aren't present.

Visiting the child

Make your visits cheerful. That may sound obvious. But some parents find it difficult not to bring worries and concerns with them from home.

In some hospitals, parents are given opportunities to participate in caring for hospitalized children. The opportunities may be limited to extended visiting hours or overnight stays with a child who has had a minor operation. In some cases, as at the University of Kentucky Medical Center and Indiana University's Riley Hospital for Children, there are parent-care units where a parent, given instructions as needed by a nurse-specialist or other staff member, rooms with a child and cares for him after surgery.

Children tend to bounce back after surgery and to recuperate more quickly than adults. Still, a child may need reassurance that all is going well, that he is progressing and recovering. Surgeons recognize this and offer reassurance, sometimes even going to the extent of deliberately reducing the size of bandages from day to day as visible "proof" that the child is getting better and better.

A complication may occur. More often that not, it isn't serious, but if there is any undue parental anxiety about it, a child, quick to sense the anxiety, may become despondent. If a complication should occur, it can be important for you to reassure yourself about it, accept it matter-of-factly, and display no anxiety.

Going home

When the child is ready to go home, you should, of course, get complete instructions from the doctor—on diet, medication, any temporary limitations on the child, how much activity he can be permitted.

Many parents tend to worry and be overly protective after a child has had an operation and are fearful of allowing the child to engage in activities the doctor indicates are within his capabilities. For a while, you may have to make a conscious effort to stop worrying excessively and stop being overprotective. It is well worth the effort, for the child needs to take advantage of all the opportunities open to him to be active, regain strength, and grow and develop. Activity within allowable limits is good for him—mentally as well as physically.

Years ago, when there was much less understanding of the needs of children undergoing surgery, some children bore not only the physical scars of operation, which in due course became less apparent and even virtually invisible, but also psychological scars that lingered.

Surgery for children today is far safer. Operations for conditions beyond hope not many years ago are now being done effectively and safely. Children are recovering swiftly from even the most complex procedures, including open-heart surgery, to become healthier than they ever were before. And they are coming through operations psychologically sounder as well.

PART ONE

Stomach and Intestinal Operations

Stomach and intestinal operations are relatively common and the success rate for them is high. We are endowed with an efficient and generously sized digestive system. It can become disordered and very often the disorders are readily treatable by medical means. When medical measures are inadequate and surgery becomes necessary, the system is ample enough so that even extensive operative remodeling can be carried out; if need be, large sections of diseased tissue can be removed, and life can go on and very often go on well.

A View of the System

The digestive tract is a 30-foot tube in which food is subjected to both mechanical and chemical changes.

Food is first chewed and mixed with saliva—and thus softened and lubricated—in the mouth. It then enters the esophagus, or gullet, which carries it downward a distance of nine or ten inches to the stomach.

The stomach

The stomach is a baglike structure about one foot long and six inches wide that can hold about 2½ pints. It has layers of muscles that contract in different directions. As a result, the stomach can squeeze, twist and churn food to break it up mechanically and to mix it with digestive secretions. The stomach's thick mucous lining acts like a chemical

15

factory. It produces hydrochloric acid to help in the digestion of proteins and various enzymes to split up fats and other food substances.

While fluids, including water and various beverages, can pass through the stomach in minutes, solid foods spend from three to six hours there. Sugars and starches pass through most quickly; proteins take longer; fats require the most time.

When once-solid foods leave the stomach, they are in the form of a semifluid called *chyme*.

Where esophagus and stomach join, there is a ringlike muscular valve, the cardiac sphincter. And where the stomach at its lower end joins the small intestine, there is a similar valve, the pyloric sphincter. During digestive activity in the stomach, both valves are closed. When chyme is ready to move on to the intestine, the pyloric sphincter opens and closes several times to allow the stomach to empty gradually.

Small intestine

The small intestine, into which the stomach empties, is a coiled tube about one inch in diameter and twenty feet long. It has three parts: the first, the duodenum, is about twelve inches long; the second, the jejunum, extends about eight feet; the third and longest section, about twelve feet, is called the ileum.

When chyme enters the duodenum, more digestive juices are added—by the intestine itself and also by the pancreas and liver, which empty secretions into the duodenum. Enzymes in pancreatic fluid break proteins down into their amino acid constituents, complex sugar molecules into simple sugars, and fats into fatty acids. Bile, coming either from the liver where it is produced or from the gallbladder where it is stored, emulsifies (converts) fatty foods so they become easier to absorb and also reduces the acidity of chyme.

Only a little absorption takes place in the stomach. The bulk of it occurs in the small intestine, which has millions of little fingerlike projections called villi that do the absorbing.

After a meal has spent several hours in the stomach followed by about five hours in the small intestine, what remains to enter the large intestine is a combination of indigestible waste and water.

Large intestine

Also known as the colon, the large intestine is two to three inches in diameter and about five feet long. The first portion ascends along the right side of the body; then comes a curved section which is located under the liver on the right side of the body; next, there is a transverse section across the top of the abdomen. After a sharp curve, the colon descends on the left side of the body. There is also an S-shaped section, called the sigmoid colon, which comes next and ends in the rectum, where waste is held by a sphincter muscle until it is discharged through the anal opening.

It takes twelve to twenty-four hours for waste to pass through the complete length of the colon. The colon has no digestive function but does serve the vital purpose of absorbing water from the material passing through so it is taken into the blood to maintain the body's fluid balance.

On the average, about twelve ounces of chyme may enter the colon daily and from this, after the water is removed, will be derived about four ounces of feces.

Peptic Ulcer (Ulcer of the Stomach or Duodenum)

An ulcer is an open sore, a break in a surface. While it can occur anywhere in the body, including the tongue and skin, most people think of ulcer in connection with the stomach, or duodenum. More specifically, a stomach or duodenal ulcer is known as a peptic ulcer; the word peptic comes from pepsin, an enzyme in stomach juice that helps digest protein.

Peptic ulcer is the most common organic gastrointestinal disease in the United States. It affects at least 10 million people (according to some estimates, 20 million). It is most common in men between the ages of twenty and sixty, and occurs in the duodenum four times more often than in the stomach. A peptic ulcer may vary in size from a barely visible sore to a crater as wide as an inch or more and as deep as half an inch.

Symptoms

If you have the typical symptom of a peptic ulcer, you experience a gnawing or burning pain in the upper abdomen, which is relieved by eating. You may be awakened at night by pain. For some weeks before this characteristic warning sign, you may have experienced frequent heartburn and belching. In some cases, there may also be a regular occurrence of "water brash," which is the feeling experienced when stomach juice regurgitates upward and mixes with saliva. Sometimes nausea and vomiting occur.

Diagnosis

A peptic ulcer can be diagnosed by X-ray and fluoroscopic studies of the stomach and duodenum after barium has been swallowed. The barium helps to visualize the ulcer. In some instances, a special lighted tube or gastroscope may be inserted to permit observation of the ulcerated area. Removal of gastric juice for analysis may also be used for diagnosis. In most ulcer patients, gastric juice flow is increased and the fluid has more than the usual acidity.

Causes

How did you get your ulcer? Normally, when food is eaten, messages are sent through a nerve, the vagus, to stimulate cells in the soft inner coating of the stomach to secrete juices which aid digestion. The juices contain hydrochloric acid and enzymes. After a few hours, the secretions are turned off as the stomach empties. Normally, too, at the times when no food is taken and the stomach is at rest, no juices are secreted. And, at all times, the coating of mucus in the stomach serves to keep the juices from digesting the stomach itself.

Ulcer may develop if, for any reason, there is an excess secretion of juices or if the mucus coating is altered so that it becomes less viscid and protective. Thus, excessive nerve impulses that keep the stomach secreting juices at virtually all times may lead to ulcer formation. Some ulcer patients have two to four times as many juice-secreting cells as normal, either because of hereditary influences or because excessive nerve impulses have led to extra cell formation. Sometimes diseases elsewhere—for example, diabetes or chronic lung disease—may stimulate the vagus nerve which in turn stimulates excessive stomach juice production. Acid formation also is increased with smoking and drinking alcohol. Nervousness, tension, rage, and fear may lead to excessive acid production. The mucus coating of the stomach may also be detrimentally affected by various agents, including alcohol, aspirin and cortisone-like drugs.

Medical treatment

For most ulcer patients, medical treatment is effective. Medication and diet give the body a chance to heal the ulcer much as it would heal an open sore elsewhere, provided there is no continued irritation. The aim of medical management is to reduce or eliminate the irritation by reducing the amount of acid formed, neutralizing already present acid, and calming the patient if necessary. Certain drugs called anticholinergics may be used to partially block vagus nerve stimulation of stomach secretions. Antacids may be employed to neutralize excess acids.

Once, special "bland" diets were almost universally accepted by physicians as of prime importance for ulcer patients. But their necessity is no longer taken for granted. The American Heart Association has pointed out that diets rich in cream and milk may be potentially harmful over long periods because such diets may affect blood fat levels and possibly influence development of atherosclerosis, or the building up of clogging deposits in arteries, that may lead to heart attacks and strokes. The American Dietetic Association recently published a position paper on the bland diet and concluded it has no known advantage over regular diets. More and more physicians now advise ulcer patients that eating regular meals to help buffer stomach acids is probably more important than the contents of the meals.

Frequently with such treatment, combining regular eating with antacids and other medication, symptoms disappear within a week or so. But to ensure complete healing of an ulcer, the treatment should be continued for four to five weeks.

When surgery may be needed

There are several reasons why surgery may sometimes become necessary.

For one thing, despite persistent medical treatment, some ulcers stubbornly refuse to heal and may continue to cause pain, which may go beyond the merely annoying and seriously interfere with the patient's life and work.

If a resistant, nonhealing ulcer is in the stomach rather than in the duodenum, there is an added possible reason for surgery. A true ulcer does not change to cancer no matter how many years it persists or how often it may heal and recur. But when a supposed ulcer of the stomach does not heal readily, it could be a cancer masquerading as an ulcer. And while special X-rays and other studies may solve the problem of diagnosis, of distinguishing ulcer from cancer, sometimes accurate diagnosis can be made only by examination of the area through surgery. Duodenal ulcers, however, are almost never cancerous.

Ulcer complications sometimes occur. When they do, surgery may be required.

Perforation. An ulcer may bore through the wall of the stomach or duodenum. Stomach juices may then spill into the sensitive abdominal cavity. The pain is severe and inflammation (peritonitis) also develops. Immediate surgical repair is indicated.

Bleeding. An ulcer may hemorrhage. This may occur when a nearby blood vessel is eroded, its wall eaten away. The amount of bleeding will depend on both the size of the vessel and of the hole in it. In some cases, the bleeding may become apparent through the vomiting of bloody or dark brown stomach contents or by passage of stools that look black and tarry or may even be visibly bloody. In other cases, bleeding may not be apparent to the patient; the only symptoms may be weakness, dizziness, and sometimes fainting. Medical management—including stomach washout and blood transfusions to replace the lost blood—may help; in some cases, the bleeding stops. But if the bleeding continues, an immediate operation may be performed to stop it.

Obstruction. An ulcer may lead to obstruction when it produces inflammation or scarring at the outlet of the stomach or in the narrow duodenum. Symptoms may include vomiting of food and foul, gaseous belching. In some cases, in which the obstruction is due to inflammatory swelling, medical treatment may suffice to eliminate it. Other cases require corrective surgery.

Types of operations

There is no one "best" or generally preferred operation for peptic ulcer. Any one of several operations may be used. Results from all have been shown to be satisfactory. The choice of operation will be influenced by many factors: the site and extent of the ulcer; the degree of excess acidity; the presence or absence of severe complications; and the individual surgeon's success experience with particular procedures.

Partial gastrectomy. In this operation, introduced more than half a century ago, half or more of the stomach—the lower portion which contains most of the acid-secreting cells

—is removed. In addition, about an inch or two of the duodenum is taken out. Then the remainder of the stomach is stitched to the small intestine at a point beyond the duodenum. Thereafter, food no longer goes through the sensitive duodenum but moves directly from stomach to intestine. The duodenum is no longer exposed to any acid, yet it still functions to pass along to the intestine the digestive materials it receives from the pancreas and liver.

With half or more of the stomach removed, there is a period of time—perhaps three or four months—when smaller, more frequent meals are eaten to limit food intake at any one time. Thereafter, the stomach distends enough to permit virtually normal eating.

Gastroenterostomy. When the end of the stomach is obstructed by scar tissue and the ulcer is not active, it is possible to relieve the obstruction with a much simpler operation than gastric resection—gastroenterostomy. This procedure entails joining the small intestine to the stomach, using a new opening which makes it possible for food to pass through.

Nerve-cutting. An operation to cut the vagus nerves that influence stomach acid formation is now more than thirty years old and has been used for tens of thousands of patients all over the world. The operation is called vagotomy. With vagotomy, the ulcer itself can be left alone; after the operation, with the markedly reduced acid secretion, the ulcer heals on its own.

The surgeon takes into account another aspect of vagotomy. Once stimuli from the vagus nerves are no longer present, the pylorus muscle at the stomach outlet tightens up. As a result, food passage out of the stomach can be slowed. To avoid this, the surgeon cuts the pylorus muscle while performing the vagotomy, thus enlarging the stomach outlet. The enlarging procedure is called pyloroplasty.

Correcting perforation. When an ulcer perforates, immediate surgery is required. Because the patient is very sick, the operation usually is limited simply to stitching the perforated area and sucking fluid or pus from the abdominal cavity. If further surgery is indicated, it may be delayed, but when possible, one of the procedures already noted is carried out.

Anesthesia

Stomach operations are performed under general anesthesia.

Length of operation

Operating time may vary from two to four or five hours, depending upon the type of operation and any special problems that may be encountered. A gastrectomy takes longest. In no case is speed essential.

Special preparation

A patient who is to have ulcer surgery may be prepared for it by admission to hospital a day or two in advance so the stomach and intestine can be emptied and put to rest. If the stomach has become dilated because of obstruction, a longer time may be needed to deflate the stomach through a tube.

Postoperative care

There will be discomfort—moderate abdominal pain— for a few days after the operation. Usually it is not severe, and most patients bear it well. For the first two or three days, food is withheld and nourishment is given intravenously (through a vein). During surgery and for a few days afterward, a thin plastic tube inserted through the nose is used to keep the stomach empty.

Many surgeons now encourage patients to get out of bed for a short period the day after operation. Usually, the surgical wound heals in one to two weeks, and often the patient may leave the hospital after about ten days.

There will be a scar after healing. To reach the operative site, various types of incisions can be made. Some surgeons use a midline incision from the breastbone to about the navel or a little beyond. Some make an incision to the left or right side of the midline. Others make the incision across the upper part of the abdomen. Usually, in any case, the scar is not markedly disfiguring.

Bathing can be resumed after the wound is healed, usually about two weeks after operation. Generally, the surgeon advises about eating before the patient leaves the hospital. He may suggest a soft diet and small frequent feedings for the first several months. Several weeks after you return home, he may want to see you to check the incision and your general progress.

Some patients develop a "stomach dumping" problem after partial gastrectomy, with symptoms that may include weakness, dizziness, sweating, nausea, and warmth after meals. The symptoms, which arise from the fact that the stomach, after the operation, tends to empty food into the intestine more rapidly than before, may come on shortly after eating and may last up to thirty minutes. Usually they can be minimized or avoided by frequent small, rather than infrequent large, meals; often, lying down for ten or fifteen minutes after a meal that proves to be too large is helpful. Drugs—including those known as anticholinergics, which block certain nerve impulses—may be of value. Generally, dumping symptoms tend to disappear after several months.

Recovery time. After getting home from the hospital, you can usually go out immediately, but it may be about six weeks before you are ready to go back to work full-time.

Success rate. The success rate for ulcer operations is high. The likelihood of coming through an operation is better than 98 percent. The likelihood of complete relief of all symptoms is better than 80 percent—and in those cases in which complete relief is not obtained, the symptoms that do recur are usually mild and fleeting.

Surgery does not completely eliminate the possibility of further ulcer formation. The chance for that is about 10 percent. But it can be minimized further by reasonable diet, by restrained use of alcohol and cigarettes (ideally, smoking should be avoided), and by increased attention to relaxation and to avoidance of excessive nervous tension.

Are you left with any limitations?

Very likely, no—just the reverse. Ulcer surgery is not to be entered into lightly. In some cases, as in perforation, for example, there is no choice; surgery is immediately necessary. In many instances, surgery is indicated when medical management proves to be inadequate. Successful operation may then remove previous limitations. Even when partial stomach removal is involved, there need be no fear that inevitably this must interfere with normal living or affect life span. The remaining stomach accommodates after a time. Nor need there be fear that loss of acid-secreting cells in the removed portion of the stomach must have a debilitating effect. The fact is that as many as 10 percent of all people produce no acid in their stomachs and yet live normally.

SEE ALSO PART II for pertinent information about choice of surgeon, preoperative and postoperative care, anesthesia, tests, costs, and other aspects of your operation.

Pyloric Stenosis (Stomach Obstruction in Infants)

Very early in life, usually by about the second or third week, some infants develop pyloric stenosis, an obstruction at the stomach outlet, the pylorus. The ringlike sphincter muscle at the pylorus, which normally opens to allow food to move from stomach to intestine, become swollen and stiff, unable to contract and relax properly, and emptying of the stomach is impeded. Pyloric stenosis (stenosis means narrowing or contraction) is about three times as frequent in boys as in girls and there is a familial tendency toward it. Its estimated occurrence is about once in every 700 babies.

Symptoms

The initial symptom is vomiting, which may be mild at first but becomes increasingly forceful. Curdled milk shoots out from the mouth and if the condition were allowed to continue, the baby would suffer marked weight loss and depletion of fluids.

Diagnosis

The projectile vomiting itself is a significant clue to diagnosis. Often, too, the overgrown, tight sphincter muscle can be felt as a lump in the upper right portion of the abdomen. X-ray examination, using barium, may be made to confirm the diagnosis.

Cause

Unknown.

Medical treatment

In some cases, an infant with pyloric stenosis responds to antispasmodic drugs which act to relax the sphincter muscle. A trial with such medication may be carried out for a few weeks, and if the infant responds, there may be no need then or later for surgery; recovery may be complete.

But many infants do not respond to medical treatment and after an unsuccessful trial period, delay in correcting the condition surgically can be harmful to the child, producing weight and fluid loss and general deterioration of health.

The operation

The surgical procedure to correct pyloric stenosis is relatively simple and has been used effectively since shortly after the turn of the century.

A small incision, about two inches long, is made in the right upper part of the abdomen. Without need for opening the stomach itself, the surgeon can slit the sphincter muscle fibers. The muscle is left this way; later, on its own, it will grow and reunite and when it does, it will function normally. The infant's abdomen is then closed with sutures or stitches.

Anesthesia

Light gas anesthesia—often ether—is used.

Length of operation

The whole operation is over in less than an hour, often within thirty minutes.

Postoperative care

Within twelve to twenty-four hours after the operation, the infant can be fed and will retain the feedings. No special nursing is usually needed. The child may be home from the hospital in less than a week. The wound is usually healed within seven to ten days, and the child may then be bathed.

Success rate

The operation for pyloric stenosis is not dangerous and is almost certain to cure the condition.

Is the child left with any limitations?

None. There are no aftereffects, for there has been no alteration in food pathway or digestion. Rarely, if ever, does the sphincter muscle become abnormally tight again. The child can expect to lead a completely normal life. The scar is not disfiguring.

SEE ALSO PART II for pertinent information about choice of surgeon, postoperative care, anesthesia, tests, costs, and other aspects of operation.

Appendicitis

The vermiform appendix, as its name suggests (vermiform means wormlike), is a narrow, hollow, blind tube, about three inches long, that looks much like an earthworm. It is located at the juncture of the large and small intestines. It serves no known purpose. Appendicitis is an inflammation of the appendix. It is rare before the age of four years, has it highest incidence between ages six and twelve, but may appear thereafter at any time of life.

Symptoms

Typically, at the beginning, there may be pain in the umbilical or navel area of the abdomen. Loss of appetite, nausea, and vomiting may follow. Although constipation is usual, about 10 percent of patients have diarrhea instead. After several hours, the pain usually shifts to the lower right abdomen over the appendix, is continuous, and may be dull or severe. Usually the pain is sharpened by movement, coughing or sneezing. There may be mild fever (up to 102°) in adults, sometimes high fever in young children.

But because the tip of the appendix in some cases may be located other than where it is expected to be in the lower right part of the abdomen, symptoms may vary. The tip may sometimes be on the left side, producing pain there.

Diagnosis

Appendicitis is not always easy for a physician—let alone a lay person—to diagnose definitely. The physician looks for positive evidence of inflammation. Tenderness may be felt over the appendix when pressure is applied there. Pushing down on the area and then suddenly letting go often produces very sharp pain. Sometimes pain is felt in the appendix area during an examination through the rectum. A

laboratory test—the blood leukocyte, or white cell, count
—is helpful in diagnosis.

The physician also may have to consider and rule out by
history or examination other conditions that sometimes may
be mistaken for appendicitis, such as pelvic inflammatory
disease in women, gallbladder disease, kidney infection, pancreas inflammation, and spastic colon.

Causes

Appendicitis starts when the appendix becomes obstructed
by fecal material or a foreign body, or when the appendix
becomes kinked. The obstruction may be followed by bacterial infection. The infected, inflamed appendix, filled with
pus, may enlarge to six or eight, or even more, times its
usual size.

When surgery is needed

Beyond the discomfort appendicitis produces, it brings
with it the risk of complications: One complication is perforation. The appendix may burst. Infection then may
spread throughout the abdominal cavity, leading to peritonitis, with protracted vomiting, generalized pain, and finally shock. While peritonitis often may be controlled by
antibiotics, some deaths do occur. Another possible complication is an appendix abscess, which may develop within
days after onset of appendicitis. The abscess is around
the appendix, and when it develops, two operations may be
needed: first, one to drain the pus out of the abscess; then,
about six weeks later, a second operation to remove the
appendix.

Early operation to remove the appendix is recommended
not only when the diagnosis of appendicitis is proven but
even when appendictis cannot be definitively diagnosed and
is only suspected—because it is safer to operate than to risk
rupture and peritonitis. Years ago, operations generally
were much more dangerous because the risk of wound infection and postoperative pneumonia was high. Unless the
diagnosis of appendicitis was certain, surgeons hesitated to

operate because of the risk. Today, every effort should be made to confirm the diagnosis beforehand, but when some doubt remains, the rule generally is to operate, since the operation in uncomplicated appendicitis carries very little risk.

The operation

An incision about two to five inches long is made in the lower right part of the abdomen. It may run straight up and down, crosswise, or at an angle. The appendix is lifted into the wound, its base is tied, and it is then cut away. The incision is stitched closed. The abdominal wound may be drained if pus is present. This is called delayed closure; gauze soaked in penicillin is placed in the wound and later is gradually taken out.

Anesthesia

General or spinal anesthesia may be used.

Length of operation

The complete operation—from opening to closing—may require from just a few minutes to an hour or two, depending upon the disease condition of the appendix. An expert surgeon, in a case of uncomplicated appendicitis, can remove the appendix in as little as ten minutes.

Postoperative care

An appendectomy involves virtually no blood loss, and blood transfusion is rarely needed. In uncomplicated appendicitis, no special postoperative care is usually required. You can generally expect to be out of bed the day after surgery. For the first two or three days, you're likely to experience some discomfort from the incision. If fluid collects in the wound a few days after operation, this is no cause for alarm; the surgeon will drain it off with little if any discomfort for you.

You can expect to return to a normal diet within a few

days. Usually the wound will heal in seven to ten days, at which point you can bathe or shower. Usually, too, you can go home from the hospital in five to seven days.

If there has been a complication, if the appendix has ruptured with or without peritonitis, the time in bed after surgery may be extended several days and the hospital stay may be lengthened to two weeks to a month. Special measures may be used, including antibiotic therapy and intravenous medications.

Recovery time

If your appendicitis was uncomplicated, you can expect to return to work in two to three weeks. If peritonitis occurred, you may get back to work in 1½ to 3 months.

Success rate

The results of appendectomy are excellent. It is not considered a serious operation and ranks as one of the most frequently performed of all operations. Even those suffering from other ailments such as heart disease usually come through the surgery and anesthesia very well. Once the appendix is removed, there is no possibility of recurrence of appendicitis.

It is seldom that death follows appendicitis now, except in some of those who wait too long, who seek help only after the disease has been present for a long period and serious complications have developed. Before modern antibiotics became available, as many as 5 percent of those with complicated appendicitis died. Now the death rate has been reduced to well below 1 percent.

Deaths from appendicitis and its complications could be reduced to practically zero if people did not delay in seeking medical help and did not indulge in improper treatment. The guidelines are few and simple: if any abdominal pain lasts for three or four hours, consult a physician as soon as possible and don't attempt self-treatment with cathartics, enemas, or heat. Cathartics and enemas increase contractions of the large intestine and cause pressure to develop in the appendix, increasing the chance of rupture. With each dose of cathartic or laxative, the rupture risk goes up. Local heat may both obscure symptoms and hasten rupture.

Are you left with any limitations?

None. Nor is the scar likely to be disfiguring. In some cases, it may be just barely noticeable after a year or so.

SEE ALSO PART II for pertinent information about choice of surgeon, preoperative and postoperative care, anesthesia, tests, costs, and other aspects of your operation.

Hiatus Hernia

The diaphragm is a strong, dome-shaped muscle which separates the chest from the abdomen. It has several openings through which pass blood vessels, nerves, and also the esophagus. When the normal opening, or hiatus, through which the esophagus passes is enlarged, part of the stomach may be pushed up, out of place, into the chest, either intermittently or constantly, by the pressure within the abdomen.

This is called a diaphragmatic hernia, or hiatus hernia. It is said to be the most common cause of upper gastrointestinal symptoms, which often mimic many other conditions. The condition has been called the "great masquerader."

Symptoms

A hiatus hernia may cause pain under the breastbone and the burning sensation, "heartburn," with reflux or regurgitation of stomach juices. The symptoms are usually worse after eating and with lifting or stooping. Sometimes the pain may resemble the anginal chest pain associated with heart disease. Hiatus hernia symptoms also may sometimes be confused with those of peptic ulcer or gallbladder ailments. On the other hand, in many cases—and it has been estimated that hiatus hernia occurs in as many as 50 percent of all people—there may be no symptoms at all.

Causes

A hiatus hernia may be present at birth, the result of not quite normal development of the diaphram. It may appear as the result of an injury to the diaphragm, often in connection with rib fracture, and may make its presence known weeks or months later. In most cases, the hernia develops as the result of relaxation and stretching or widening of the hiatus or opening for the esophagus.

Diagnosis

The diagnosis is made by X-ray study. The protrusion of the stomach through the diaphram can be seen on X-ray film taken after barium, a radio-opaque material, is swallowed. The esophagus itself may be looked at directly to see whether it has become inflamed as the result of regurgitation of stomach juices; this can be done with a lighted instrument, an esophagoscope, inserted through the mouth under local anesthesia.

Medical treatment

In the ansence of symptoms—and a hiatus hernia is sometimes discovered during even routine chest X-ray in a person who has never experienced any discomfort—no treatment at all may be needed.

When symptoms are present, a number of measures may be used. In the obese, weight loss to reduce upward pressure from the abdomen is helpful. Avoidance of bending over, lifting, and straining at stool also helps to reduce that upward pressure. Elevation of the head of the bed on eight-inch blocks often is very helpful, because it reduces the likelihood of regurgitation of stomach acids into the esophagus. Often, antacids taken after meals and sometimes midway between meals are useful in reducing stomach acidity. Such measures usually are sufficient.

When surgery may be needed

Hiatus hernia rarely causes serious complications. Most patients respond favorably to medical treatment. If medical treatment fails, however, and symptoms are intolerable and it is certain that they are caused by the hiatus hernia and not by other conditions such as gallbladder disease, then surgery is the definitive method of treatment.

The operation

A hernia of the diaphram may be repaired either through an incision in the chest or in the abdomen.

There are many operative techniques, which vary somewhat in detail. All, however, aim at returning the stomach to its proper position and repairing the hiatus or hernia hole. No absolute superiority has ever been shown for any one particular technique.

Anesthesia

The operation is performed under general anesthesia.

Postoperative care

There will be some discomfort, but not intolerable, for a few days after surgery. The surgical wound usually heals in one to two weeks and the patient may go home in about ten days. Bathing can be resumed after the wound is healed. There will be a scar, but not a markedly disfiguring one.

Recovery time

After getting home from the hospital, you can usually go out immediately and after a few weeks return to full-time work.

Success rate

The results of hiatus hernia operation are usually excellent. Recurrences develop in less than 20 percent of patients.

Are you left with any limitations?

No.

SEE ALSO PART II for pertinent information about choice of surgeon, preoperative and postoperative care, anesthesia, tests, costs, and other aspects of your operation.

Diverticulitis

Diverticulum comes from the Latin *divertere,* meaning "to turn aside"—and a diverticulum is an outpouching or sac that protrudes from the intestinal lining into the intestinal wall. There can be scores and even hundreds of such outpouchings or diverticula, especially in the colon. *Diverticulosis,* the presence of many such diverticula, occurs in as many as 10 percent of Americans over age forty and, according to some estimates, in as many as 30 percent over age forty-five. Diverticulosis is always benign at the outset and usually remains so. Although the pouches provide traps for feces, they seem to fill and empty efficiently in most people who have diverticulosis and remain free of all symptoms. But in a minority, about 20 percent, inflammation develops—and when the inflammation is severe, the result is acute *diverticulitis.*

Symptoms

The symptoms of acute diverticulitis are much like those of a "left-sided appendicitis." Along with pain in the left lower part of the abdomen, there may be nausea, vomiting abdominal distention. Bowel habits may be drastically changed, usually by severe constipation but occasionally by diarrhea and sometimes by alternating constipation and diarrhea. Chills and fever occur in accordance with the degree of inflammation.

Diagnosis

Diverticulitis is one of the first possibilities to be considered by a physician in a patient, particularly one over forty or forty-five, who has left-sided abdominal pain or experiences fluctuating bowel habits. It is also considered as a possibility when there is recurrent fever that cannot be explained. The diagnosis can best be established by X-ray examination of the intestine after a barium enema.

Cause

What causes the formation of the diverticula, the pouches, is unknown. There are theories that they may be the result of aging and weakness; possibly, too, some people have an inherited predisposition for them. Diverticulitis occurs when a pouch becomes obstructed by feces or tissue swelling. The obstruction favors the multiplication of bacteria and infection, as a result of which the diverticulum and nearby colon become inflamed.

Medical treatment

Acute diverticulitis is treated with bed rest and antibiotics to control the bacteria and infection. If the pain is severe, a drug such as meperidine may be used for relief. The bowel is rested: mild cathartics may be used to eliminate hard, irritating stool. Feeding may be limited to clear fluids until improvement begins. Other medication, including antispasmodics, may be used if the bowel is overly active as indicated by cramps or frequent bowel movements. Medical treatment may succeed in relatively mild cases of acute diverticulitis.

When surgery may be needed

Surgery is often necessary. It may have to be considered if obstructive symptoms of a first episode do not subside within twenty-four to forty-eight hours. If obstruction is complete, surgery is essential.

Surgery is also essential when there is a dangerous complication—perforation. A swollen, inflamed diverticulum may burst. When this happens, an abscess may form and not resolve, or intestinal contents may spill into the abdominal cavity and produce peritonitis.

Sometimes surgery is essential when there may be a suspicion that a cancer is present. In most but not all cases, X-ray studies can distinguish between diverticulitis and cancer. But particularly when diverticulitis is accompanied by complications, it is difficult to exclude the possiblity that a cancer may be present.

The operation

Removal of the severely inflamed, diseased area of the intestine may be done in stages.

In the first stage or operation, a loop of healthy, disease-free intestine is moved onto the abdomen outside the body. An opening is made in the loop so that temporarily, stool can come out through that opening rather than go through the rest of the bowel and rectum. This is called a colostomy. It is certainly not a pleasant experience and takes some adjusting to. But it diverts the stool from the inflamed portion of the bowel.

In a second operation, the diseased area of intestine is removed and the remaining healthy portions are joined together. Because the stool is still being rerouted via the colostomy, the joined portions of healthy intestine have a chance to heal and usually do so readily.

Finally, in a third operation, the colostomy is eliminated. The opening in the healthy intestinal loop that has been out on the abdomen is closed, the loop is returned inside, and the abdominal incision is closed. Now stools again take their normal route.

Anesthesia

General anesthesia is usually used.

Length of operation

The procedure for colostomy requires about an hour; for bowel removal, two to four hours.

Special preparations

Antibiotics may be given when surgery can be delayed long enough for them to have time to work. Feedings and medications may be administered by vein and the intestinal tract may be emptied and given a rest.

Postoperative care

Usually you can expect to be up within one to three days after each procedure. For each procedure, a hospital stay of about ten days may be needed and, with an interval of perhaps three to four weeks at home between stages, the total surgical treatment may require three to four months.

Once the surgical wound has healed—which takes about two weeks if drainage is not required, two to three times as long if drainage is needed—you can bathe. Usually, convalescent care is not required and social and marital life may be resumed in about six weeks or less. Return to work is possible about two weeks later.

Success rate

Surgery for diverticulitis is major. Yet the chances for recovery and cure are well over ninety-five out of a hundred. Once the diseased section of bowel has been removed, there is little likelihood of recurrence.

Are you left with any limitations?

Typically, many patients experience years of discomfort from diverticulitis before an operation is considered essential. During that time, they may become trapped in a morbid life style governed by what happens in their colons. With successful surgery, they become less limited.

In fact, their diets may become even freer. In recent

years, evidence has been accumulating that lack of fiber in the diet may contribute to the development of diverticular disease. As recently as five years ago, it was customary to place all patients with diverticulitis, including those undergoing surgery for the disease, on a bland, low-bulk diet. Now, more and more physicians and surgeons advocate a normal, well-rounded diet with emphasis on having it include not only vegetables but also unrefined cereals such as those containing the word "bran" in their names. Many physicians go further and advocate the addition, too, of unrefined bran, a natural part of cereal that is removed in processing cereal grains into breakfast cereals and bread meals. Such bran usually can be obtained at health food stores and may be available elsewhere as well.

More and more physicians and surgeons believe that it is essential for patients to have a high-fiber diet (rich in vegetables and in unrefined cereals) as a means of helping to assure that surgery for diverticulitis, once done, will not have to be repeated.

SEE ALSO PART II for pertinent information about choice of surgeon, preoperative and postoperative care, anesthesia, tests, costs, and other aspects of your operation.

Ulcerative Colitis

A serious, inflammatory disease, ulcerative colitis may affect the entire length of the colon and the rectum. It may occur at any age but most frequently it attacks young adults aged twenty to forty.

Symptoms

Usually, there are attacks of bloody diarrhea, with freedom from symptoms in between. The attacks may range from mild to severe and may vary in duration. An attack may come on suddenly with violent diarrhea, high fever, severe cramps. More often, onset is slow and insidious, starting with increased urgency to move the bowels, mild lower abdominal cramps, and appearance of bloody mucus in the stools. There may be loss of appetite, moderate malaise, mild elevation of temperature at night. But as the inflammation becomes more extensive, stools become looser, more frequent (ten to twenty a day), sometimes consisting entirely of blood; high fever may develop; and there may be severe loss of appetite, nausea and vomiting, and anemia.

Diagnosis

The diagnosis can be suspected from the symptoms and from examination of the stool. It can be confirmed by proctosigmoidoscopy—inspection of the lower colon and rectum with an instrument—and by X-ray study which will show ulcers and typical changes in the lining of the colon and rectum.

Cause

The cause is not known. There have been theories that ulcerative colitis is basically a bacterial infection. There is some evidence that, instead, it may be an allergic type of disease. In many cases, emotional factors seem to play a role.

Medical treatment

In 10 to 20 percent of patients with ulcerative colitis, there may be complete recovery after a single attack. More typically, the disease is one of repeated attacks.

Although there is no single specific treatment, various measures are often helpful. To lessen cramps and stool frequency during an attack, various drugs, including opiates, may be prescribed. Antibiotics or sulfa drugs may be used.

Cortisonelike drugs, although not curative, may bring remission of an attack in two-thirds or more of all cases, sometimes with dramatic speed. They may be given by injection, by mouth, or by enema.

When surgery may be needed

Surgery has to be considered when there is no response to medical measures and when the disease becomes so severe that the patient no longer can function usefully. Surgery also has to be considered and used more promptly if there is massive uncontrolled bleeding or if there are other complications such as perforation of the colon and peritonitis, or obstruction, or cancer development (cancer of the colon may develop in 5 to 10 percent of patients who have ulcerative colitis for ten years or more).

The operation

The usual operation is called a proctocolectomy and involves removal of the colon and rectum. A permanent abdominal opening called a stoma through which bowel evacuation can take place is made. The end of the small intestine, the ileum, is diverted into this opening.

This is drastic surgery, but it can be lifesaving. Compromise surgery—in which only an area of diseased colon is removed—has often failed because another area of the colon later becomes involved.

Depending upon the condition of the patient, the operation may be done in one or several stages.

Anesthesia

Either general or spinal anesthesia may be used.

Special preparations

For several days before operation, a low-residue diet may be used. Antibiotics and sulfa drugs may be administered, and blood transfusions may be used if marked anemia is present.

Postoperative care

It is possible for a patient to be out of bed within one to three days after surgery. For the first several days, he will usually get nourishment by vein, not by mouth, along with antibiotics, and a rubber tube inserted through the nose into the stomach may be used to help keep the abdomen from becoming distended with gas. The in-hospital stay may run as long as four to six weeks, sometimes longer. During that time, the patient will learn how to manage his new bowel opening, called an ileostomy. It begins to function within a few hours after operation.

Recovery time

It may take six months or more before the patient is fully recovered, in the sense that he has regained his strength and has become expert in the care of the ileostomy opening, and can carry on with school or work, and married life.

Success rate

Although surgery for ulcerative colitis appears to be formidable and is often undertaken for patients who are very sick and in danger of losing their lives, the success rate is over 90 percent.

Are you left with any limitations?

It may seem difficult to imagine getting along without the colon, yet the fact is that the colon plays no vital part in digestion; that work is carried out in the small intestine. The colon, as we noted earlier, absorbs water. After a time, the small intestine takes over that function.

The patient with an ileostomy wears an unobtrusive, odor-sealing, specially fitted appliance. Appliances have been greatly improved recently, as has instruction in their use provided by hospitals. More and more hospitals now employ specialists, called enterostomal therapists, who have been trained in Enterostomal Training Schools in Cleveland, Harrisburg, Grand Rapids, and Buffalo. An increasing number of hospitals are also establishing outpatient stoma clinics, with attending enterostomal therapists, where patients may come later for practical solutions to their problems and for information on the latest techniques and equipment.

Emotional support as well is provided by the clinics—and also by ileostomy clubs, one of which is Ileoptimists at 3813 West 56th Street, Chicago, Illinois. The patient with an ileostomy, cured of ulcerative colitis, can expect to live as long as others who have not had the disease. He can expect, after a period of adjustment, to live a normal life in every area—career, marital, social, recreational.

Preparing yourself psychologically

If you face surgery for ulcerative colitis, you will do best to face it realistically, not blinking at the problems and readjustment it will entail, but also not blinking at the great likelihood that, with all the problems and readjustment, it will free you of a disease that has tortured you and ruled your life.

You will be in large and growing company. Advances in surgical techniques in recent years have pushed the number of new patients with intestinal stomas to 86,000 during the year 1971 and the ostomy population, now about half a million, is certain to increase in coming years.

For any operation, it is important to choose a good surgeon in whom you can have confidence and with whom you can establish rapport. For no operation perhaps is the rapport more important than for this one.

If you have the opportunity to do so, get in touch with an ileostomy club, talk to one or more members so you can get the feel of what your life afterward will be like. Your surgeon may be able to help put you in touch and will be glad to do so.

If you feel anxious or depressed, you deserve and will benefit from help for the anxiety or depression, and you may get such help from your surgeon or personal physician or from a psychiatrist either may recommend. In some cases now, hospitals have such psychiatric help available and you may use it in the days before as well as after your operation.

SEE ALSO PART II for pertinent information about choice of surgeon, preoperative and postoperative care, anesthesia, tests, costs, and other aspects of your operation.

Ileitis (Regional Enteritis)

This is a slow, recurring form of inflammatory disease of the lower part of the small intestine, the ileum. In about half of all cases, it begins between the ages of twenty and thirty, has equal incidence in men and women, tends to be more common among Jewish people.

Symptoms

These may include mid-abdominal cramping pain and several loose, nonbloody bowel movements daily, along with mild fever, loss of appetite, and weight loss. In some cases, the abdominal pain may be steady and, additionally, there may be acute attacks of superimposed pain that may resemble that of appendicitis. In some cases there may be partial intestinal obstruction with abdominal distention and vomiting.

Diagnosis

A definite diagnosis requires X-ray studies. A barium enema-X-ray examination may be performed first. Additional X-ray studies usually will show the problem in the ileum.

Cause

For an unknown reason, a section of the ileum becomes swollen, red, and hard. Ulcers may develop on the ileum wall, followed by abscess formation. The effected section of ileum may stick to another loop of the ileum. A fistula, or abnormal, tubelike passage between the loops may develop. Other fistulas—to the bladder or skin—may develop.

Medical treatment

In some cases complete recovery may follow a single acute attack. In most cases, however, there are repeated attacks with remissions in between. Although there is no single specific treatment, various measures may be helpful. During acute attacks, bed rest is indicated. Medication, including mild sedatives and cortisone-like drugs by mouth, may reduce fever, improve appetite, lessen the number of bowel movements, and help foster normal absorption of nutrients by the small intestine. A high-calorie, low-residue diet excluding whole or raw fruits and vegetables may be prescribed.

When surgery may be needed

Surgery is often essential when intestinal obstruction, fistulas, or abscesses develop. It may be needed, too, in some cases when the possibility of acute appendicitis cannot be ruled out without operation, when massive bleeding occurs, or when medical treatment fails.

The operation

In surgery for ileitis, diseased areas of the small intestine are removed and the remaining healthy portion is connected to the colon. An alternative procedure which may sometimes be used leaves the diseased areas in place and bypasses them by connecting a healthy loop of ileum to the colon. The hope is that with intestinal contents no longer passing through the diseased areas, healing may take place.

Anesthesia

Spinal or general anesthesia may be used.

Length of operation

Either procedure may require one to three hours, depending upon conditions found within the abdomen.

Special preparations

Prior to surgery, fluids and other materials may be administered by vein to return body chemistry as much as possible toward normal. Stomach tubes may be used to overcome distention of the bowel.

Postoperative care

For several days after surgery, feeding will be by vein and the stomach tube will remain in place to help prevent distention. A patient who has been very ill may remain in bed several days after operation; if he has not been too ill, getting out of bed the day after may be encouraged.

The incision, which may be just to one side of the navel, extending four to six inches above and below it, will usually heal in about two weeks and bathing can then be resumed. The total hospital stay can vary considerably from patient to patient, depending upon preoperative conditions as well as postoperative progress, and may run anywhere from two or three weeks to two or three months.

Except for spicy foods and alcohol, a full diet may be recommended.

Recovery time

The time to full recovery is variable from patient to patient. In some cases, several weeks of convalescent care after leaving hospital will be helpful. While it may be possible for some patients to return to work in six to eight weeks, others do best by postponing the return until several months after surgery.

Success rate

Virtually all who undergo operation come through it and experience complete relief of all symptoms. Surgery does not cure ileitis; it does control complications. In many cases, there will be no further difficulty following operation. But about 30 percent of patients experience recurrences after some years. Recurrence is least likely in patients over the age of fifty.

Are you left with any limitations?

Removal of a section of ileum is well tolerated. There is small intestine to spare; even with less than ten of its original twenty feet, food can be assimilated, and you can expect to live normally. One well-known sufferer from ileitis was Dwight Eisenhower. The former President underwent surgery in 1956 and had an excellent recovery.

SEE ALSO PART II for pertinent information about choice of surgeon, preoperative and postoperative care, anesthesia, tests, costs, and other aspects of your operation.

Intestinal Obstruction

Intestinal obstruction, which may be either partial or complete, interferes with or completely stops the passage of intestinal contents.

Symptoms

Symptoms vary depending upon whether the obstruction is in the small or large intestine and whether complete or partial.

When the small intestine is completely obstructed, around the area of the navel there usually is severe, cramplike pain, that may come and go. Vomiting develops. The vomiting becomes fecal. There is abdominal distention; no feces or gas is passed. With partial obstruction of the small intestine, symptoms are similar but often less severe, and diarrhea may follow cramps.

When the colon is completely obstructed, symptoms often come on insidiously. Vomiting is not frequent; pain may be less severe than with small bowel obstruction; the abdomen becomes distended slowly. With partial obstruction, there are lower abdominal cramps and constipation; in some cases, constipation alternates with diarrhea.

Diagnosis

Plain X-ray films of the abdomen aid diagnosis by showing dilated loops of intestine. A barium enema X-ray film may be used to reveal the presence or absence of obstruction in the colon.

Causes

There are numerous possible causes of intestinal obstruction. One is adhesion, sometimes from an old operation. Normally, the intestinal tract lies in the abdomen coiled like a hose and the loops, with their smooth, moist surface, move easily over each other. With infection or injury, an area of surface may become dry, scarlike tissue may develop, and the area may stick to other tissue, including another loop of intestine. This is an adhesion. There may then be twisting and knotting, with resulting obstruction.

Obstruction of the small intestine may occur when a loop of it becomes caught in an inguinal hernia sac in the groin region. Adhesions and hernias are the most common causes of mechanical obstruction.

Among less common causes is *volvulus*. The mesentery is a tissue that attaches the intestine to the back wall of the abdomen, thus supporting it. If the mesentery becomes twisted, one or several folds of the intestine may be turned abnormally, producing obstruction. When volvulus occurs, it is mostly in the elderly.

Another less common cause is *intussusception,* which is limited primarily to infants and children under three. In this condition, one part of the intestine, the ileum, telescopes into another part, the colon, and obstruction results.

Medical treatment

This may be limited to relieving pain and other preliminary steps prior to surgery. If an obstruction is partial, an attempt may be made to overcome the obstruction by passing a long tube into the small intestine but if not successful, continued attempts, which delay surgery, may not be advisable.

When surgery is needed

Surgery is almost invariably needed when obstruction is complete and it is very often required when obstruction is partial. Usually, the sooner the surgery, the better.

Failure to relieve obstruction may not only lead to a dangerous toxic state; the distended intestine may rupture, producing peritonitis and possibly fatal consequences. Also, with obstruction, there is the danger of strangulation, in which blood supply to the area is cut off. This may result in gangrene in a few hours.

Types of operations

The surgical procedures used depend upon the cause of obstruction.

If small bowel obstruction is due to adhesions, merely cutting the adhesions may be all that is needed.

When blood circulation to a segment of bowel has been impaired, the surgeon may relieve the obstruction of the bowel and then wait, allowing as much as half an hour, to see whether, with the bowel obstruction relieved, circulation returns to normal. If it does, nothing further may be needed and the incision can be closed.

If circulation has been hopelessly damaged by prolonged strangulation, the affected segment must be removed. The remaining healthy portions above and below the removed segment are then firmly stitched together.

When a hernia has been responsible for obstruction, the bowel will be freed. If there has been strangulation, the affected portion will be cut out and the remaining healthy portions joined, and the hernia will be repaired.

When volvulus is the cause of obstruction, the surgeon may choose between straightening the loop of intestine and attaching it to the abdominal cavity or removing it. The chances that volvulus may recur are great. The chances are reduced when the attachment procedure is used, but if the patient is strong enough for the loop to be removed and the remaining sections united, recurrence is much less likely. When strangulation has occurred, removal of the affected section of intestine may be essential.

When a child has an intussusception, the telescoped loop may slip free on its own, but most often it does not. Usually, if operation is not unduly delayed, the loop can be readily freed and restored to normal position. With delay, the loop may become gangrenous and will have to be removed, with the healthy sections then rejoined.

In some cases, when the colon is obstructed, a *colostomy* may be performed. An opening is made in the colon ahead of the blocked segment and the opening is brought outside of the body onto the abdomen and a special pouch is placed over it to receive bowel movements. (A colostomy differs from an ileostomy; in the colostomy, a portion of colon or large intestine is brought to the outside; in the ileostomy, it is a portion of the ileum, or small intestine.)

A temporary colostomy allows the patient to pass feces, and gas; his nutrition and general condition improve; and the removal of diseased colon can be undertaken in a subsequent operation two or three weeks later. When the diseased section of colon is removed, the colostomy may be left for several more weeks, giving the intestinal repair opportunity to heal. Thereafter, the colostomy is closed and bowel movements are again passed in the normal fashion by rectum.

Anesthesia

General anesthesia is usually used; occasionally, spinal may be.

Length of operation

A temporary colostomy can be accomplished in less than an hour. The more extensive operations for obstruction, particularly those which involve removal of segments of bowel, may require two to four hours.

Special preparation

Before operation, a rubber tube passed through the nose into the stomach is used to suck out gases and fluids and help relieve distention. Fluids and medications may be given by vein. If necessary, blood transfusions may be administered.

Postoperative care

For several days after operation, there will be discomfort. The stomach tube will remain in place to help avoid distention. Medication to relieve pain may be administered.

If obstruction has been relieved by cutting an adhesion, the patient may be out of bed the day after surgery. In other cases, he may be up after a few days. Feeding may be by vein for several days. Once gas can be passed normally, indicating a return of normal intestinal function, food may be taken by mouth.

Recovery time

This will vary considerably, depending upon the type of operation that was needed. If the operation is performed in one stage, the hospital stay may range from about ten days to four weeks. If two or three operations are needed, they are usually done several weeks apart and several hospital admissions may be needed, with each stay running from two to six weeks or more.

Once the incision has healed, which may be in about two weeks, bathing can be resumed. Within two weeks, normal eating may be resumed if all goes well. Normal work, marital, and social life may be resumed in some cases within a month or six weeks.

Success rate

The success rate for operations to relieve intestinal obstruction has been remarkably high, considering the problems. The shorter the lapse of time between onset of obstruction and corrective surgery, the greater the likelihood of successful outcome. Yet some patients, out of failure to realize the seriousness of their symptoms or because of stoical acceptance of abdominal pain, have sought medical advice only when the disease process was far advanced.

Even so, overall, 91 percent of patients have been saved. Even further saving of life can be expected now, as the concept that intestinal obstruction is one disease in which surgery is indicated upon suspicion is increasingly accepted by physicians.

At age extremes, too—in the very young and in the very old—technical advances are now making it possible for surgery for obstruction to be lifesaving in the great majority of cases.

Are you left with any limitations?

When a child requires surgery for obstruction due to intussusception, there are no aftereffects in later life. When a portion of bowel must be removed, there is usually plenty to spare and the remaining bowel can carry on and allow normal living.

SEE ALSO PART II for pertinent information about choice of surgeon, preoperative and post operative care, anesthesia, tests, costs, preparing yourself for surgery, and other aspects of your operation.

Megacolon

Also known as Hirschsprung's disease, megacolon is an abnormal enlargement of the colon present from birth.

Symptoms

Symptoms include severe constipation, with an infant sometimes going for several weeks without a bowel movement, loss of appetite, vomiting, and abdominal distention. The child may also be anemic and fail to thrive.

Diagnosis

Along with symptoms, the doctor has as aids to diagnosis certain signs: the rectum is empty; the enlarged colon can be felt. Biopsy specimens—little snips of tissue from the colon which can be taken fairly readily—show a characteristic absence of nerve fibers.

Cause

The great majority of infants with megacolon are boys. They are born lacking normal nerve supply in a portion of the colon; these nerves are needed to allow normal propulsive waves to continue and move waste material along. Without the nerves, the waves stop at this area of the colon. Material stays and stagnates there, and the bowel ahead of the affected area becomes overgrown.

The operation

Cure for megacolon now can be achieved by surgery.

Through an incision usually in the left lower part of the abdomen, the rectum is cut inside the anal opening, the part of the colon lacking nerve supply is cut away, and the remaining colon is securely stitched to the rectum.

Anesthesia

Anesthesia may be general.

Length of operation

The time required from start to finish may extend from two to four or five hours.

Special preparation

Prior to surgery, the bowel may be emptied as much as possible with enemas and irrigations; a fluid or low-residue diet may be used; if needed, transfusions may be administered; antibiotics may also be given.

Postoperative care

There will be some discomfort for several days following the operation and for a week or more a special diet may be used. Normal bowel function may be established within several weeks, sometimes within a week. The wound will usually be completely healed within two weeks, at which point the child can be bathed.

Recovery time

The child may remain in the hospital for three to four weeks. If he is of school age, he may return to school not long afterward and to all other activities within three months or less after the operation.

Success rate

Children come through the surgery well. The great majority are cured. In a small percentage, there may be a recurrence; if so, removal of additional affected colon may produce permanent cure.

Is the child left with any limitations?

On the contrary, a child's development after successful surgery is stimulated, and any previous lag may be overcome.

Preparing yourself psychologically

Because parents can communicate anxiety even to infants, it is important for both you and the child to prepare yourself psychologically for the operation. You will have some natural anxiety; this may be reduced by your understanding of exactly what is involved in the operation, the very great odds in favor of its success, and the reassurance that with success the child can expect to live a normal, healthy life and be a far happier child than he has been up to now. If you have a need for additional details about the operation, you have every right to ask your surgeon for them and to expect him to supply them. You may wish to communicate with other parents whose children have undergone the operation, and the surgeon may be able to supply their names.

SEE ALSO PART II for pertinent information about choice of surgeon, preoperative and postoperative care, anesthesia, tests, costs, and other aspects of the operation.

Stomach Cancer

Cancer of the stomach has been declining in incidence for some years. It affects twice as many men as women and is concentrated largely at ages over forty.

Symptoms

Symptoms, which can occur either singly or in combination, include upper abdominal discomfort often, but not invariably, worse right after eating; pain in the region over the pit of the stomach which may be irregular; loss of appetite; vomiting; weight loss; anemia.

Diagnosis

A major aid in diagnosis is X-ray examination of the stomach. The X-ray can reveal a tumorous growth or a type of ulcer that could be cancerous. The tumorous growth may be benign but more often is likely to be malignant. Another aid to diagnosis is gastroscopy: under a local anesthetic, a lighted tube is inserted into the stomach through the mouth so the tumor may be examined and a small piece of it may be removed for microscopic study (biopsy).

The need for surgery

When a definite diagnosis of stomach cancer is established, surgery is essential. It is also strongly advisable in cases where there is doubt. Sometimes, when a stomach ulcer is present, X-rays and tests may not be able to rule out the possibility that it is cancerous. Duodenal ulcers rarely if ever are malignant, but stomach ulcers sometimes are. Thus, it is often wise to operate for stomach ulcer rather than using medical treatment, since surgery increases the chances that if the ulcer is cancerous, the malignancy will be discovered early when there is greater likelihood of cure.

Even when a growth appears extremely large on X-rays, surgical cure may be possible. The growth itself may be small but may have produced a significant inflammatory reaction around itself which makes the growth appear larger than it actually is. In some series of patients, 15 to 20 percent of stomach cancers that seemed from X-ray studies to be inoperable, proved to be curable by surgery.

When a stomach cancer is too far advanced to be removed, surgery may provide a new route for food through a rerouting procedure. While this may only make life a little more comfortable and not prolong it, a few patients do live for prolonged periods, and some may be helped with anti-cancer drugs and with radiation treatment.

The operation

Much or all of the stomach may be removed, depending upon the extent of the cancer. In addition, lymph nodes and nearby membranes and fat are taken out.

When a tumor turns out to be benign (a piece of it can be examined microscopically during the operation), only the stomach area containing the tumor may be removed and there is little sacrifice of stomach function.

When the entire stomach must be removed, the first part of the small intestine may be connected to the esophagus so that food goes straight from the esophagus to the intestine.

Anesthesia

General inhalation anesthesia is used.

Length of operation

The time depends very much on the specific conditions found. It may range from two or three hours to five or more.

Special preparations

A patient who is to undergo stomach surgery may be admitted to hospital several days in advance to be placed on a liquid diet, to have the stomach washed out, to receive medication by vein and, if necessary, blood transfusions.

Postoperative care

For a few days after surgery, there will be abdominal pain which is bearable. Feeding for several days will be by vein. The patient may be encouraged to get out of bed briefly a day or so after operation. The incision—which may be from the breastbone to or a little beyond the navel in the center or to one side, or alternately may run across the upper part of the abdomen—will take about two weeks to heal, after which bathing can be resumed. If all goes well, the hospital stay may be approximately two weeks.

Recovery time

If all goes well, the convalescent time may run about two months.

Success rate

The chances for cure of cancer of the stomach seem gloomy at first glance. For stomach cancer of all stages, far advanced as well as early, the survival rate at the end of five years has been only 11 percent for men and 14 percent for women. For stomach cancer operated on relatively early, when still localized, the five-year survival rate has been 37 percent for men and 43 percent for women, and the ten-year survival rate has been 33 percent for men and 36 percent for women.

There is now increasing hope that earlier and earlier recognition of stomach cancer and earlier and earlier surgery for it can increase the odds in favor of life-saving and that new methods of medical treatment now being explored could, when added to surgery, increase the odds still more.

Are you left with any limitations?

Yes, but they are tolerable limitations.

With the stomach removed, meals must be small, perhaps half the usual size, and taken half a dozen times a day. Slow eating and a diet made up of easily digestible foods may be prescribed. To make up for the loss of a material, called intrinsic factor, which is normally produced by the stomach lining and is needed for properly assimilating vitamin B12 which in turn is required for producing antianemia factor, injections of the vitamin may be required at first and thereafter it may be possible to take the vitamin by mouth. The fact is that patients with pernicious anemia have the same problem and do well with the same treatment.

Preparing yourself psychologically

Anyone facing surgery for known or suspected stomach cancer may understandably feel anxious or depressed. It may not be enough to try to combat the feelings by suppressing them or by determinedly seeking to look on the bright side. There is a bright side: it may not be cancer but only a stomach ulcer or a benign tumor; if it is cancer, it may be well localized and readily curable and even if it is somewhat advanced, it may still be curable.

If you feel anxious or depressed, do seek help. Talk out your feelings with your surgeon, or family physician, or with a psychiatrist either may suggest or who may be available as part of the hospital's service. Bottling up your feelings is not helpful; talking them out, ventilating them, bringing them out into the open, very often is—and to a remarkable degree.

SEE ALSO PART II for pertinent information about choice of surgeon, preoperative and postoperative care, anesthesia, tests, costs, and other aspects of your operation.

Intestinal Cancer

There has been a marked rise in recent years in medical and public understanding about, timely detection of, and survival rates for intestinal cancer. For reasons unknown, it is rare that cancer occurs in the small intestine. On the other hand, cancer and nonmalignant tumors are common in the large bowel or colon. The colon, in fact, is one of the areas in which cancer occurs most commonly.

Symptoms

A tumor of the colon may manifest itself by blood in the stool, by a change in bowel habits from few movements to many or from many to few, by cramps. In some cases, there may be anemia, weakness, and weight loss.

Diagnosis

A large proportion of colonic tumors can be seen with a sigmoidoscope, an instrument which is inserted through the rectum for a distance of ten or more inches. The sigmoidoscope is being, and should be, used increasingly today in routine checkups to find early cancer of the bowel. A stool sample for determination of the presence of hidden, or occult, blood is another useful aid to diagnosis.

A new aid to diagnosis is the colonoscope, an instrument which is slender and flexible and, when inserted through the rectum, permits examination of the whole five-foot length of the colon.

Another diagnostic procedure is to instill barium into the intestine by enema and take X-ray films. The barium makes the growths show up on the film.

Cause

The cause of cancer of the colon is unknown. It is more common in the United States and other Western countries and rarely appears in blacks in Africa but is as frequent in

American blacks as in whites. In the African diet, a large amount of roughage, which is often missing in the American diet, is used. This lends some support to a theory that bowel cancer incidence might be reduced by consumption of more whole-grain cereal products and fewer refined ones.

The need for surgery

Surgery is the only definitive treatment for bowel cancer.

Surgery also is often considered wise when benign growths, called adenomas or polyps, are found in the large bowel. Such growths extend outward from the mucous membrane lining and may be attached to the lining by long stalks.

Polyps occur in 10 percent or more of the population. They may appear at any age. Because they may cause few symptoms, if any, they are often discovered only during periodic checkups. When they do produce symptoms, the most common of them is painless rectal bleeding. Because some polyps have a tendency to become cancerous, their removal is advocated by many doctors.

Types of operation

Polyps lower down in the colon near the anus, often can be removed through the sigmoidoscope, a minor procedure. Recently, with the development of the colonoscope, there have been successful results in removing polyps higher up in the colon, the procedure requiring only light sedation. Through sigmoidoscope or colonoscope, a polyp may be electrically burned or snared off. If the polyp has only a short stalk, a short section of bowel will be removed and the ends joined.

When a cancer is found, operation consists of removing the growth and the section of bowel containing it, plus a segment on each side, plus the mesentery or suspending membrane in that area, for the mesentery can be a pathway through which cancer cells may spread. The two remaining ends of the colon are then joined together.

If, prior to surgery, a bowel cancer has reached the point of causing obstruction, it may be necessary first to relieve the obstruction through a temporary colostomy. The colon above the growth is cut across and brought up to an opening in the abdomen so bowel movements can be received in a pouch placed over the opening. This allows the taking of nourishment and buildup of strength. Several days or weeks later, depending upon progress of the patient, the cancerous segment of intestine is removed, after which the temporary colostomy is closed and, with the ends of healthy bowel joined, bowel contents are routed normally again.

A permanent colostomy is required when the cancer is located less than three or four inches above the anus, because its removal does not leave enough of a rectal stump to allow reestablishment of the normal pathway.

Currently under investigation is a technique of electrocoagulation—burning out a bowel cancer with electric current—instead of surgical removal.

Anesthesia

General anesthesia may be used; sometimes, spinal may be.

Length of operation

This varies considerably, depending upon type of operation. For a simple colostomy, the time required may be less than an hour; for removal of a benign tumor through the abdomen, two hours or less; for removal of a section of bowel, up to five hours.

Special preparation

In the hospital, for several days prior to operation, the bowel will be sterilized with intensive antibiotic or other medication and a liquid or low-residue diet will be used. Cleaning out and sterilizing the intestine is of great value in avoiding suturing difficulties and complications. If anemia has developed, measures will be instituted to help correct it.

Postoperative care

The removal of a simple polyp through the rectum produces little if any discomfort afterward and may in fact be done as an office instead of hospital procedure.

After removal of benign tumor or cancer through the abdomen, there may be several days of discomfort. Stomach and intestinal tubes may be required to deflate the intestinal tract. Feeding may be by vein rather than mouth for two to four days. Unless the patient has been unusually sick because of obstruction or an unusually severe operation has had to be performed, he may be out of bed within a few days, possibly the day after surgery. The abdominal incision, which may be about five to eight inches long over the tumor site, usually heals within two weeks and bathing may be resumed at that time. Bowel function usually returns within seven days after surgery, sometimes in half that time. Depending upon the progress of the patient, he may go home from the hospital within two weeks, unless there has had to be extensive surgery done in stages. Usually, normal marital and social life may be resumed within about two months and work not long afterward.

Success rate

Any benign tumor is curable. Moreover, most cancers of the colon are curable when found at early stages, and some are curable when found at later stages. At all ages and for all stages, the survival rates among women run 52 percent at the end of three years, 47 percent at the end of five years, and 44 percent at the end of ten years. The corresponding rates where the disease is not widespread run 79, 74, and 71 percent respectively. For men, at all ages and with all stages, the survival rates run 49 percent at the end of three years, 42 percent at the end of five years, and 39 percent at the end of ten years. The corresponding rates where the disease is not widespread run 76 percent, 70 percent and 66 percent respectively.

Currently, it is believed that more than three of every four patients with bowel cancer could be saved by early diagnosis and prompt surgery. And some recent studies indicate that 88 percent of patients who undergo surgery while they are still free of symptoms do not die of their cancers. There is reason for increasing hope now, too, that more and more patients with advanced bowel cancer can be saved with newer treatments to augment surgery, including therapeutic radiation and anticancer drugs.

Are you left with any limitations?

After successful surgery, you can eat what you wish. Even after removal of a large part of the bowel, if that is necessary, you can live a full and active life. If a permanent colostomy is essential, you can still live a full, active, and happy life. It has been possible for scores of thousands of people to do so, to learn how to empty their bowels each morning, regulate diet, take routine care of their colostomy, and have no worries about or discomfort from it.

SEE ALSO PART II for pertinent information about choice of surgeon, preoperative and postoperative care, anesthesia, tests, costs, and other aspects of your operation.

Rectal Operations

Although a majority of all people have no problems at any time in life associated with the rectal area, a sizable minority, perhaps as many as one-third, do. The area is often the site for hemorrhoids, fistulas, and other disturbances. Many disturbances commonly can be managed well with medical measures but when these are inadequate, surgery may be required, and very often surgery is highly effective in correcting the disturbances.

The Rectal Area

The large bowel or colon ends in the rectum. The rectum, about six inches in length and two inches or more in diameter, acts as a temporary storage area for waste awaiting elimination. The waste is held there by a sphincter, a circular muscle which remains contracted or closed except during elimination. Just belowe the rectum is the inch-long anus into which the rectum empties.

Hemorrhoids (Piles)

Hemorrhoids are stretched veins—varicose veins—under the mucous membrane lining of the anal and rectal area. When they occur in the wall of the rectum above the sphincter muscle, they are classified as *internal;* those below, in the anal canal, are called *external.* Often, both internal and external hemorrhoids may be present.

Symptoms

External hemorrhoids may be soft and seldom painful although they may produce a sense of fullness at the anus. Sometimes, under acute local stress such as is produced by straining at stool, the veins may enlarge suddenly, become filled with blood clots, and inflamed, and may break down and bleed. The condition, especially during defecation, is painful, usually for about five days until the clots begin to be absorbed and the mass disappears. After such an attack, there may be no symptoms or there may be severe itching.

Internal hemorrhoids may bleed as the result of minor injuries and bleeding is the main symptom but, if the hemorrhoids are large, there may be a feeling of incomplete evacuation of the rectum.

Cause

During defecation all parts of the anorectal area, including the veins, are stretched but, after passage of the stool, they return to a normal relaxed state. If the veins are somewhat weak, as seems to be the case with some people, they may remain permanently stretched. Also; increased pressure within the vein system may lead to hemorrhoids. Such pressure increase may be produced sometimes by pregnancy, obesity, coughing, sneezing and straining at stool because of constipation.

Diagnosis

External hemorrhoids can be diagnosed by direct vision; internal hemorrhoids by symptoms and also by examination through an instrument, the proctoscope. Rectal bleeding most often is caused by hemorrhoids and the bright red blood is seen on toilet paper and may even drip into the toilet bowl.

Hemorrhoids do not become cancerous and do not cause cancer, but they are so common that they may exist along with cancer. Because cancer of the colon and rectum may also cause bright red blood in stools, it is a cardinal rule of diagnosis that rectal bleeding must never be assigned to hemorrhoids without first considering other possible causes.

Medical treatment

Small, uncomplicated hemorrhoids which cause only slight bleeding on relatively rare occasions may yield to medical measures. If the patient changes his habits of defecation, does not attempt elimination unless there is an urge and evacuates only without attempting to strain, bleeding and protrusion may be eliminated. The use of mineral oil to soften any large, hard stools may be helpful. Correction of contributing factors such as obesity, chronic cough, excessive cleansing of the anus may also help. Internal hemorrhoids which appear during pregnancy often disappear after childbirth.

When external hemorrhoids become clotted, the pain usually stops within three to five days and the mass is gone within three to four weeks. If the pain is intolerable, the clots may be removed by incision for quicker relief.

Simple, small, bleeding internal hemorrhoids may sometimes be treated with injections of irritating solutions that scar and obliterate them. External hemorrhoids have been found to be unsuitable for injection treatment.

66   THE PATIENT'S GUIDE TO SURGERY

When surgery is needed

Surgery for hemorrhoids may be needed when bleeding is severe enough to cause anemia, when the pain is disabling or the itching becomes intolerable, or when there is a large, protruding mass.

The operation

Called hemorrhoidectomy, the operation for removal of hemorrhoids is relatively simple and not considered major surgery. It involves tying off the hemorrhoids close to their origin, carefully dissecting them out from surrounding structures, and removing them.

Anesthesia

Spinal, caudal, or general anesthesia may be used.

Length of operation

The operation on the average may require half an hour or less.

Special preparation

No special preparation before operation may be needed unless the hemorrhoids are severely swollen and inflamed, in which case several days of bed rest and cold applications may be needed.

Postoperative care

For as long as five days after operation, there may be considerable pain. For relief, local anesthetics may be applied and daily sitz baths—sitting in warm water—may be used. The first bowel movements, which may begin within the first few days after operation, may be especially painful. The patient may be out of bed as early as the day after operation, and home from hospital in four to seven days. At home, to keep bowels moving, mineral oil or another lubricant may be used and sitz baths several times daily be taken to relax the rectal area and cleanse it. It may be necessary for the surgeon to gently finger-manipulate the rectal area about once a week in his office for a time to make certain that the rectum is kept stretched.

Recovery time

Usually the rectal area becomes painless in ten to fourteen days, and the patient can return to normal life, including work and marital relations.

Success rate

Hemorrhoids that have been removed cannot recur again and surgery provides permanent cure for more than 90 percent of the patients. Sometimes, however, other veins may enlarge; only in a small percentage of cases is the second operation needed.

An alternative treatment

For internal hemorrhoids they consider suitable, some surgeons now employ a nonsurgical technique called "rubber-band ligation."

It involves placing a special latex band over the neck of a hemorrhoid. The band ties off the hemorrhoid, which then gets no blood, dries up, and falls off in one to fourteen days. No general anesthesia is needed; the procedure is essentially painless. Usually only one ligation is done in the office on each occasion since it may be difficult to do a second one with the first obstructing the view. Subsequent ligations may be done at two-week intervals or sooner.

Afterward, it is uncommon for the patient to have any real pain although there is usually some discomfort. The ligated hemorrhoid produces a sensation of rectal fullness and an urge to defecate. No special diet is required unless the patient is constipated. It may be quite uncomfortable to sit in a car for a drive of any great length on the day of a ligation. When the hemorrhoid drops off, there may be some brief spotting of blood; rarely is there serious bleeding.

Itching may be aggravated for a time when the hemorrhoid drops off.

There have been reports both in this country and Canada of thousands of patients treated successfully without need for hospitalization and only rarely with significant pain or loss of time from work.

Some surgeons have modified the rubber-band ligation technique further; after the band has been applied to the hemorrhoid, the pile is touched briefly with an extremely cold instrument that freezes it and, in so doing, both minimizes later discomfort and shortens the period of discomfort.

Rubber-band ligation may not be suitable for all hemorrhoids, particularly complicated ones.

SEE ALSO PART II for pertinent information about choice of surgeon, preoperative and postoperative care, anesthesia, tests, costs, and other aspects of your operation.

Anal Fissure (Fissure-in-Ano)

A fissure-in-ano is an ulcerated crack in the anal canal. It may originate as a superficial crack caused by passage of large, hard stools. When the crack does not heal because of the distention and contraction of the canal with stool passage, it may deepen and become inflamed. A fissure leads to marked spasm, or involuntary contraction, of the anal sphincter muscle and can be very painful. Distress can be intense when the anus is stretched during defecation.

Cure for a fissure is frequently possible in two or three weeks with medical measures which may include a low-residue diet, use of stool softeners and anesthetic ointments, and sitting in warm water in a tub (sitz bath) after bowel movement to help relax spasm.

When a fissure becomes chronic, it can be removed surgically. The operation, which may be performed under spinal, caudal or general anesthesia, takes half an hour or less, and is considered minor. The hospital stay may be five days or less. Healing occurs in two to three weeks. There will be discomfort during the first few days. Almost invariably, the operation is successful, with relief of pain and without after-effects. Only occasionally does a fissure recur.

SEE ALSO PART II for pertinent information about choice of surgeon, preoperative and postoperative care, anesthesia, tests, costs, and other aspects of your operation.

Fistula-in-Ano

A fistula-in-ano is an abnormal tunnel from inside the rectum to the skin outside. Usually it results from an infection that may start in the wall of the rectum or anus and form an abscess or painful "boil" that breaks through the skin near the anal opening and discharges pus. The abscess opening may seem to heal but then may open and discharge repeatedly over a period of weeks or months. A fistulous tunnel becomes established.

A fistula-in-ano never heals spontaneously but must be surgically removed. Symptoms consist of a pus-containing discharge near the anus, often with skin irritation, itching, and repeated abscess formation.

Surgery consists of unroofing the fistula, removing all the tissue that overlies it. The operation may be simple or complex, depending upon how the tunnel runs, whether it is single or multiple, and whether it goes through the sphincter muscle. It sometimes is necessary to cut the sphincter muscle in order to lay open the tunnel. When the muscle must be cut, it may be necessary to do the operation in two stages to prevent incontinence. In the first stage, the tunnel is unroofed and the muscle, after careful cutting, is lassoed with a heavy suture so it keeps its circular shape. In a second operation several weeks later, the muscle is divided so it may heal and retain its function.

Fistula operations may be done under spinal, caudal, or general anesthesia. Operative time may range upward from twenty minutes depending upon complexity. There is discomfort for several days after operation. The hospital stay may be a week or less.

In the vast majority of cases, surgery is curative. Occasionally, a hidden branch of a fistula may not be detectable during surgery and may cause a recurrence, necessitating reoperation.

In about 10 percent of patients, when the sphincter muscle has had to be cut, there is some degree of fecal incontinence after surgery, but with expert surgery the risk of this can be further minimized.

SEE ALSO PART II for pertinent information about choice of surgeon, preoperative and postoperative care, anesthesia, tests, costs, and other aspects of your operation.

Rectal Polyps

Polyps of the anus and rectum are very common. The soft growths, which may be pea-size or larger, often cause no symptoms. Sometimes, however, they may cause concern by producing painless hemorrhages from the rectum. Frequently they are discovered during periodic examinations.

Polyp removal is usually simple and because there is a possibility that in time certain polyps may become cancerous, it is common practice to advise removal. Very often, polyps can be removed in an office procedure without any need for anesthesia because there is no pain sensitivity in the area where they grow.

Through a proctoscope, a lighted tubelike instrument used for rectal examinations, an electric needle or cutting forceps is inserted and the polyps are destroyed electrically or snipped off. If the polyps do not lend themselves to removal in the office, only an overnight hospital stay may be required. There are no aftereffcets.

SEE ALSO PART II for pertinent information about choice of surgeon, preoperative and postoperative care, anesthesia, tests, costs, and other aspects of your operation.

Pilonidal Cyst

A cyst is a liquid-containing sac or capsule. A pilonidal cyst, which may be present in as many as one of every twenty people, is located in the middle of the lower back just above the cheeks of the buttocks. It is present at birth and is believed to result from an infolding of skin in which hair continues to grow. It may remain entirely symptomless and unnoticed until adolescence or adulthood when, as the result of irritation and entrance of bacteria, it may become a small lump exuding a slight yellowish discharge. Sometimes a cyst may become severely abscessed and require lancing to permit excape of pus. This may be done as an office procedure under local anesthetic, provides immediate relief of pain, and a few days later inflammation subsides.

After that, the cyst can be removed surgically in hospital. The operation, which may be performed under low spinal anesthesia, is considered minor and without danger. The objective is to remove all of the affected tissues. The incision may be two to four inches long and an inch wide or less, and all the tissue beneath the skin, including the cyst, is removed. There are variations in the technique and also in wound closure. The deep hole left by the operation may be sutured shut or the hole may be packed with gauze and, without suturing, allowed to heal from the bottom up. While the nonsuturing method leads to slow healing, requiring as long as five or six weeks, some surgeons believe it produces the smallest number of recurrences.

After operation, the patient may get out of bed next day, go home in four days or a little longer, return to work in two or three weeks. For two or three days after operation, there is some discomfort localized to the area of incision. The bowels may not move for a day or two, and in some cases there is also difficulty in voiding for a day or two, which may necessitate catheterization for urine removal.

Showers and tub baths can be taken after about two weeks even though the wound is still healing The surgeon may change dressings about twice a week until healing is complete.

Pilonidal cysts do recur in perhaps 5 to 10 percent of cases, requiring a second operation.

SEE ALSO PART II for pertinent information about choice of surgeon, preoperative and postoperative care, anesthesia, tests, costs, and other aspects of your operation.

Rectal Cancer

Rectal cancer is one that is readily diagnosable. Most of the growths are within reach of the examining finger.

Symptoms

Rectal bleeding, although often due to other causes, can be an important symptom of rectal cancer. Any change in bowel habit—in the nature and amount of bowel movements—may signal malignancy.

Diagnosis

Diagnosis is made by microscopic examination of a piece of tissue removed during internal rectal examination (biopsy).

Cause

Cause is not known.

The need for surgery

When a definite diagnosis of rectal cancer is established, surgery is essential. If offers a good chance for cure—the earlier the cancer is discovered, the better the chance, but even in advanced cases cure may be possible.

The operation

Surgery for rectal cancer must involve complete removal of the malignancy. The nature of the operation will depend upon the site of the cancer. The rectum is only six inches long. If the cancer is three or more inches inside the rectum, away from the anal opening, it may be removed and enough healthy rectum may be left to preserve the sphincter muscle function. Most rectal cancers, however, are nearer to the anal opening and their removal means that too much of the rectum must be sacrificed to preserve sphincter function.

If the sphincter can be preserved, the operation involves one incision through the abdomen. A portion of the rectum, the cancer, and a section of colon just ahead of the cancer are removed. The ends of the colon and rectum are then securely sutured together to reestablish a passageway for waste.

If the rectum must be removed completely, the operation —called abdominoperineal resection—requires, in addition to the abdominal incision, another in the perineum, the region between the legs from vaginal orifice to anus in women and from scrotum to anus in men. The rectum is removed and the space left in the perineum is sutured closed. The end of the colon, cut above the rectum, is brought to a circular opening usually in the lower left part of the abdomen, forming a colostomy or abdominal anus.

Anesthesia

General or spinal may be used.

Length of operation

From two to four or five hours, sometimes a little longer.

Special preparations

For several days before operation, the bowel may be sterilized with antibiotics or other drugs, and a liquid or low-residue diet may be used.

Postoperative care

For four or five days after operation, there will be discomfort. Feedings may be by vein. Bowel function returns gradually; four to five days may be required before a colostomy begins to function and a similar period of time may be needed for return of function after ends of colon and rectum are rejoined.

Often the patient is out of bed within one to three days, may go home in about two weeks, resume a normal diet in a few weeks, bathe when the wound has healed completely in about two weeks, take up normal marital and social life in two months or less, and return to work shortly afterward.

Success rate

Overall, for rectal cancers of all stages, the survival rate for women is 50 percent at the end of three years, 43 percent at the end of five, and 38 percent at the end of ten; when the cancer is still in early stages, the rates, respectively, are 75 percent, 68 percent and 63 percent. For men, overall, for all stages of rectal cancer, the survival rate is 46 percent at the end of three years, 39 percent at the end of five, and 34 percent at the end of ten; when the cancer is still in early stages, the rates, respectively, are 69 percent, 63 percent and 59 percent.

There is now increasing hope that earlier diagnosis and aggressive surgery, plus careful, regular follow-up examinations, can increase the saving of lives.

Are you left with any limitations?

There may be virtually none when a colostomy is not required.

If a colostomy is needed, it may seem limiting at first but not for very long. A plastic bag to collect stools is fitted over the opening. Usually, a special nursing team expert in colostomy care instructs you and demonstrates care. There will be no odor; the colostomy will not be apparent, and no one will know you have one unless you inform them.

Over a period of a few months, you can train the colostomy so that there is a bowel movement only once a day. Alternatively, you can use a special appliance to irrigate the colostomy—in effect, take an enema—every other day, producing a movement which goes directly into the toilet bowl.

You will be able to eat what you like, carry on every activity you carried on before, bar none. Many well-known personalities in business, entertainment, politics, and other professions have colostomies which do not limit them in any way.

An alternative procedure

When a rectal cancer is such that a standard surgical procedure cannot be used, an alternative is to freeze the malignancy with extreme cold (cryosurgery). Usually, this is done by inserting the freezing instrument through the rectum, without an incision. The technique is showing promise but, since it is relatively new, long-term results in quantity are not yet available. At this point, therefore, many surgeons consider it an alternative rather than a primary procedure.

Preparing yourself psychologically

Any operation for cancer is likely to produce anxiety. In the case of rectal cancer, the odds in favor of cure are good, best when the cancer is found early, but still good even for more advanced malignancy. There is reassurance in this.

Still, if you feel anxious or depressed, you deserve and will benefit from help for the anxiety or depression, and you may get such help from your surgeon or personal physician or from a psychiatrist either may suggest. In some cases now, hospitals have such psychiatric help available and you may use it in the days before as well as after your operation.

If you require a colostomy, you will be much more cheerful about it if you can talk with someone who has lived for years with one and see for yourself how well it can be adapted to. Your surgeon may be able to put you in touch with such a person or with several even before operation. Many people with colostomies volunteer eagerly for such meetings out of awareness, from personal experience, of how forbidding a colostomy may seem at first.

SEE ALSO PART II for pertinent information about choice of surgeon, preoperative and postoperative care, anesthesia, tests, costs, and other aspects of your operation.

Abdominal Operations

Gallbladder Operations

The gallbladder, which is located in the upper right part of the abdomen under the liver, is a pear-shaped sac that stores bile coming from the liver. It holds an ounce or two and discharges the bile through the gallbladder duct (cystic duct) into the common bile duct, from which it enters the duodenum, or first part of the small intestine. Bile is discharged when food, especially greasy food, leaves the stomach and enters the duodenum. Bile helps in digestion. The gallbladder is not an essential organ; when it is removed, the liver supplies bile directly to the duodenum.

Most common gallbladder diseases are associated with the presence of stones which, for reasons not clearly understood, often form out of the fluid content of the gallbladder. Commonly they contain cholesterol, although no relationship between cholesterol level in the blood and gallstone formation has been established.

An estimated 32 percent of women and 16 percent of men at age forty have stones in the gallbladder and the numbers increase after forty and with obesity. Some people with gallstones never develop symptoms; others suffer enough from them so that some 750,000 gallbladder operations are done each year in the United States.

Symptoms

Many patients have upper abdominal discomfort, bloating, belching, and are unable to tolerate fried food and

77

various vegetables. Attacks of pain, called biliary colic, may develop; the pain is very severe, knifelike, occurs in the upper right part of the abdomen and may radiate to the back or the right shoulder. In some cases, jaundice—yellow discoloration of the skin—may be a complication as bile pigments, unable to flow freely because of the presence of a blocking stone, back up into the bloodstream.

Diagnosis

The symptoms may suggest the diagnosis and often the stones can be seen on X-ray film. The X-ray is made after a dye is administered in the form of pills taken by mouth or by injection into a vein. Sometimes stones are not seen on X-ray but the gallbladder itself also does not appear, suggesting that stones are present and the gallbladder is diseased. This is the case about 95 percent of the time.

Cause

Gallstones are formed from salts and cholesterol that crystallize and precipitate or drop out of bile fluid. As the crystals clump together, they mix with other materials, such as bile pigments or calcium, and form hard masses. The stones may range in size from sandlike grains to pebbles and larger.

Gallstones are silent and generally harmless until they get caught in the gallbladder duct or common bile duct. Then, as pressure increases behind the obstruction, pain develops; the gallbladder swells and becomes inflamed. If the pressure becomes excessive, gangrene may develop. Acute inflammation of the gallbladder is known as acute cholecystitis.

Sometimes, acute cholecystitis may subside if the stone manages to drop back into the gallbladder or works its way through the cystic duct into the common bile duct and from there into the intestine. If the stone should become lodged in the common bile duct, all bile flow is obstructed, and jaundice develops.

Repeated attacks of acute cholecystitis, even though the

stones are eventually passed in each case, may lead to chronic cholecystitis in which the gallbladder becomes shrunken and scarred, often producing abdominal discomfort, bloating, and flatulence.

Medical treatment

There is no established medical treatment for gallstones. During an acute attack, such measures as bed rest, administration of fluids by vein, and of pain-relieving agents may be used. Antibiotics may be administered to treat or prevent infectious complications, and abdominal distention may be relieved by means of a tube passed through the nose into the stomach. For chronic cholecystitis, if no stones are apparent on X-ray, medical treatment which may include a low-fat diet or antispasmodic drugs may be helpful.

When surgery may be needed

Surgery may be advisable when there is an acute attack of cholecystitis and the diagnosis is quickly and clearly established. If the diagnosis cannot be established clearly within forty-eight to seventy-two hours after onset but is established later, surgery may be performed at least six weeks later. Surgery sometimes may be performed even later than that, when the patient's physical condition or the presence of other medical complications makes a delay wise.

Surgery is also considered essential when a patient has repeated attacks of pain caused by gallstones, when jaundice traceable to an obstructing stone is present, and when the patient suffers from chronic indigestion, nausea, and flatulence definitely established as being due to gallbladder condition.

It is often considered wise to remove the gallbladder when stones are detected even though the stones may be causing no problems of great concern; they may well do so later.

Gallstones are so common that their presence does not rule out the possibility that another cause of trouble may be present. To be certain that an ulcer or other stomach or duodenum problem is not causing or contributing to the symptoms, X-rays of these organs often are made before surgery.

The operation

The operation, called cholecystectomy, removes the entire gallbladder with the stones it contains. An incision, below the ribs and to the right of the navel, is made and may be vertical, horizontal or slanting. During the operation, a solution is introduced in the main bile (common) duct and X-rays are taken to see if there may be any stones there. If so, the duct is opened and cleaned.

Anesthesia

General anesthesia is used.

Length of operation

Gallbladder surgery usually can be completed within an hour, sometimes in half that time. In complicated cases, more than an hour may be required.

Special preparation

Little preparation before operation, except for possibly limiting fatty food intake, may be needed when the problem is chronic cholecystitis. When the problem is acute, preparation may include use of antibiotics and administration of medications by vein. It is sometimes necessary, when very severe infection is present, that an operation limited to draining pus and bile to the outside be done, followed some weeks or months later, once severe infection and inflammation have subsided, by a second operation to remove the gallbladder.

Postoperative care

Usually a gallbladder incision is painful for several days and pain-relieving medication is needed. Body movement need not be limited and the patient may be out of bed the day after surgery. Frequently after gallbladder surgery, a rubber tube is inserted through a half-inch incision to drain the operative site; it is removed after several days. The average hospital stay is about eight to fourteen days.

Recovery time

Bathing usually may be resumed in about two weeks, marital relations in about four weeks, work in about five to six weeks. For some months after surgery, it may be wise to use some caution about diet, keeping fat intake low, but foods previously avoided may be introduced gradually, until almost anything can be eaten without difficulty.

Success rate

Gallbladder surgery is major surgery. In the hands of an experienced surgeon, the odds are better than 90 percent that the surgery will be successful, with cure of major problems, and in about 80 percent of cases, with elimination of all digestive difficulties due to gallbladder disease. In up to about 10 percent of patients, occasional minor discomfort may persist and may be due to spasm, or involuntary contraction, of the common bile duct; usually the discomfort can be relieved with antispasmodic medication.

Once, in a fairly substantial minority of patients, a second operation was required because of a stone overlooked the first time. With more care now taken during surgery and the use of special X-rays at the operating table, the incidence of overlooked stones has dropped to about 5 percent and may drop further. A second operation, when necessary, is usually successful.

Are you left with any limitations?

After successful surgery, you can expect that, if anything, the chances for a long and healthy life will be increased. Within three to four months, the functions of the gallbladder are taken over by the bile ducts and the gallbladder is not missed. There is no interference with normal pregnancy in women who wish to have children after gallbladder surgery.

SEE ALSO PART II for pertinent information about choice of surgeon, preoperative and postoperative care, anesthesia, tests, costs, and other aspects of your operation.

Liver Operations

The human liver, which looks very much like beef liver, is one of the most vital organs in the body. The body's largest organ, the bulk of it lying in the upper right abdomen, it produces bile which aids digestion. In addition, it receives digested food materials through a *portal* system of veins from the digestive tract, chemically processes the materials, then sends them on through the general bloodstream to reach all tissues of the body. The liver produces and stores body proteins, stores sugar and regulates the amount of sugar in the blood, stores and uses fats, chemically detoxifies or breaks down any harmful materials that may be circulating in the blood, and produces a material called prothrombin which is needed for normal blood clotting.

Liver surgery may be necessary under several circumstances: to take a biopsy, or tiny sample, of liver tissue for microscopic examination; to repair accidental liver injury; to treat a liver abscess; when a liver cyst or tumor is present; and in some cases of cirrhosis of the liver.

Liver Biopsy

Like any other organ, the liver is subject to diseases that may begin there—for example, cirrhosis or hardening, and the inflammation called hepatitis. Moreover, because it is a way station for blood returning to the heart, diseases from elsewhere in the body may spread to the liver. A piece of tissue from the liver may be studied microscopically to determine whether the liver has been affected by disease.

Often, under local anesthesia, a needle biopsy can be performed by inserting a five-inch needle between the ribs or through the front of the abdomen into the liver, after which an instrument can be moved through the needle to a little beyond the needle tip, and can take a small section of liver for examination.

Sometimes, it is necessary to use general anesthesia and make an incision in the upper right abdomen, through which a wedge of liver tissue can be removed for examination. Such an *open* biopsy entails little risk.

Liver Injury

The liver may be cut or torn in automobile or other accidents, leading to bleeding which, even though small, may be fatal if it continues. The need for surgery may be indicated by swelling and tenderness in the right upper abdomen and by signs of internal hemorrhage with a fall in blood pressure caused by the disturbance in circulation.

If the internal bleeding stops quickly, surgery may not be needed. When surgery is required, an incision is made in the right upper abdomen, and the liver is sutured to stop the bleeding. In some cases, special gauze or a plastic material may be used to pack the liver and stop the bleeding; both the gauze and the plastic are later dissolved and harmlessly absorbed.

General anesthesia is used; the operation may take about an hour; a drain may be left in place. After a liver injury, a patient may have to remain in bed for several days or even weeks to help liver healing and minimize the risk of further bleeding. A hospital stay of several weeks or even several months may be required depending upon the progress of the patient. Discomfort after surgery is relatively mild. When the wound must be drained, healing may require several weeks or months.

Liver Abscess

Liver abscesses are far less common today than they once were. In the past, they were relatively frequent occurrences after gallbladder, appendix, or other abdominal surgery when infection spread to the liver. The use of antibiotics has markedly reduced the incidence of such abscesses. Liver abscesses in the past often developed in people with amebic dysentery but modern drugs to control the dysentery have greatly reduced the incidence of these abscesses as well.

When a liver abscess does occur, it may yield to medical treatment with antibiotics or other drugs. When surgery is required, depending upon where on the liver the abscess is located, an incision may be made in the upper right abdomen or the lower right part of the back of the chest, and the abscess is opened and drained. The operation may require one to two hours. The postoperative period is not markedly uncomfortable and the patient may get out of bed within a few days. A drained wound may require several weeks or even months before it heals completely. More than nine of every ten patients recover from surgery.

Liver Cysts and Tumors

A cyst is a sac or capsule containing a liquid or semisolid substance. Occasionally a liver cyst may be caused by a parasitic organism and may grow to grapefruit size, requiring removal. Occasionally, blood and lymph cysts develop and may cause some swelling of the liver but often they may be left without surgery, because they are difficult to remove, cause no great harm, and do not become malignant.

Cancer may sometimes arise in the liver and is called primary cancer of the liver. The liver is also the most common site, because of its key position in blood circulation, for the deposit of malignant cells from organs elsewhere in the body.

It is the unfortunate fact that as of now most cases of cancer of the liver are fatal; the malignancy is scattered throughout the liver and cannot be successfully removed. Sometimes, however, a cancer is well-localized, confined to one of the two lobes of the liver, and cure may follow removal of the whole affected lobe.

Operation for removal of a cyst or tumor, which may require from about one and one-half to four hours, is carried out under general anesthesia. An incision is made in the upper right abdomen; the cyst or tumor is cut out; bleeding is controlled with sutures. Usually after surgery, pain from the incision is not great. The patient may be out of bed after several days to a few weeks. When drainage is not needed and the incision can be tightly sutured, it usually heals in about two weeks; if drained, it may require up to several months for complete healing.

When a cyst or tumor can be removed successfully, the patient thereafter may live normally. As much as four-fifths of the liver can be taken out if necessary, and the remaining fifth is enough to take care of all needs.

Cirrhosis

Surgery sometimes can be helpful in cirrhosis of the liver. In this disease, which may be caused by severe malnutrition, virus infection, or the effects of alcohol, the liver becomes hard, overgrown with scar tissue. Blood flow through the veins of the liver may be impeded, and the back pressure may lead to development of internal varicose veins in the stomach or esophagus as well as elsewhere. Those in the esophagus may be especially pronounced and are called esophageal varices and can be the source of repeated hemorrhages.

A shunt operation may help. Sometimes the portal or entrance vein to the liver is connected to the inferior vena cava, the major vein returning blood to the heart from the lower part of the body. In some cases, a connection may be made between the vein of the spleen and a kidney vein.

The aim is to reduce the amount of blood that must flow through the obstructed vein system of the liver and to allow more blood to bypass the liver and go directly into the general circulation. In that way, the backup of blood and the backup pressure are reduced, and hemorrhages from the varicose veins in the esophagus may be stopped.

The operation is carried out under general anesthesia, through an incision in the upper right abdomen, and may require from two hours up to five or six hours. The hospital stay runs from ten days to two weeks or more.

The operation is a major one. Delicate surgery is involved. Because a severely diseased liver can lead to complications and may interfere with proper healing afterward, not all patients with cirrhosis can be operated on with any reasonable hope of success. If liver tests show very severe damage that cannot be remedied by a period of in-hospital treatment before operation, surgery may be inadvisable.

From one-fourth to one-half of patients with cirrhosis may benefit from shunt surgery. The cirrhosis itself is not cured, but with regular medical management and discontinuance of alcohol, return to previous work may be possible.

SEE ALSO PART II for pertinent information about choice of surgeon, preoperative and postoperative care, anesthesia, tests, costs, and other aspects of your operation.

Pancreas Operations

The pancreas, a large gland which lies high up in the abdomen, deep behind the stomach, serves two purposes. Much of the gland is made up of cells which produce juices that help to digest protein, fat, and carbohydrates. It also contains cells found in clusters called islets of Langerhans that produce the hormone *insulin* needed for the proper utilization of sugar. Insulin is secreted into the bloodstream, and an insufficiency of it leads to diabetes. The digestive juices produced by the pancreas move through the pancreatic duct, which joins the main bile duct to enter into the duodenum.

For several diseases that attack the pancreas, surgery may be needed.

Acute Pancreatitis

An inflammation of the pancreas, acute pancreatitis produces severe abdominal pain, usually steady and boring, which may radiate to the back and chest. Nausea and vomiting are common, and either constipation or diarrhea may occur but constipation is more usual. There is usually a fever of up to 102°.F.

All causes are not yet known. In about 40 percent of cases, gallstones are associated with the inflammation; in another 40 percent excessive intake of alcohol; in 10 percent pancreatitis appears to develop in association with injury, peptic ulcer, mumps, or other infectious disease; in the remaining 10 percent no cause can be found.

In acute pancreatitis, digestive juices that ordinarily go into the duodenum to work on food may be released into the pancreas itself and may digest some of the gland tissue or they may escape and attack surrounding tissue, inflaming the abdominal caviety.

Occasionally, the diagnosis of acute pancreatitis cannot be definitely made without an exploratory operation. But usually blood and urine tests showing an increased amount of the digestive juice amylase along with X-rays of chest and abdomen indicate the problem.

In most cases, acute pancreatitis can be made to subside by helping body defenses. To put the pancreas at rest and reduce its secretions, no food is given by mouth, only by vein. With a tube introduced through the nose into the stomach, acid may be sucked out before it can stimulate pancreas secretion. Antibiotics may be used.

Surgery is rarely used to treat acute pancreatitis. Sometimes large cysts may form because of the inflammation. They may grow to grapefruit size or even larger and press on surrounding structures. A cyst may lend itself to surgical removal, but usually the cyst is opened and its edges are attached either to the abdominal wall or to the stomach or small intestine and after several weeks or months it dries up and disappears or remains as only a scarred remnant.

The operation for a cyst, which usually relieves the pain, gaseous distention, and appetite and weight loss caused by the lump, is performed usually after inflammation has subsided. The operation, which may require one to two hours, is performed under general anesthesia through a 4- or 5-inch-long incision in the upper abdomen. The wound, which is drained and may take several weeks or even longer to heal, causes discomfort for several days. Often the patient may be out of bed within two or three days and may return to work about two months after complete healing of the wound.

Chronic Pancreatitis

More common in men than in women, chronic pancreatitis may follow repeated acute attacks or may develop insidiously. About one-third of repeaters are alcoholics. It is associated with the formation of stones within the pancreatic duct and there may be scar tissue formation in the gland.

The symptoms include constant or intermittent pain in the upper abdomen which may spread out toward the left shoulder and the back, fever, and some jaundice or yellowing of the skin during acute flare-ups. About one of five patients develops mild diabetes. Commonly, nausea, and weight and appetite loss occur.

The diagnosis of chronic pancreatitis may be made on the basis of past acute attacks (incidence of recurrence is about 50 percent) and X-rays which may show stones within the pancreas may help. Some cases, however, can be diagnosed only by exploratory operation.

Medical treatment may be helpful. It may include a ban on alcohol; a high-carbohydrate, low-fat diet; vitamin B supplements; pain-relieving agents; correction of any anemia;

treatment for diabetes if necessary; and in some cases use of pancreatin, a preparation containing pancreatic juice compounds.

When symptoms are persistently severe, surgery may be performed. In one procedure, subtotal pancreatomy, a small portion of the pancreas, about an inch of the tail, is removed, any stones in the pancreatic duct are removed, and the remainder of the tail is attached to a loop of intestine. In an alternative procedure, the pancreas is split lengthwise along the duct, stones are removed, and the split surface is attached to the small intestine. In either case, the previously restricted pancreatic juices can flow freely into the intestine, improving digestion and relieving pressure-caused pain.

Surgery is performed under general anesthesia through a 4 to 5-inch-long incision in the upper abdomen and may require up to two or three hours. There is some discomfort afterward for a few days; the patient may be out of bed in one to three days; the incision usually heals in two weeks; the patient may go home then, and work may be resumed about two months later. A low-sugar and low-fat diet may be recommended.

Benign Tumors and Cancer

Nonmalignant tumors sometimes affect the insulin-producing cells of the pancreas, leading to excessive insulin production. Because of the excess insulin, blood sugar level is held very low and this may lead to attacks of trembling, fainting, mental confusion, and in some cases convulsions. Very often now, to produce cure, such tumors can be removed without great difficulty.

When cancer occurs in the pancreas, a prime symptom is abdominal pain that ofter radiates to the back. Jaundice is common, as are weight and appetite loss, nausea, and vomiting. Various laboratory procedures, including blood and urine tests, tests for blood in the stool, and X-rays may suggest cancer.

About three times as many cancers occur in the head of the pancreas as in the body and tail. When the cancer is localized in the tail, cure may possibly be achieved by removal of the tail or the gland and the spleen which joins the pancreas at the tip.

When the cancer is in the head of the pancreas where it may press upon the bile duct and produce jaundice with its yellowish skin, and when the cancer has progressed so far that it cannot be removed entirely, a short-circuit operation may be performed. The gallbladder is connected to the small intestine or stomach so that bile can bypass the obstructed bile duct and enter the gastrointestinal tract, relieving the jaundice and the severe itching that may accompany it.

Sometimes the short-circuit operation is performed first to make possible enough of an improvement in the patient's condition so that a more heroic but sometimes life-saving operation can be performed. In other cases, the latter operation may be used the first time. It is extensive. The entire portion of the pancreas containing the cancer, and sometimes even the entire pancreas, is removed, along with all of the duodenum to which the cancerous pancreas has become adherent. The stomach is attached to the small intestine in the area beyond the duodenum, and the common bile duct is attached to the small intestine.

The operations are performed under general anesthesia through an abdominal incision. Up to three hours may be required to remove a localized tumor; as long as six hours to remove the pancreas. Following removal of much or all of the pancreas, diabetes develops, but this can be controlled with diet and medication, and administration of substitutes for pancreatic juices provides control of digestive disturbances.

The extensive operation for cancer of the pancreas carries a risk that is high—operative mortality may run 15 percent or so, several times greater than for the short-circuit procedure, but it holds some hope for cure if the malignancy has not spread beyond the pancreas.

SEE ALSO PART II for pertinent information about choice of surgeon, preoperative and postoperative care, anesthesia, tests, costs, and other aspects of your operation.

Spleen Surgery

Roughly fist-shaped and about six inches long, the spleen lies high up behind the stomach. In the unborn baby, it plays an important role in producing red and white blood cells. After birth, it no longer makes red cells but still produces white cells. In adult life, it makes neither but does serve a purpose by doing the opposite—destroying old blood cells.

The spleen is not vital. It can be removed without harm. While it is a useful organ, its functions can be taken over elsewhere in the body. Normally, the spleen cannot be felt from outside unless it enlarges considerably. It usually does so when affected by disease and in extreme cases may increase fifty-fold in size. Enlargement may carry some hazard since an ordinarily innocuous bump or knock of the spleen, when it is engorged with blood, may lead to severe internal hemorrhage.

Surgical removal of the spleen may be advisable for any of a number of problems.

A severe blow, fall, or other accidental injury may rupture the spleen, leading to severe bleeding into the abdominal cavity. Diagnosis is usually obvious from the history of the accident, the abdominal pain and tenderness and the patient's pallor. Immediate surgical removal is essential if life is to be saved.

Tumors, cysts, and abscesses of the spleen are rare, but when they occur, they may require removal of the spleen.

Overactivity of the spleen may lead to excessive destruction of blood cells and may cause anemia or mild jaundice with yellow discoloration of the skin. Excessive spleen activity may destroy elements in the blood called platelets needed for clotting and this may lead to thrombocytopenic purpura with bleeding from nose or gums and into the skin, producing bruiselike spots in the skin. Spleen removal may end such problems.

A wide variety of diseases—including blood disorders, tumors, infections and cirrhosis may lead to excessive spleen activity. While spleen removal may produce some temporary improvement, permanent improvement depends upon controlling the underlying disease.

Except for rupture, spleen removal, or splenectomy, is not an emergency operation. There is time for consultation with internist and hematologist (blood specialist) before a decision to perform splenectomy need be made.

The operation is performed under general anesthesia. An incision up to about eight inches long may be made in the upper left abdomen. Blood vessels to and from the spleen are tied off and cut. The organ is then cut away from its attachments to stomach, diaphragm, and colon. Sometimes little accessory spleens are found in the abdominal cavity and these, too, must be removed or they may grow, following the operation, and duplicate what the removed main spleen has been doing. The length of operation may range from an hour or a little less to two hours or a little more depending upon the accessibility of blood vessels and how the spleen is attached.

There is some discomfort from the incision for a few days. In some cases, a rubber drain may be left in place for a few days. For a day or two, a stomach tube may be used to deflate the stomach. Often the patient can be out of bed the day after surgery, can resume bathing in two weeks when the incision has healed, and may leave the hospital within about two weeks; no convalescent care is needed, and work may be resumed within two months.

Once removed, the spleen does not grow back and, since its normal functions are taken over by other body tissues, absence of the spleen does not interfere with normal living. Spleen removal is a major operation but the operative risk is very low. Although it is not possible to tell in advance in every case whether splenectomy will be beneficial, in most cases it is and improved health can be counted on.

SEE ALSO PART II for pertinent information about choice of surgeon, preoperative and postoperative care, anesthesia, tests, costs, and other aspects of your operation.

Adrenal Gland Surgery

The tiny adrenal glands, one atop each kidney, perform many vital functions through the hormones they produce and pour into the bloodstream. Each gland has an inner core, the medulla, and an outer shell, the cortex. The medulla produces the hormone epinephrine, more commonly called adrenalin, which serves, when you become fearful, angry, or excited, to speed up the heartbeat and produce other chemical changes that prepare the body for action. The cortex secretes about thirty hormones that help to control salt and water content of the body, and the handling of sugar and protein.

Occasionally, cancer may originate in the adrenal glands; occasionally, too, cancer originating elsewhere may spread to the adrenals. Much more common are benign tumors.

Tumors of the medulla, called pheochromocytomas, can be a cause of high blood pressure. In some cases, they may lead to headache, abdominal cramps, trembling, palpitation, and excessive sweating. Removal of the tumors can be curative.

Tumors of the cortex are of several types. One, an aldosterone tumor, increases blood pressure, produces blood changes and loss of potassium salts, and leads to painful muscle spasms and weakness. Another type, gluco-corticoid, produces Cushing's syndrome, a set of symptoms that includes rounded, moonlike face, pot belly, excessive fat that makes the upper back humplike. The third type, adrenogenital, causes excessive sex hormone production which may lead to abnormal sexual development in a child or masculinization of a girl or woman and feminization of a boy or man.

Sometimes overgrowth of one or both adrenal glands may produce the same effects as tumors.

Surgery may be used to cut back an overgrown gland or

glands and to remove tumors. Because some cancers elsewhere in the body, such as breast cancer, seem to be influenced to some extent by adrenal gland secretions, the adrenals may sometimes be removed in an effort to prolong life for some months or years.

For adrenal gland surgery, an incision may be made across the upper abdomen or across the back, allowing both glands to be reached. Another incision, such as half on the back and half on the side, may be used to reach one of the adrenal glands.

Adrenal gland surgery is major but most patients recover well and benefit. Usually the patient is out of bed within a day or two after surgery, experiences some discomfort from the wound for several days, has complete healing within about two weeks, and may go home from hospital within two or three weeks.

Some time will be needed to adjust to the new level of hormone secretions. A patient can lead a normal, healthy life if one adrenal gland has to be removed and the other is healthy. If both glands must be removed in their entirety, the patient will need adrenal hormone treatment.

Some adrenal gland cancers can be controlled or destroyed by radiation treatment. Radiation treatment may sometimes be used to supplement surgical removal of a cancerous adrenal gland.

SEE ALSO PART II for pertinent information about choice of surgeon, preoperative and postoperative care, anestheisa, tests, radiology, costs, and other aspects of your operation.

Hernia Operations

Except for tonsillectomy, no operation is performed so frequently as that for hernia or "rupture." About half a million hernia operations are done each year in the United States. On a worldwide basis, it is estimated that hernia affects 10 to 15 percent of the population.

Common hernias occur when internal organs push through

the normally strong wall of the abdomen. Abdominal organs are contained within a thin but tough membrane called the peritoneum. The membrane has a number of passageways in it—for femoral arteries on their way to the legs, for ligaments that support the uterus, for the umbilical cord that nourishes the unborn baby, for the spermatic cords that transport sperm cells from the testes, and others. At any of these passageway areas, the muscles and connective tissue supporting the peritoneum may weaken.

With the weakening, anything that puts added strain or stress on the abdomen—a sudden muscle pull, gain in weight, pregnancy, heavy lifting, repeated coughing attacks, or constipation—may cause a rupture. The peritoneum pushes out through the weakened area, forming a sac with a lump under the skin, and the sac may be filled by abdominal organs.

Hernias can occur at any age. They sometimes occur in babies. They occur in women but far more commonly in men. The common types include inguinal hernias in the groin, femoral hernias just below the groin, umbilical hernias through the navel, incisional hernias through the scar of a surgical incision.

Inguinal Hernia

This is the most common type, accounting for more than two-thirds of all hernias, much more frequent in men than in women. In the unborn male, testes are in the abdomen until about a month before birth, when they discend to the outside through inguinal canals. A tight seal of tissue then normally forms around the spermatic cords which occupy the canals and carry sperm from the testes up through the abdominal wall to the prostate gland and seminal vesicles.

In many men there is no seal, or it is weak and may give way. The opening at first may be no bigger than the little finger and the protruding sac about olive-size. But the opening may grow and the protruding sac sometimes may become as big as a cabbage. Usually, protruding abdominal organs tend to slip out and into the sac after a day's work, while walking or standing or straining; they may return to normal position when the patient lies down. As many hernia sufferers know, a coughing fit will force the organs out and this often can be prevented by using a finger to block the weak spot during a coughing seizure.

Women develop inguinal hernias much less often because there is a tighter bond in their inguinal canals.

A hernia bulge may be present without symptoms, but discomfort is usual. A truss or abdominal support may be worn to hold in the abdominal contents but this method may not be adequate and never produces cure. Many victims learn to manipulate the hernia back but this can be an activity-limiting and uncomfortable way of dealing with the condition. As long as protruding organs move freely in and out, a hernia presents no immediate danger. But at times the organs may become "incarcerated." The neck of the opening may narrow or the contents of the sac may swell and this can lead to strangulation, cutting off of blood supply to the protruding intestine. Gangrene, which follows quickly, produces an emergency situation requiring immediate surgery if life is to be saved.

In surgical repair, the neck of the sac may be tied and the sac itself then cut away after loops of intestine are returned to the abdomen. Muscle and fibrous tissues are overlapped to provide support. If the muscles are not strong enough, a fine wire or plastic mesh may be sewn in to provide additional support. The mesh is strong yet so flexible that its presence is never noticed by the patient.

A hernia repair operation may be carried out under general, spinal, or in some cases local anesthesia. For the usual uncomplicated repair, about forty-five minutes may be needed. There may be some discomfort for a few days in the operative region but it is not great enough to require narcotics. Often the patient is up the following day and may be home a few days later. The wound is usually healed within ten days. After about six weeks, the abdominal wall should have normal strength and there is usually no need to restrict activities. A truss is not needed postoperatively, nor is there interference after the healing period with marital relations or pregnancy.

Hernias can recur but improved surgical techniques have reduced the recurrence rate and more than 90 percent of operations result in permanent cure.

Femoral Hernia

This hernia, much more frequent in women than in men, occurs high up in the thigh, about an inch or so below the groin. Sometimes a femoral hernia may not be noticed until the intestine is trapped and the operation then becomes an emergency one.

Surgical repair may be made through an incision, about three inches long, either in the groin or upper thigh. The repair procedure, including replacement of the intestinal loop in the abdomen, is essentially the same as for repair of an inguinal hernia, and after a six-week period for strengthening of the repair, there is usually no limitation on physical activity.

Umbilical Hernia

This herniation or protrusion through the navel occurs most often in infants and may also develop in women after pregnancy. As weak muscles pull away, the abdominal membrane protrudes under the skin and the navel may appear to be inflated.

Many small umbilical hernias require no surgery. They tend to disappear gradually over the first few years of life and adhesive tape to help hold the muscles together or other support may be used during that time.

When a child is about one year old, if an umbilical hernia remains or has become large enough to admit an adult little finger, its repair may be advised. Repair may be advised especially for girl infants since unrepaired umbilical hernias may enlarge later during pregnancy and require repair after childbirth. There is also some tendency for the intestine to become caught in umbilical hernias in women.

For surgical repair, which may be carried out under general, spinal, or local anesthesia, the navel is lifted, the sac removed, the muscles are pulled together, and the navel is then repositioned. After umbilical hernia repair, as after other hernia surgery, about six weeks are required in adults for strengthening of the repair, after which there need be no limitation on physical activity. Usually, in infants, no special limitations are required.

Incisional Hernia

An incisional hernia, a protrusion through the scar of a surgical incision, can occur shortly after surgery or many years later. When it occurs, it is almost always in the abdomen. The cause often is poor healing in very sick and weakened patients.

The patient may notice a swelling about or through the incision and development of a hard lump which sometimes disappears when he lies down. Intestine, stomach, or liver may be present in the hernia.

For repair, the incision is reopened, the sac removed, and the muscle layers overlapped. If the muscle layers are weak, a plastic fabric mesh may be inserted for support. Because of its flexibility, it will be unnoticeable after surgery. The incision is then stitched securely.

Usually the patient is out of bed next day, pain is only relatively mild and readily relieved for a few days, and hospitalization may run about a week. Usually the repair is successful, for now, in comparison with the time when the original operation was done, the patient may be far better nourished and stronger, greatly increasing the likelihood of healthy healing of the incision. If there should be a recurrence, a second repair operation may still be permanently successful.

The "one day" hernia operation

The patient may check into the hospital the evening before surgery, undergo routine blood and other tests. Early next morning he is wheeled into the operating room, gets a pain-less injection of a local anesthetic in his abdomen, and the surgeon and his assistants go to work. The patient can't see what the surgeon is doing but can talk to him. Half an hour later, the first line of sutures is in place. The surgeon asks the patient to cough, raise his shoulders, testing the strength of the incision. If not satisfied, the surgeon puts in more stitches. Forty-five minutes after the operation began, the patient is told it is over and to "lift yourself off the table." Handed his robe and slippers, he is told to walk back to his hospital room and keep walking all day! If necessary, he may be given a mild analgesic.

Next day, after a hearty breakfast, he spends hours walking miles through hospital corridors, gets a second night's sleep in the hospital. The following day, early in the morning, the surgeon checks him, removes the dressing, and home he goes, even driving his own car.

Such can be the scenario for a procedure which, because of the short hospitalization, has become known as the "One Day" hernia operation. And the patient may be back at work a couple of days later.

The procedure is based on research findings indicating that if strong sutures, such as Dacron-Teflon, are used instead of the conventional type, a wound has 70 percent of normal tissue strength when tested immediately after surgery and may be as strong then as two months later. It is also based on better understanding of the use and possible advantages of local anesthesia. With local anesthesia, the surgeon can test the strength of a hernia repair before final stitches are put in place and strengthen the repair if necessary. According to some reports, the success rate has been better than 97 percent.

While some surgeons—perhaps about a hundred across the country—are enthusiastic about the one-day procedure and use it almost routinely, others have reservations and pre-fer to use traditional methods. They prefer to observe pa-tients in hospital for several days, some for at least five days, for any indications of possible postoperative complications.

SEE ALSO PART II for pertinent information about choice of surgeon, preoperative and postoperative care, anesthesia, tests, costs, and other aspects of your operation.

Undescended Testicle

An undescended testicle very often is accompanied by a hernia. During fetal life, the testicles are in the abdomen, but usually by the time of birth they have descended into the scrotal sac. Sometimes there may be some delay and a normal descent may occur in infancy or childhood. But failure of descent of either one or both testicles may be the result of mechanical interference or inadequate hormone secretion.

Since many testicles do descend spontaneously at about the time of puberty when hormone secretions increase greatly, it is often possible to delay surgery until a child reaches the age of nine or ten or even eleven, especially if the accompanying hernia is small and causes no problems. If the hernia is large and producing symptoms, hernia repair may be required, and during the repair the testicle can be brought down into the scrotum.

In the operation, carried out under general anesthesia, an incision is made in the groin, as for inguinal hernia. By snipping away fibrous tissue which tends to shorten the spermatic cord, the surgeon can lengthen it to permit the testicle to be brought down. To hold the testicle in place long enough to overcome its tendency at first to pull back into the abdomen, the surgeon may use either of two methods. In one, the testicle is slipped through a hole made in the bottom of the scrotum, and anchored to the thigh, buried in a pocket under the skin. After some weeks, the testicle is removed from the thigh and placed in normal position within the scrotum. Alternatively, the testicle, after being brought down within the scrotum, may be anchored there with a suture which is brought out from the bottom of the scrotum and attached to adhesive tape around the thigh. After about a week or so, the suture and tape can be removed. The child is often fully recovered within ten days after the operation.

SEE ALSO PART II for pertinent information about choice of surgeon, preoperative and postoperative care, anesthesia, costs, and other aspects of the operation.

Exploratory Operation

An exploratory operation, also called an exploratory laparotomy, is an abdominal operation performed when there is no definite diagnosis. The hope is that the operation may reveal what is wrong and that the condition, when found, can be treated successfully during the operation.

Exploratory operations are often necessary in emergency situations. After accidents, for example, it can be obvious to the skilled eye that the victim is bleeding internally or has suffered internal injury. There may be no time for delay until repeated X-ray and other studies can be done. The abdomen is opened, a search is made, the bleeding stopped, the injury repaired if possible.

There are also elective exploratory operations. A patient may, for example, have abdominal pain or prolonged weight loss. All X-rays may have been normal and other tests may have provided no definite clues. There may be a tumor.

In some cases, X-ray studies may reveal a definite abnormality but its nature can be determined only by direct vision during exploratory operation. The patient may have known cancer in some cases but operation may be needed to determine the extent of the cancer. In some cases, a patient may have what is called FUO—fever of undetermined origin. The fever persists in the absence of other symptoms or signs, and vigorous search may have failed to produce reliable indications of the real cause.

With diagnostic techniques constantly improving, and with the development of increasingly sophisticated new diagnostic tests, fewer elective exploratories may be needed, but some still remain essential.

An exploratory operation in and of itself carries no great risks. The same type of anesthesia may be used and the same types of incisions may be made as for other abdominal operations. How effective the operation will be depends, of course, upon the problem for which the exploratory is performed. Often the problem becomes quickly apparent and can be corrected, and the operation is a success. Sometimes when the problem turns out to be one that requires no surgical treatment, doubt is removed and medical management thereafter, more aggressive in the absence of lingering doubt, may be successful.

When an elective exploratory operation is advised, consultation is in order. The Joint Commission on Accreditation of Hospitals (see page 360) calls for consultation when a diagnosis is not clear. That regulation should, but may not always, be followed. You have the right to have consultation. It sometimes happens that the consultant can clarify the diagnosis and an unnecessary operation may be avoided.

SEE ALSO PART II for pertinent information about choice of surgeon, preoperative and postoperative care, anesthesia, costs, tests, and other aspects of your operation.

Chest (Thoracic) Surgery
Esophagus, Lungs, and Heart Operations

Thoracic surgery includes operations which involve entrance into the chest or thorax—operations on the esophagus, lungs, and heart. Thanks to special methods developed for them, such operations today are practical and are used increasingly.

The chest, the part of the body between the neck and abdomen, is separated from the abdomen by the diaphragm, a strong dome-shaped muscle which is used in breathing and which forms the floor of the chest cavity. The walls of the chest are formed by the twelve pairs of ribs, attached in back to the sides of the spine and curving toward the front. The upper seven ribs are attached to the sternum or breastbone. The next three ribs connect with cartilage below the sternum and the last two (the floating ribs) are unattached in the front. The ribs surround and guard the lungs and the heart, and also the trachea, or windpipe, the air passage tube extending from the throat and larynx toward the lungs, and the esophagus, which travels through the chest to connect with the stomach below the diaphragm.

Special Measures for Chest Surgery

Until special measures for anesthesia were developed and perfected, chest surgery was very dangerous because of the possibility of lung collapse. The chest cavity is like a closed box. Its walls, being airtight, protect the lungs from atmospheric pressure so they can inflate and deflate during breathing.

The lungs do not suck in air. All the work is done for them by the diaphragm and muscles of the rib cage. When you inhale, muscle fibers of the diaphragm contract and the diaphragm is drawn downward; at the same time, rib muscles pull the ribs upward and outward. This expands the chest cavity, reduces the pressure within it, allows the lungs to expand, and air can rush into the lungs through the air passages. When you exhale, just the opposite series of events occurs. The diaphragm and rib cage muscles relax, the chest becomes smaller, the elastic tissue of the lungs returns to its original shape, and air is driven out.

During surgery, when the chest is open, air enters the chest cavity and the atmospheric pressure on the lungs can make them collapse, shutting down normal breathing. Now, however, with a technique called endotracheal anesthesia, the anesthesiologist can assist the lungs while the chest is open. A tube is inserted into the windpipe and is connected at its outer end to a rubber bag containing oxygen and anesthetic gases. When the bag is squeezed, the lungs are inflated with the oxygen and anesthetic gases. In between squeezes, the lungs can relax and get rid of carbon dioxide through the tube.

With completion of a chest operation, the bag can be squeezed to inflate the lungs and keep them inflated until the ribs have been brought together and the incision has been sutured tightly closed. When the patient comes out of surgery, long rubber catheters or drainage tubes have been left in place. They emerge from the chest cavity and go to bottles of water on the floor at the bedside. This is a closed drainage system. It allows drainage while preventing air from being sucked back into the chest. As the operative site heals, the lung surfaces become sealed to the chest cavity lining and cannot collapse, and the catheters can be slipped out without difficulty. An airtight bandage is then applied.

After operation, the patient may go to an intensive care unit or in some hospitals a special-care nursing unit for chest surgery patients. There, trained nurses and aides can make certain that drainage tubes stay open. The patient will be encouraged to cough in order to remove phlegm from air passages and throat. When the patient has difficulty coughing enough, the phlegm may be sucked out through a tube.

Various types of incisions may be used to enter the chest cavity and the incisions may be lengthy, occasionally, extending fifteen inches or more. One type of incision, on the side, starts in the back at about the middle of the shoulder blade, curves below the blade and then frontward toward the nipple. A rib may be removed or a cut may be made between two ribs. Another type, an incision in the back, may run between shoulder blade and spine. A third, in front, may start under the armpit and extend to the breastbone.

The Esophagus

The esophagus, or gullet, which has no digestive function but carries food from the mouth downward through the neck, chest, and diaphragm to connect up with the stomach, is occasionally subject to disorders which may require surgery.

Relatively rarely, a child may swallow a harsh caustic which may burn part of the esophagus, and the scarring that follows may obstruct the food passage. Often the scarred area can be dilated with instruments. When this is unsuccessful, surgery may be required. It is sometimes possible to remove the scarred section of esophagus through a chest opening and reunite the healthy sections. When the scarred section is long, it may be removed and the stomach then may be brought up enough into the chest so the remaining length of healthy esophagus can be connected to it.

Sometimes, foreign bodies—pins, bones and the like—get caught in the esophagus and must be removed through an instrument, the esophagoscope. Usually this is all that is needed, but if the object has torn or perforated the esophagus, the chest may be opened to allow the tear or perforation to be stitched together.

Congenital deformities, or birth defects, of the esophagus are rare. A short section may be cordlike instead of tubelike so food cannot get by. Or there may be a fistula, an abnormal connection, between esophagus and windpipe, so that some milk gets into the lungs. X-ray films identify such defects, and emergency surgery is needed. Through a chest incision, under general anesthesia, the abnormal opening is closed or the abnormal length of esophagus is removed and the healthy portions reunited. If the baby recovers—and the chances are now better than 50-50 that he will—he will swallow and breathe normally.

More common esophageal problems for which surgery may be required are diverticula, spasm or achalasia, and tumors.

Diverticula of the Esophagus

A diverticulum is a pouchlike deformity produced when the membrane lining the esophagus protrudes through the muscular wall of the esophagus. Pouches may occur anywhere in the esophagus but most commonly form in the neck region.

Symptoms

When diverticula enlarge, sometimes to several inches in diameter, food and liquids may collect in them. There may be peculiar bubbling sounds during food swallowing. Some food or liquid may be regurgitated to the mouth in original form. With sufficient enlargement, diverticula may interfere with swallowing.

Diagnosis

Diverticula can be seen clearly on X-ray films when the patient has taken barium.

When surgery may be needed

When diverticula produce obstruction or severe symptoms, surgery is necessary. Rarely do pouches in the chest area of the esophagus cause any serious difficulty, and surgery is rarely needed. Diverticula in the neck region are removable through an incision about three inches long that may be made at about Adam's apple level.

The operation

The pouches are carefully dissected and removed, and the openings into the esophagus are tied.

Anesthesia

General anesthesia is used.

Recovery

Usually the patient is out of bed the day after surgery. Swallowing is uncomfortable for some days and except for clear liquids, foods by mouth may be banned for as long as a week. Usually, quick recovery takes place.

Achalasia or Esophageal Spasm

This is a condition in which the lower end of the esophagus, the area around the point where the esophagus joins the stomach, is in continuous spasm or contraction. The exact cause is unknown.

Symptoms

There may be progressive difficulty with swallowing and finally inability to swallow at all. Foods stick in the lower end of the esophagus and may be regurgitated. Particularly when prolonged and acute, achalasia can be dangerous be cause of starvation and possible spillage of food into the breathing passages with resulting lung complications.

Medical treatment

Often medication and dilatation, or stretching, of the contracted section of esophagus with tubes provide effective relief.

When surgery may be needed

If medication and dilatation fail to help, surgery can be used.

The operation

Under general anesthesia and through an incision between ribs, the wall of the lower end of the esophagus and sometimes of the upper end of the stomach is cut. The slit may be about four inches long and it is the muscular layers of the wall, not the inner lining, which are cut.

Recovery

The patient without complications may be out of bed within a day, allowed liquids in a day or two, soft foods a few days later, and may be able to go home from the hospital in little more than a week. Most patients are completely relieved of spasm and symptoms.

Cancer of the Esophagus

About 1 percent of all cancers occur in the esophagus, most often in men after the age of fifty.

Symptoms

Because malignant tumors of the esophagus tend to start in the lining membrane, an early symptom may be the sensation of food, particularly meat and soft bread, sticking somewhere behind the breastbone. Pain, sometimes of a fleeting, burning type, may occur with swallowing, or there may be a persistent, boring discomfort.

Diagnosis

A cancer of the esophagus usually shows up on X-ray films. If can also be viewed directly through a tubelike instrument, and a piece of it can be removed for microscopic examination.

When operation is needed

Surgery is the only definitive treatment for cancer of the esophagus.

The operation

The operation, called esophagectomy, is performed under general anesthesia through a chest incision. The earlier the disease is detected, the more likely it is to be confined. The entire cancerous area must be removed, if possible. Improved methods of surgery have made this possible in more and more cases.

It is sometimes possible to have enough remaining healthy esophagus so it can be connected to the stomach. For this, the diaphragm may be cut through and the stomach brought into the chest. In other cases, a portion of intestine may be taken and used to replace the diseased chest part of the esophagus. In some cases, a plastic tube may be used as a replacement.

Recovery time

Surgery for cancer of the esophagus is, of course, very major surgery. There is an uncomfortable period for days afterward. The chest is drained for several days. During the early period, feeding may be by vein, sometimes by way of a tube passed into the stomach. The hospital stay may run two to four weeks, sometimes longer.

SEE ALSO PART II for pertinent information about choice of surgeon, preoperative and postoperative care, anesthesia, tests, costs, and other aspects of your operation.

The Lungs

The lungs, which supply the blood with oxygen inhaled from outside air and dispose of waste carbon dioxide in exhaled air, lie on either side of the heart within the chest cavity. The lungs are divided into lobes: the left lung has two lobes, the right has three. Each lobe has independent subdivisions or segments. There are several diseases of the lungs for which surgery may be needed.

Surgical procedures performed on the lungs include removal of an entire lung, which is called pneumonectomy; removal of a lobe of a lung, called lobectomy; and removal of only a segment, called segmental resection. The procedure utilized depends upon the size of the area involved and the nature of the disease.

Lung Abscess

Lung abscess is an infection of a lung with a localized accumulation of pus. It may be a complication of pneumonia or tuberculosis, or of food going the wrong way and lodging in a lung area, or of lung cancer (in up to 10 percent of cases).

Symptoms

The first symtoms may be cough with purulent sputum, sweats, chills, fever, loss of appetite. Chest pain may be present.

Diagnosis

Such symptoms, and especially purulent sputum, suggest abscess. X-rays and examination of air passages through an instrument, the bronchoscope, may be used to aid diagnosis.

When surgery may be needed

About 85 percent of patients respond to medical measures, including use of antibiotics. When medical treatment fails, an incision may be made in the chest; the abscess may be opened and drained for a few days while antibiotic medication is continued. Usually, when medical treatment fails, the lobe of the lung containing the abscess is removed. In some cases, only a segment of a lobe may be removed; in other cases, when many abscesses are present, an entire lung may be removed.

Recovery

The chances of recovery from removal of a complete lung are now better than 90 percent; from removal of a lobe, better than 95 percent and from removal of a segment, still better. The operation may take two to four hours; the patient may be out of bed in one to three days. The incision heals in about two weeks, and it is possible for the patient to be out of hospital in two weeks or a little less. There is lung to spare, and loss of a segment or lobe is of little consequence. When necessary, a whole lung can be removed and the patient can get along well on the one remaining lung, capable of ordinary exertion though not of extremely vigorous exertion.

Lung Cyst

A lung cyst is a sac that may be filled with fluid or air and may be present at birth or develop at some point later. If a cyst becomes infected, an abscess may form. If a cyst should burst, air may enter the chest cavity and lung collapse may follow, with pain and breathlessness.

When a cyst causes symptoms, surgery similar to that for lung abscess may be used to remove the cyst or the part of the lung containing it.

Tuberculosis

Modern drug treatment for tuberculosis is so effective that surgery is rarely needed. When such treatment fails, surgery may be used to supplement it.

In some cases, a localized diseased segment of lung may be removed to speed cure and help insure against recurrence. The procedure is similar to that for lung abscess.

In some cases, it is not feasible to remove the diseased area because it is large or because it adheres to chest lining or large blood vessels. Then thoracoplasty, or collapse surgery, may be used. All or portions of two or more ribs over the affected lung may be removed. With their removal, the chest wall can sink in against the diseased lung and cause it to collapse. The collapsed lung is motionless, at rest, and, with continued intensive medical treatment, the chances for eradication of infection and healing are increased.

With thoracoplasty, there is a better than even chance that the disease will be halted. Almost all patients recover from the surgery itself.

Bronchiectasis

Bronchiectasis is a chronic disease in which there is a widening of the bronchial airway in a single area or throughout as the airway wall loses elasticity. Infection sets in.

Symptoms may include persistent cough, usually in spells; foul-smelling sputum; unpleasant breath odor; expectoration of blood; recurrent attacks of acute respiratory infection.

In most cases, treatment is medical and aimed at controlling infection. If the diseased area is sufficiently localized in one portion of the lungs, marked improvement may follow removal of the diseased area. The procedure may be similar to that for removal of a lung area containing an abscess.

Lung Tumors

Benign tumors of the lungs occur but are relatively rare; most lung growths are cancerous. Ninety percent of patients with lung cancer complain of a cough and in 50 percent it is the first symptom. Often the chest X-ray provides the first indication of abnormality in a patient with lung cancer who does not yet have symptoms. About two-thirds of cases of lung cancer can be diagnosed from examination of sputum.

The diagnosis is usually established definitively by bronchoscopy. Under either general or local anesthesia, a thin, tube-like, illuminated instrument is inserted through the throat into the windpipe and bronchial tubes. When the tumor is seen, a tiny bit of it can be snipped with scissors through the bronchoscope and examined with the microscope.

An additional diagnostic aid is scalene biopsy. The scalene area, which is just above the collarbone on each side of the neck, contains lymph nodes to which a lung cancer may spread. Under local anesthesia, a two-inch incision is made above the collarbone, and the scalene nodes are removed for microscopic examination.

When surgery is possible, it is the treatment of choice.

If the cancer has not spread, lobectomy to remove an affected lobe or pneumonectomy to remove an entire affected lung may be used. The incision and anesthesia (general through an endotracheal tube) are the same as used for lobectomy or pneumonectomy for other lung problems such as lung abscess. The patient may be out of bed within one to three days; the chest will be drained for several days; and it may be possible for the patient to go home in about two weeks.

Unfortunately, only about one-fourth of patients with lung cancer come to operation early enough, with the cancer still localized enough, to permit surgical removal. Hopefully, growing attention to earliest possible detection of lung cancer, including yearly chest X-rays of people over forty who smoke, will make possible more surgical cure.

X-ray treatment may be used before or after surgery or when surgery is not feasible. By shrinking the tumor, irradiation may permit surgery on a previously inoperable growth. Treatment with various anticancer drugs may produce some temporary improvement in patients with inoperable cancer. Early experimental results with new techniques of massive administration in pulses of anticancer medication and with methods of immunotherapy aimed at increasing the body's defense mechanisms give some promise of improving the outlook for lung cancer in the future.

The overall five-year survival rate as of now is less than 10 percent. But this, it must be remembered, is an overall statistic. Any individual patient can be hopeful of possibly much greater chances for successful treatment particularly with early diagnosis.

SEE ALSO PART II for pertinent information about choice of surgeon, preoperative and postoperative care, anesthesia, tests, costs, and other aspects of your operation.

Heart Operations

Man has always been fascinated by the heart, once regarded as the seat not only of life but of intelligence and reasoning power. We know now that the heart is a pump, a remarkable one, but just a pump. And surgical advances have made correctable disorders of the pump which once were inevitably debilitating or deadly.

Among the beneficiaries are the 30,000 to 40,000 babies born each year in the U.S. with heart defects—defects in the main blood vessels connecting directly to the heart; defects in the valves between the chambers of the heart and between the heart and its outlets; and defects in the inner heart walls. The beneficiaries also include children and adults with defects acquired later in life. Additionally, in very recent years, surgery has opened up new hope for many people with coronary heart disease in which the coronary arteries feeding the heart muscle become clogged, leading to chest pain, restricted activity, and heart attacks.

Reaching the heart

The heart's location in the chest makes it as readily reachable as the lungs and other organs in the chest. The chest can be opened and the heart brought into full view. The type of incision used depends upon the part of the heart to be repaired. In some cases an incision may be made through the side of the chest under the arm, right or left. In other cases, a middle-of-the-chest incision is made and the breastbone is split with an electric saw. The breastbone is drawn together after the operation.

Anesthesia

Endotracheal anesthesia is used. The anesthetic is administered through a tube inserted into the windpipe, as for most operations in the chest area.

Closed-heart surgery

Some heart operations can be carried out while the heart remains closed and continues to pump blood.

Open-heart surgery and the heart-lung machine

One of the major advances in surgery was the development of the heart-lung machine, which made it possible to still the heart and open it for complex repairs. The machine, also known as a pump-oxygenator, can take over both the pumping work of the heart and the work of the lungs and can do this for several hours when necessary while surgery is performed on the heart.

There are variations in the way the machine may be used, but generally the method is this: Blood, which returns from the body to the heart through the two great veins, the venae cavae, is instead brought temporarily through tubing into the machine. In the artificial lung part of the machine, oxygen is added and carbon dioxide is removed much as the lungs would do the job. This is done by exposing the blood to oxygen or air on large flat disc surfaces or by bubbling oxygen through the blood, or by other means. The machine then pumps the blood into tubing that connects with the artery system of the body, through which it is then sent to all body tissues. By thus taking over the work of heart and lungs, the machine allows the heart to be stopped temporarily and opened up. Then repairs can be made in a dry and motionless heart.

A view of the heart

To understand the surgical procedures that may be used for heart problems, it is helpful to know a few facts about the heart and its functioning.

When fully grown, the human heart is a little larger than a clenched adult fist and weighs less than a pound. It roughly resembles a ripe eggplant in shape and is located in the front (part) of the chest, under the breastbone in the center, with its apex pointed to the left. It is a hollow organ. Its wall is made up of thick muscle called the myocardium. Inside are four hollow chambers, two on the right side and two on the left. The top chamber on each side is the atrium, or receiving chamber for blood; the bottom chamber on each side is the ventricle, or pumping chamber. A solid partition of muscle, the septum, separates right atrium and ventricle from left atrium and ventricle, so the heart functions as two separate pumps, side by side. The right side of the heart sends blood that has circulated throughout the body to the lungs to be freshened with oxygen; the left side sends the blood freshened in the lungs back through the body again.

Blood returning from the body to the heart enters the right atrium through the great veins, the venae cavae. As the atrium fills, it passes the blood through a valve, the tricuspid, into the right ventricle below. The right ventricle contracts and propels the blood into the pulmonary artery, which carries it to the lungs. In this process a valve, the pulmonary, opens to let the blood flow into the artery and closes behind the blood to avoid backflow.

After freshening in the lungs, blood returns via the pulmonary veins to the heart and enters the left atrium. As the atrium fills, it contracts to send the blood through a valve, the mitral, into the left ventricle below. With a strong contraction, the left ventricle pumps the blood into the aorta, the body's great trunkline artery, and in this process a valve, the aortic, opens to let the blood through and then closes to avoid backflow.

Like all other body tissues, the heart muscle itself must have oxygen replenishment and waste removal. A special coronary circulation system takes care of this. From the aorta, near the point at which this great vessel comes out of the heart, two coronary arteries branch off. Each has a diameter about the size of a thin pencil. The left coronary artery supplies mainly the left side, part of the front and the back of the heart muscle. The right coronary supplies mainly the right and back sides of the ventricle areas. Each artery branches. The left coronary divides into two major divisions, which is why it is sometimes said that there are three main arteries that nourish the heart.

Congenital Heart Defects (Defects Present at Birth)

There is still no clear-cut answer to why some children are born with heart defects. If a mother has German measles early in pregnancy, her baby's heart development may be affected—and, since German measles is a virus disease, the possibility that other virus diseases early in pregnancy may account for some defects is under study. The role of heredity is uncertain. While more than one child in a family may have a congenital heart defect, such cases are rare. Also under study is the possibility that some drugs taken in early pregnancy may cause malformation of the baby's heart.

Patent Ductus Arteriosus

Because an unborn baby gets oxygen from the mother, and not from his own lungs, he has a short blood vessel, a ductus, that bypasses blood around his lungs. The channel is not needed after birth and normally within a few weeks after birth, the ductus closes off and begins to shrivel away.

If the ductus continues open or patent, some fresh blood, already circulated to the lungs, is needlessly circulated back again to the lungs. In some cases, as much as half of the blood leaving the left ventricle to go to the body—head, trunk and limbs—may be shuttled needlessly back to the lungs again.

Then, with so much blood being returned to the lungs, in order to maintain adequate circulation for the body, the heart effort has to increase. The heart accommodates to the job, but over a period of time it may pump less efficiently, the child's growth may be slowed, and there is risk that infection may develop in the ductus.

A child with a patent ductus arteriosus may have no symptoms or he may have blueness of the lower half of the body. The condition can be diagnosed by the whirring noises heard through a stethoscope during medical examination.

Surgery to close the ductus is relatively simple. The duct is located outside the heart and no heart-lung machine or other special equipment is required. The duct is tied off and cut for permanent correction. Within two to three weeks after the operation, the typical child thrives and is normal in every way and has a normal life expectancy.

Coarctation of the Aorta

Coarctation is a pinching or constriction of the aorta, the great artery coming out of the heart. The pinching may be minor, or so great that only a tiny channel for blood flow remains. Usually the pinching occurs at a point in the aorta just beyond where arteries to the head and arms branch off. Because of the pinching and obstruction, blood pressure increases much like water pressure does when you tighten a garden hose nozzle. The pressure increase occurs in vessels of arms and head before the point of narrowing in the aorta and long-continued excessive pressure may lead later in life to damage to blood vessels in head and eyes with possible stroke or visual disturbance. The heart, too, forced to work harder because of the pressure against which it must pump blood, may begin to fail.

Usually, a child with coarctation has no troublesome symptoms. The condition is detected during physical examination when blood pressure is found to be high in the arms and a check of pressure in the legs shows it to be lower than in the arms.

Surgery for coarctation, as for patent ductus arteriosus, does not require going into the heart. The pinched section of aorta is cut out and the healthy ends of the aorta are joined. If a long section must be removed, a synthetic graft may be placed between the healthy sections.

The operation usually produces complete cure, and after a stay of about two weeks in the hospital, the child is usually ready to go home in good health.

Atrial Septal Defect

This is an abnormal opening in the upper septum, the part of the wall that separates the left and right atria, or upper chambers of the heart. It allows some blood to flow abnormally from the left to the right atrium, the amount depending on the size of the septal opening. Usually the amount is substantial.

The blood from the left atrium has already been to the lungs, but the right atrium sends it to the right ventricle which pumps it back to the lungs again. Right atrium and right ventricle must work harder, increase in size, and later in life the heart may weaken. In childhood, increased flow through the lungs may lead to reduced resistance to respiratory infections and a child with an atrial septal defect may have repeated colds and pneumonia. There may be some shortness of breath and a tendency to tire easily.

Diagnosis can be made on the basis of a heart murmur, X-ray examination showing enlargement of the right side of the heart, changes in the electrocardiogram indicating strain on the right half of the heart.

Generally, the most suitable time for surgery, which can cure the defect, is between ages six and twelve. The heart-lung machine is used so the surgeon can open the heart. If the septal opening is small, he can stitch it closed; if large, a patch can be used to close it. The closing is permanent.

The operation takes two to three hours, the patient is in hospital for ten to fourteen days and back in school within four weeks, with a normal life expectancy.

Ventricular Septal Defect

In this condition, the abnormal opening is in the lower septum, the part of the wall that separates the left and right ventricles or lower chambers of the heart. The defect may be so small that no treatment is needed and occasionally a small defect may close on its own, but with a large defect, blood is shunted from the left ventricle to the right ventricle. Pressure in the right ventricle then goes up abnormally and the increased pressure is transmitted to the lungs, sometimes producing abnormalities in the blood vessels there.

With a large defect, the usual symptoms are labored breathing and fatigue with exertion. In infants, there may be breathing difficulty even at rest, and increased susceptibility to upper respiratory infections. Children with large defects often are undersized because more blood flows to the lungs than to the rest of the body.

Diagnosis is much the same as for atrial septal defect: a typical heart murmur, X-ray examination, electrocardiographic changes. Surgery, too, is much the same, using the heart-lung machine. The opening is closed by stitching or, if too large for that, by inserting a patch. The operation takes two to three hours, the patient is home from hospital in about two weeks, and a normal, healthy life can be expected.

Surgeons usually prefer to postpone permanent procedures until a child is two or three years old, when the likelihood of success is greater; in some infants with a large defect, a temporary surgical procedure may be needed. It consists of opening the chest and placing a band around the outside of the pulmonary artery. This reduces blood flow to the lung and also increases pressure in the right side of the heart; the increased pressure there helps to lower the amount of blood shunted into the right ventricle from the left ventricle. The temporary procedure can be life-saving and later, when the defect is closed permanently, the band can be removed.

Pulmonary Stenosis

Some children are born with a stenosed, or narrowed, pulmonary valve. The amount of blood that can go to the lungs is then reduced and body tissues get less than an adequate supply of fresh blood. The strain of pumping blood through the narrowed valve may also cause the right side of the heart to enlarge.

Some children have no symptoms; others experience fatigue, light-headedness, and shortness of breath. Diagnosis can be made without difficulty. A harsh murmur can be heard over the lung area; X-ray examination may show enlargement of the right ventricle and changes in pulmonary artery and lung vessels; and there are usually electrocardiographic changes.

The constricted valve can be cut and dilated while the patient is on the heart-lung machine and thereafter more blood can flow through. In some cases, there may also be a thickening of the heart wall near the valve, and a portion of the wall can be cut away. The operation takes several hours and is successful in the great majority of cases, making possible normal life expectancy. The patient may be home from hospital in about two weeks.

Aortic Stenosis

Stenosis, or narrowing, of the aortic valve which regulates flow of blood from the heart into the great aorta makes it difficult for the heart to pump blood to the body.

Many children with aortic stenosis do well in the early years, have no symptoms, and develop normally. In time, however, the obstruction may increase, seriously interfere with heart function, and produce fatigability and chest pain with effort.

Diagnosis can be made from the loud murmur that can be heard over the aortic area, X-ray studies showing enlargement of part of the aorta, and electrocardiographic changes.

Surgery is done with the aid of the heart-lung machine. Sometimes the valve can be opened up sufficiently for normal flow. In other cases, the valve may be removed and replaced with a plastic substitute. The outlook after such surgery is excellent.

Tetralogy of Fallot (Blue Baby)

Some congenital heart defects can lead to mixing of fresh and used blood so the blood flowing from the heart to body tissues is poor in oxygen and bluish-red in color. This is known as cyanotic (from the Greek word for "blue") heart disease and the baby is said to be a "blue baby" because of bluish color in fingernail beds, lips, nose tip, and other areas.

The most common such defect with which a child can live for any length of time is Tetralogy of Fallot. It really consists of four defects. The pulmonary valve or area below it is narrowed and impedes blood flow to the lungs (pulmonary stenosis). An opening in the wall between the two ventricles (ventricular septal defect) permits used blood in the right ventricle to mix with fresh blood in the left. The aorta, instead of emerging from the left ventricle, straddles both ventricles and leaves the heart at a point just over the septal defect so it receives an unhealthy mix of oxygen-rich and oxygen-poor blood for the body. The right ventricle is enlarged because of the extra work it has to do to pump blood through the narrowed pulmonary valve.

The degree to which the child is affected depends on the obstruction to blood flow to the lungs. When obstruction is great, much of the oxygen-poor blood from the right ventricle bypasses the lungs and goes to the body and the child may be cyanotic or blue from birth. When obstruction is relatively slight, which is often the case in early infancy, much of the oxygen-poor blood moves past the obstruction to the lungs, only a small proportion goes to the aorta, and there may be no blueness except when the baby cries or is physically active. Occasionally, with very mild obstruction, blueness never develops. Except in the mildest cases, a child with Tetralogy tends to be underweight and underdeveloped for lack of adequate oxygen supply to body tissues.

Diagnosis can be made by the child's appearance, the murmur that can be heard through a stethoscope, X-ray study of the heart, and electrocardiographic studies. And although the outlook for a child with a combination of four defects may seem poor, today it is excellent.

In most cases, complete cure is achievable with surgery, which usually is best performed in an older child or young adult. Until then, medication can be used if necessary to strengthen the heart muscle. To compensate for blueness, the body often increases the number of oxygen-carrying blood cells; if excessive cells are formed, they can be removed by careful bleeding. In a child too ill to wait for curative surgery, a special palliative operation can be used for temporary relief.

In a palliative operation, which is designed to increase blood flow to the lungs, an artery coming off the great aorta, usually the subclavian, is connected to the pulmonary artery, thus bypassing the pulmonary valve obstruction. In this way, some of the mixture of oxygen-rich and oxygen-poor blood coming into the aorta from the heart moves through the pulmonary artery to the lungs for oxygen enrichment, and more oxygen can reach body tissues. Although the palliative operation corrects no defects, it is safe, does not require opening the heart, and decreases blueness and breathing difficulty.

Later, often when the child is between five and twelve, the permanently corrective operation may be performed, using the heart-lung machine. After opening the chest, an incision in the right ventricle is made, the pulmonary valve is repaired, and the opening in the wall between the ventricles is closed. Often, results are dramatic as a healthy pink look takes the place of blueness, and activity tolerance increases greatly. The child may be home within two to three weeks.

Transposition of the Great Vessels

In this defect, which also causes blueness, the pulmonary artery is located where the aorta should be, and vice versa. Normally the pulmonary artery comes out of the right ventricle and carries blood to the lungs. In transposition, the artery comes out of the left ventricle instead and so takes blood, which has already been to the lungs, back there again. And the aorta, which normally comes out of the left ventricle and takes fresh blood to body tissues, is attached to the right ventricle and so gets and takes used blood to body tissues.

Blue at birth or within a few days, babies with transposition live only if they have an additional heart defect which actually helps counter the transposition. It may be an opening in the wall between ventricles or between atria (ventricular or atrial septal defect), or a connection between pulmonary artery and aorta (patent ductus arteriosus). With one such defect present, there is some mixture of fresh and used blood and the child may receive enough oxygenated blood to survive.

Murmurs, X-ray and electrocardiogram, and other studies allow diagnosis of the problem. Surgery consists of inserting a catheter into a body vein, maneuvering it into the heart, and using the catheter to make an opening in the septum between the atria. The opening increases the amount of oxygenated blood that can reach body tissues and although the technique is only palliative, not curative, it can be lifesaving. There is increasing hope that a curative technique for transposition may be found before very long.

Combinations of Defects

Tetralogy of Fallot, as we have seen, is one combination. Others may occur. There may be an atrial defect associated with a ventricular septal defect or with patent ductus arteriosus. There may be a patent ductus arteriosus associated with a ventricular septal defect or with coarctation of the aorta.

Diagnosis usually can be made quickly from symptoms and from X-ray, electrocardiogram, and other studies. And the surgical treamtents used for the individual defects can be used to correct the combination. The results are often excellent.

Overall Care for a Child
with a Congenital Heart Problem

If your child is born with a heart defect, you have reason now to be more optimistic than you could have been several years ago.

There may be no urgent need for surgery during infancy. Many babies with defects are otherwise healthy; even a blue baby may do well. Unless the child is doing very poorly, gaining no weight and showing signs of heart enlargement or other deterioration, your physician may counsel watchful waiting to see how his body and circulation may adjust and compensate for the defect. Even with blueness, the brain has priority on blood supply and there is little likelihood of interference with mental development.

If the child has a minor defect, avoid treating him as an invalid. Only rarely is limitation of activity necessary. It's as if, guided by nature, the child will be only as active as his condition permits. If he wants to engage in some activity the chances are great that he has the capacity for it. Allowed to enjoy childhood, the child will be better for it. An older child who becomes so competitive in sports that he overexerts himself may need some restrictions, and your physician will indicate the need.

With good care, a child with a defect can come through the usual childhood diseases. He should, of course, have periodic checkups for his heart condition. Medication may not be needed at all. In some cases, it may be used to relieve symptoms or help avoid complications, and to keep the condition under good control until a suitable age for surgery is reached.

The best time for surgery

If a child's growth and development is not seriously affected by a defect, it is often wise to delay surgery at least to age two and preferably to age five or beyond. It does sometimes happen that a defect repairs itself in the first several years of life. If it doesn't, surgical results are more likely to be excellent when a child is a little older. When a defect is so severe that surgery must be performed very early, even immediately after birth, the risk is greater than it would be later—but it is still justified, since there is no real alternative and often such early operations are successful.

The risk

There is always some risk in any kind of surgery, as there is in almost any activity in life. The risk in connection with congenital defect correction, once high, has been lowered greatly and is constantly being lowered further. Now, even for a very complex defect, there is less than a 5 percent chance that an operation will fail, that a child in good surgical hands will succumb in the operating room or soon afterward—and for some of the simpler defects, the risk is less than 1 in 100.

Still, even a 1 in 100 chance that a child will not come through makes a parental decision for surgery no light one. In deciding, you have every right to answers from your family doctor, the child's cardiologist, or the surgeon, or all three, to these questions: Is the child's life threatened immediately? If not, is the defect sooner or later going to lead to irreparable heart damage? Are the chances good that surgery can mean that the child will have a normal or near-normal life expectancy?

Preparing the child

Your doctor will have suggestions about how to do this.

Generally, the truth is less frightening to a child than what he may imagine. Without excessive detail, you can tell the child that his heart is not working exactly as it should and it can be repaired so it will work properly. You can tell him that the repair can be made more easily in the hospital, and while it is being made he will be asleep and will not feel anything. Afterward, he may hurt a bit for a while but he'll not care too much about that because he'll know he is getting better, and the pain will go away before long. You can tell him, too, that he'll stay in the hospital for a few weeks so doctors and nurses can help him get better faster, he'll meet other children in the hospital, and you will be coming to see him.

You won't be able to obliterate all his fears, but by

giving him a true picture, not excessively detailed, you will lessen them.

After the operation

The length of hospitalization after surgery for a heart defect averages about two weeks but may run longer, depending upon the type of defect, its severity, and the type of operation. The same considerations determine the length of convalescence at home. You'll get a good idea, usually from the hospital staff cardiologist, just before you take the child home or when you bring the child back to the hospital for a follow-up visit, about the likely length of convalescence, what the child can and cannot do while convalescing.

After convalescence, the outlook for the child's future is good. When a defect can be completely cured, the child can engage in all normal activities after convalescence. With partial correction, he can be—in most cases—much more active than in the past. Rarely is there a recurrence of a defect after correction.

Adult Congenital Heart Defects

The same corrective surgical techniques for congenital heart defects in children can be used for such defects in adults.

In some cases, a heart defect may produce no symptoms at all early in life but may do so in young adulthood or middle age. For lack of symptoms, a defect may not have been diagnosed early in life and, in some cases, although the defect was diagnosed early, there was no effective surgery available at that time.

When an adult has a defect that gives rise to few and relatively mild symptoms that are controllable with medication, and when there is no indication that any irreversible damage to the heart is occurring, surgery may not be needed. When it is needed, it can be used with excellent chances of success.

Acquired Heart Defects

One of the most common "minor" ailments is the sore throat, and many different disease organisms can infect the throat and make it sore. When the infection is caused by one organism in particular, Group A hemolytic streptococcus, there is a special risk. In about 3 percent of cases, particularly among children, after an interval of several weeks, a strep sore throat is followed by rheumatic fever, so-called because it produces inflammation and pain in joints such as the knees, wrists, or elbows.

Rheumatic fever may have an even more serious effect: inflammation of the heart, which may leave one or more of the heart valves damaged. Fortunately, the incidence of rheumatic fever can be reduced by closer attention to sore throats, diagnosis of the strep type, and prompt treatment with antibiotics. Moreover, rarely is such damage serious after a single attack of rheumatic fever, but repeated episodes may lead to further damage.

The valve most often affected is the mitral, less commonly the aortic. Sometimes both the mitral and aortic valves are damaged.

Mitral Valve Damage

Blood flows through the mitral valve from the left atrium, where it arrives fresh from the lungs, to the left ventricle, which pumps it out into the aorta and the body. During acute rheumatic fever, areas of the valve may thicken so it cannot close properly. Sometimes, when the rheumatic fever attack is over, the valve returns to normal size and then closes normally again, but in other cases, there is permanent impairment.

When the valve fails to close properly, blood leaks back from the ventricle to the atrium. As long as the deformity is mild and the leakage small, there may be no difficulty at all for the patient during a normal lifetime. With severe leakage, however, fatigue and weakness develop, along with a loud, high-pitched murmur that can be heard with the stethoscope. The ventricle, trying to push more blood out to the body to make up for the backward leakage, enlarges and this can be seen on X-ray pictures and can be detected in electrocardiographic studies. Such improper closure of the valve is called *mitral insufficiency*.

Alternatively, the value may be so damaged that it cannot open properly. This is *mitral stenosis*. The blood flow from atrium into ventricle is reduced. With the atrium contracting but unable to push most of its blood through the valve, pressure builds up and is transmitted back to the lungs, affecting lung functioning. Breathing may become labored, activity limited. As small blood vessels in lungs and airways become overly filled with blood from the back-pressure, they may rupture, leading to spitting of blood. Diagnosis can be made by the typical sounds of mitral stenosis heard through the stethoscope and by X-ray and electrocardiographic studies.

Aortic Valve Damage

The aortic valve, which controls blood flow from left ventricle into the great aorta, also may be affected by rheumatic fever so that it fails either to open or to close properly.

When the valve can't close completely and blood leaks backward through it, the left ventricle has to pump harder to try to maintain adequate circulation, and it enlarges. Usually, incomplete closure produces no symptoms for years until the ventricle, after being long overburdened, begins to weaken and lose ability to pump effectively. Then heart failure develops; the heart does not stop pumping, but the ventricle does not contract as forcefully and so pushes out less blood with each beat. As a result of the poor circulation, breathing becomes labored and fluids accumulate in body tissues.

Even when there are no obvious symptoms, the diagnosis

of *aortic insufficiency* can be made by the heart murmur heard through the stethoscope, the heart size, and the blood pressure.

Alternatively, as with the mitral valve, the aortic may be so damaged that it cannot open normally. If the opening is significantly reduced, pressure builds up within the ventricle and, as it works to force blood through, the ventricle thickens. Because of the extra work, the heart muscle needs much more oxygen, which must be supplied in the blood coming to the muscle through the coronary arteries which branch off the aorta. But despite the hard work of the ventricle, blood flow through the aorta may be reduced—and that means diminished flow from the aorta into the coronary arteries as well as into other arteries of the body. As a result, there may be chest pain with exertion and also fainting or light-headedness because of reduced blood flow to the brain.

Medical treatment

Valve defects from rheumatic fever can vary greatly in degree, and a defect usually must be of considerable degree to be injurious.

Slight backward leakage through a mitral or aortic valve that does not close properly is usually of no consequence. The backflow has to be large before the heart becomes greatly burdened. Similarly, the opening of either valve can be reduced to as little as one-half original size without serious consequences, and it may not be until the opening is cut by 75 percent that the heart work load is greatly increased.

Many people with mild rheumatic heart damage lead normal lives and have normal life expectancies. Some with moderate damage have only minor and nondisabling symptoms. But severe disease may produce disability early in life. Sometimes, too, disability comes on very suddenly. Mitral stenosis, for example, after producing no symptoms for twenty years or more, may in some cases suddenly lead to heart failure which may be overcome with medical treatment and the stenosis than may require surgical treatment.

Medical treatment can be used for complications of rheumatic heart disease. For heart failure, a drug, digitalis, can strengthen the heart and increase its pumping efficiency, while diuretic drugs and restriction of salt in the diet help get rid of excess fluids. In mitral stenosis, an irregular heart rhythm called atrial fibrillation, may develop. The upper chambers of the heart twitch rather than contract. Blood still moves from the upper chambers to the ventricles and atrial fibrillation is not deadly but it does reduce the heart's working efficiency. Medication such as quinidine can stop the fibrillation and lead to normal contractions.

Surgery

By no means is surgery inevitable for rheumatic heart disease. Many people do well all through life without need for operation. The need for surgery has to be weighed on the basis of the individual patient's future outlook if an operation is not performed, the benefits to be expected, and the risk and difficulty of operation. Fortunately, there have been major advances in heart valve surgery since the first successful such operation—for correcting mitral stenosis—was reported in 1949.

When a mitral or aortic valve is obstructed, it is relatively easy to correct the deformity. With the help of the heart-lung machine, the heart can be opened, the valve inspected closely, and then readily snipped apart to improve blood flow.

When leakage of mitral or aortic valve is the problem, the defective valve can be replaced with an artificial valve that consists of a small disk moving in a little cage. The operation, performed with the heart-lung machine, takes about three hours, and usually a patient is eating and drinking well within three days and is home within about two weeks. The operation to replace a valve is somewhat riskier than repair of a stenosed valve but when needed, the risk is justified since the operation can avoid invalidism and even save life.

Earlier artificial valves sometimes caused problems. The first materials used sometimes made blood clots form and these might have broken loose, traveled, and become lodged in a leg, brain, or coronary artery. With newer materials, clot formation is rare. So, too, is another complication, anemia that sometimes occurred when older artificial valves mechanically destroyed red blood cells.

SEE ALSO PART II for pertinent information about choice of surgeon, preoperative and postoperative care, anesthesia, tests, costs, and other aspects of your operation.

Pacemaker Surgery

Many thousands of people who have chronic heart disease today are doing well, their hearts kept beating properly, with the aid of electronic pacemakers.

Normally, the heartbeat is paced by electrical impulses coming from the sino-atrial node, a special area in the upper right quarter of the right atrium. The impulses from the node travel through heart muscle fibers to trigger contraction of both atria. They also travel to another area in the lower left quarter of the right atrium, known as the atrioventricular node. From this node, impulses go to the ventricles to trigger their contraction, passing through special conduction tissues.

When disease or injury has affected the conduction tissues, and therefore the impulses do not travel through them normally, the pumping activity of the ventricles is affected. The result, heart block, may vary in severity and may be either temporary or permanent. When the impaired pumping action leads to markedly diminished blood flow to the brain, there may be episodes of giddiness, fainting, and convulsions.

Some forms of heart block, milder and temporary, sometimes can be treated effectively by medication, including ephedrine, epinephrine, quinidine, procainamide, and isoproterenol. But when medication is inadequate, normal heart rate can be restored and maintained with an artificial pace-maker.

Pacemakers are compact, measuring about 2 x 2½ x 1 inches, and are powered by batteries which generally are replaced every two or three years.

An artificial pacemaker may be implanted by either of two methods:

In one method, the *transthoracic,* under general anesthesia, the chest is opened between two ribs, exposing the heart, and an electrode is sutured to the heart muscle. The pacemaker to which the electrode leads is stitched in place between the skin and fat layers of the chest or abdomen. The operation is brief, and the patient is usually out of bed the day after and home within ten days.

In a second method, *transvenous,* local anesthesia is used and a small electrode catheter is inserted in a neck or chest vein and maneuvered, with X-ray guidance, into the right ventricle. The catheter is tied securely at the point where it enters the vein and the remaining length then may be threaded under skin and fat to the chest or abdominal site where the pacemaker is implanted under the skin. The patient is usually out of bed next day and home within a week.

The first pacemakers operated at a fixed rate, firing regularly about 70 times a minute. Newer, more sophisticated pacemakers are known as "demand" types and work only when needed. As long as the heart is beating properly on its own, the pacemaker lies quiet, but the instant the heart rate becomes abnormally slow, the pacemaker automatically goes into operation to restore normal rhythm.

Once, pacemakers occasionally failed and required operation for replacement because of breaks in wires, but specially developed wires have overcome this problem. Generally, batteries are replaced every two or three years, requiring relatively simple surgery to open the skin pouch, remove the old and insert the new battery, then close up the pouch again.

Current pacemakers are highly effective. One study has shown that of more than 300 patients receiving pacemakers and followed up over a ten-year period, 73 percent remained alive at the end of that time and many of the deaths that occurred had no relationship to heart disease. Quite a few survivors had returned to jobs and near-normal living.

Under development now are nuclear-powered pacemakers which, hopefully, may run twenty years or more; others weighing less than an ounce and containing a special crystal that can change the mechanical energy from a heart contraction to electrical energy, store the electrical energy in a tiny condenser and use the stored energy as needed; and still others requiring no wires which use radio energy beamed from a transmitter worn outside the body to a tiny receiver implanted near the heart.

A new pacemaker showing great promise in trials in patients after extensive trials in animals, uses a battery that the patient can recharge for himself. The battery has reserve power for six to eight weeks, can be recharged in ninety minutes a week, and eliminates the need for periodic surgical replacement of the battery. Developed at Johns Hopkins University, this pacemaker also seems to be immune to interference from electromagnetic devices such as microwave ovens and airport weapons detectors, which sometimes produce disturbances. It is expected to have a useful life of at least ten years, possibly much longer.

SEE ALSO PART II for pertinent information about choice of surgeon, preoperative and postoperative care, anesthesia, tests, costs, and other aspects of your operation.

Coronary Artery Surgery

Coronary artery disease is the greatest scourge in Western nations, the Number One cause of premature death and among the leading causes of disability and suffering. The disease results from the gradual buildup of fatty deposits in the inner lining of the coronary arteries that nourish the heart muscle. These deposits impede blood flow to those areas of heart muscle supplied by affected arteries.

Symptoms

If coronary blood flow is seriously reduced by the fatty deposits, the patient may experience the crushing chest pain of angina pectoris whenever the blood supply is inadequate to meet the heart's requirements for oxygen and other nutrients. Most patients with angina pectoris experience chest pain during exertion. But if coronary artery disease is very severe, pain may be triggered by cold exposure, strong emotions, the mildest exercise, and may even occur at rest or during sleep.

At the extreme, a coronary artery may become so choked with deposits that suddenly one day flow is completely blocked and a heart attack, or *myocardial infarction,* develops. A part of the heart muscle, deprived of nourishment, dies. In some cases the attack is massive; the area of heart affected is very large; the attack may be fatal. Often, the heart area affected is relatively small and the patient survives.

Diagnosis

Other conditions may cause pain resembling angina pectoris. They include gallbladder disease, pleurisy, hiatus hernia, gastritis, cardiospasm, neuralgia, or neuritis. A main diagnostic aid is the typical pain with exertion and relief with rest pattern associated with angina pectoris. Prompt relief of pain after taking a drug, nitroglycerin, confirms the diagnosis.

Causes

Many factors seem to enter into the development of coronary artery disease. They include excessive levels of cholesterol and fatty materials in the blood; high blood pressure; smoking; heredity; excessive weight; too little exercise and physical activity; tension and stress; diabetes.

Medical treatment

Symptoms of angina pectoris often can be relieved by medication. Nitroglycerin is extremely useful. A tablet of nitroglycerin placed under the tongue usually gives dramatic relief in less than two minutes. Other drugs, including blood vessel dilators that are longer-lasting than nitroglycerin, may be used. In addition to use for relief of an angina attack, medication may be employed to help reduce the frequency of attacks. Mental and physical relaxation and reduction of anxiety are important in preventing attacks, and a sedative or tranquilizing drug may be used.

There is increasing hope that weight reduction, control of elevated blood pressure, reduction of levels of cholesterol and fatty materials in the blood through diet and when necessary, medication, elimination of smoking, and the wise use of exercise may help to prevent the progress of coronary artery disease which is already present and, when used early, may prevent or retard its original development.

When surgery may be considered

In patients with persistent, severe, and apparently un-yielding angina, surgery may offer hope for relief of symptoms and extended life. Not every such patient has coronary artery disease suitable for surgery. But when, as often happens, the disease is confined to relatively short segments of the coronary arteries or their branches, surgery may be considered.

Types of operation

Various surgical procedures have been developed for the relief of coronary artery disease.

In one, *endarterotomy,* fatty deposits clogging a local area of coronary artery are left intact, but the artery wall in the area is slit open and a patch of vein or other material is sewn to the wall to enlarge the caliber of the vessel so more blood can pass through.

Another technique, *endarterectomy*, involves opening a blocked artery, stripping away the clogging material with a circular knife to widen the channel, then closing the artery again. A newer version of endarterectomy makes use of gas rather than knife. A jet of carbon dioxide is injected into a blocked artery. The high-pressure jet separates the obstructing material from the artery so it can be removed.

The surgical procedure now most often used and that has shown most promise in the relief of angina pectoris is coronary artery *bypass* to detour blood around coronary artery obstructions. One bypassing method involves freeing one end of the left or right internal mammary artery, which normally supplies blood to the chest wall but can be spared, and splicing it into a diseased coronary vessel beyond the point of obstruction.

A more often used bypass method employs a length of saphenous vein taken from the patient's leg. The saphenous vein, a large vessel running the length of the leg, can be spared; it is the vein which is commonly removed in varicose vein surgery. One end of the vein is inserted into the aorta and the other end into a coronary artery beyond the point of obstruction. Thus, some of the blood coming directly out of the heart into the aorta, all freshened in the lungs, moves through the vein to the coronary artery to feed the heart muscle. Such bypasses now are used not only for single artery disease but also for multiple artery disease.

Bypass operations are performed with the aid of the heart-lung machine.

Typically, in preparation for bypass surgery—and, in fact, as a means of determining whether a particular patient may benefit from it—X-ray movies of the coronary artery circulation (cineangiograms) are taken.

For the X-ray movie study, the patient, fully conscious, lies on a table beneath an X-ray machine equipped with a special device, an image amplifier, that brightens the X-rays so they can be seen clearly and so high-speed motion pictures can be made of them. Under local anesthesia, a slender, flexible catheter or tube is inserted into a vessel at the crease of the elbow and carefully maneuvered up to a coronary artery as its progress is followed on the image intensifier. A dye is injected through the catheter. The dye quickly reaches the coronary artery and quickly is washed away by the blood. But the movie camera records the fleeting events appearing on the image screen. When the movies are carefully studied later, they reveal any areas where there is interference with the flow of the dye, a sign of arterial narrowing.

Anesthesia

General anesthesia through an endotracheal tube is used, as for most chest operations.

Length of operation

A bypass operation may take four or five hours or longer, depending upon the number of bypasses to be done.

Postoperative care

After bypass surgery, the patient may spend three days in an intensive care unit where his condition will be constantly monitored. The hospital stay may be as short as seven to ten days in some cases, and some patients may be back to work in four to six weeks.

Success rate

Bypass surgery for the coronary arteries is a recent development. It is still evolving. Because of often-dramatic immediate results in very severe coronary artery disease, its use has grown very rapidly. In 1971, for example, an estimated 20,000 coronary bypass operations were performed in the United States, many of them involving multiple bypasses. In addition to its use for patients with severe, intractable angina, it has been used in some patients who have had one to six heart attacks.

In the beginning, the mortality rate from operation ran as high as 14 percent or even more. Now, well-selected patients, those shown by preoperative studies to be most likely to benefit and most likely to tolerate the operation, can expect to have better than 96 chances out of 100 of coming through surgery well.

There appears to be general agreement that immediate results are excellent, with as many as 95 percent of patients showing substantial relief of angina, some of them freed entirely of chest pain, many of them able to live active, normal lives.

There are still unanswered questions about bypass surgery for which only time can provide answers. Vein grafts sometimes become diseased or fail for other reasons. Can such failures be prevented? How many extra years of life does operation confer?

Some evidence of bypass surgery's value, even at this relatively early stage in its development, comes from records at one major institution. Among 1,000 patients closely observed for one to three years after their operations, the death rate was 27.7 percent. This was only half as many deaths as occurred among patients with similar problems who did not have surgery, of whom 56.2 percent died within the same period.

SEE ALSO PART II for pertinent information about choice of surgeon, preoperative and postoperative care, anesthesia, tests, costs, and other aspects of your operation.

Blood Vessel Surgery

Varicose Veins

Varicose veins are abnormally dilated veins in the legs which may occur in young people but are more common later in life. Upwards of 10 percent of people over thirty-five have them, with women more often affected than men.

Symptoms

In many people, the veins can be extensively dilated and tortuous without causing any symptoms at all. Others, especially after a long period on their feet, may have muscle cramps, fatigability of leg muscles, and annoying sensations of soreness or tenderness in the calf muscles. Ankle swelling may appear, and tends to disappear overnight. Many women experience an increase in severity of symptoms during menses, and especially during pregnancy.

Diagnosis

The diagnosis that varicose veins are present is obvious. But symptoms may not all or always be due to the varicosities. Swelling, for example, can sometimes be due to other causes such as heart and kidney diseases, which will need to be checked for. Muscular fatigue or premenstrual fluid retention may cause aches, and these conditions may require consideration.

Cause

Man's upright posture may contribute to development of varicose veins. Veins are thin-walled vessels through which blood returns to the heart. In the legs and feet are two groups of veins. The femoral vein and its branches are deep inside the leg. The saphenous vein and its branches are just beneath the skin and it is this vein which becomes varicose.

Blood in the saphenous vein flows from the foot up the leg to the groin and then into the hip, where it joins blood in the femoral vein on its way to the heart. The flow is uphill all the way, against graviy, and to help there are many small valves inside the veins. When these valves are intact, pressure along a vein is evenly distributed and there is no vein bulging. When the valves break down, back-pressure on the vein causes varicosities. And while surrounding muscles give much support to the deep veins and aid in propelling blood to the heart, external support is scant for the superficial veins, especially in the obese.

Medical treatment

Elastic support of varicose veins when symptoms are not present often prevents progression of the disease. Frequent periods of leg elevation and avoidance of prolonged standing or sitting are helpful in some cases. Increased pressure within the abdomen—as the result, for example, of obesity or use of tight girdles—can contribute to varicosities, and weight reduction and elimination of such girdles can be helpful.

When surgery may be considered

When varicosities are small, not very prominent, and produce no symptoms, surgery may be unnecessary or can be delayed to see if there is any worsening. When symptoms are severe and definitely due to varicosities and when a large pool of blood is in the legs because of varicosities, surgery may be advisable. If blood pooling is persistent, there is some risk that a varicose ulcer may develop near the ankle and since this is sometimes difficult to treat, its prevention can be important. Minor ulcers often heal completely after varicose vein surgery. More severe ulcers may require pro- longed use after surgery of a medicated bandage. If an ulcer is large and deep, deep tissues may have to be removed and a skin graft used to cover the defect.

Many people wish to have varicose veins removed for cosmetic reasons.

If surgery is to be considered in any case, the deep veins must be competent and free-flowing. The saphenous vein can be removed without being missed as long as the deep veins can take over its work. When they are competent, they can do so without difficulty.

Many methods of testing to determine whether the deep veins can carry the load are available. One of the simplest involves wrapping the entire leg with elastic bandages and having the patient walk about for five minutes. With the saphenous vein compressed by the bandages, severe pain will develop if the deep veins are not competent.

Types of operation

Several forms of surgical treatment have been used for varicose veins.

Injection treatment involves introducing an irritating ma- terial into a varicose vein. Called a sclerosing solution, it produces a reaction in the vein lining that closes off blood flow. The hope is that with repeated injections the varicose vein may be obliterated. But injection treatment can be expected to be helpful only with minor varicose veins and those that may remain after other surgical treatment of major varicosities.

Cutting and ligation is another surgical treatment method. Incisions may be made at a number of points, as many as eight or ten, along the inner side of the leg and thigh, and at these points the main vein may be ligated or tied.

The tying-off serves to change the course of blood flow from the varicose veins to the deep veins, and much of the swelling and heaviness may disappear.

Ligation and stripping, a third method, is now preferred by many surgeons and has become a standard operation for varicose veins. The saphenous vein is tied off flush at its junction with the femoral vein in the groin. A long wire is inserted through the groin end of the saphenous vein and fed through to the ankle where a separate incision is made and the end of the wire is brought out. The wire is tied into the vein at the groin and then pulled through the incision at the ankle. As the wire is pulled, the vein is stripped out from above downward. In some cases, the stripping may be done upward from ankle to groin.

Anesthesia

In most cases, general anesthesia is used. In some cases, a local may be suitable.

Length of operation

Varicose vein operations, though considered to be relatively minor procedures, are tedious and may require from one to three hours.

Special preparation

No special preoperative measures may be required, but if there is swelling around feet and ankles, the patient may be admitted to hospital a day or two before the operation for bed rest to reduce the swelling.

Postoperative care

The hospital stay can be short, from three or four days to a week or so. The patient may be out of bed within a few hours after surgery. An elastic bandage is used to assist circulation for two or three weeks and a supportive bandage may be helpful for three to six months. Usually bathing can be resumed when the wounds have healed, in about two weeks; work can be resumed within the same period and all normal activities within a week or so later.

Success rate

The results of vein surgery are usually excellent. When the varicosities have been responsible for symptoms, the symptoms disappear. Usually scars become barely visible after a few months, and most patients consider the cosmetic results good.

Although varicosities which have been surgically treated rarely recur, it is possible for other varicosities to appear in what previously appeared to be normal veins.

SEE ALSO PART II for pertinent information about choice of surgeon, preoperative and postoperative care, anesthesia, tests, costs, and other aspects of your operation.

Artery Operations

Vascular surgery—operations for blood vessel problems—is carried out frequently today. As a result of major advances, these operations often save lives. In many cases, they add to comfort by improving circulation. And they prevent life-or-death emergencies.

Artery operations are required for many reasons, including injury and birth defect. Some children are born with coarctation or pinching of the aorta, the main trunkline artery, and this congenital defect today can be cured by vascular surgery (see page 119).

Hardening, or arteriosclerosis, is the most common reason for arterial disease and arterial surgery. Just as the coronary arteries may become narrowed and hardened by deposits on their inner walls, leading to a diminished flow of blood to feed the heart muscle and to heart attacks (see page 136), so many other arteries in the body, for example, those supplying nourishment to the brain or to the legs.

In some cases, as the result of arteriosclerosis or infection, a section of artery may lose its elasticity so that it stretches, thins out, balloons, and eventually may burst. Such a ballooning out, or aneurysm, very often now can be repaired.

Several methods of repair are available. In some cases, an artery may be opened, cleaned out, and stitched closed. In other cases, a vein or plastic patch can be fitted to the artery to widen it. In still other cases, the damaged area of artery can be removed and replaced with a substitute.

Endarterectomy

Endarterectomy is an operative procedure for removing thickened areas of the innermost part of an artery.

After reaching the artery through a suitable incision, the surgeon makes a slit in the diseased section of artery. The artery lining along with the deposits on it is cut away, leaving a wider passageway and a raw surface over which a new and healthy lining will form during healing. The slit is then sewn with fine silk thread.

If it is apparent that, when stitched, the artery would not be wide enough for full blood flow, the surgeon can spread the slit a bit and sew in a width of plastic material or vein, Usually the patient is up next day and home within a week.

Bypass

Under some circumstances, endarterectomy is not feasible. The obstruction may be too extensive or the hardened deposits may have extended so deeply into the wall of the artery that their removal would leave the arterial wall dangerously weak.

Then the diseased area may be bypassed. For this, a length of plastic tubing may be used. The tubing is inert and does not affect body tissues and in turn is not itself affected by them. It is crimped for flexibility, allowing it to accommodate to body movements. Alternatively, a length of saphenous vein from the thigh may be used; this is the vein often removed in varicose vein surgery and it can usually be spared.

One end of the tubing or vein is connected to the artery before the point of obstruction and the other beyond that point. Thus some blood can circulate through the old narrowed passageway and the rest of it through the new bypass or detour.

When necessary, bypasses can be lengthy—running, for example, from within the chest to arm or neck or from abdominal cavity to knee.

Bypasses are often used to improve leg circulation. It is not uncommon for arteriosclerosis to obstruct the femoral arteries in the thighs and the popliteal arteries in the knee area while lower leg arteries remain in good health. In such cases, a bypass may start above the clogged femoral artery, at the iliac artery in the pelvis, and extend down through the thigh to a point of attachment to a healthy artery in the leg. Such surgery often saves legs so poorly supplied with blood that otherwise gangrene followed by amputation would have been virtually inevitable.

Diagnosis

When a patient has artery obstruction, a special X-ray study (arteriogram) can serve as a "map," showing exactly where the obstruction is and suggesting the best means for improving the blood flow. A solution of inert material injected into the affected area can show up the artery clearly on X-ray, and the material is quickly eliminated in the urine.

Injections to visualize upper and lower limb and brain arteries can be made under a local anesthetic, although in children a general anesthetic may be used. Brain arteries can be visualized through injection into the carotid arteries in the neck; leg and thigh arteries by injection into the femoral artery in the groin.

To visualize the aorta, a needle may be inserted under general anesthesia into the middle of the back. Alternatively, a fine plastic tube may be inserted through a groin artery and maneuvered with the aid of X-ray pictures to the aorta. Such a tube may also be used for other internal arteries.

Aneurysm

Aneurysm—an abnormal bulging or ballooning out of an artery because of weakness in its wall—most often affects the aorta. Shortly after it emerges upward from the heart, the aorta makes a 180-degree turn, much like the head of a cane, and runs downward to the abdomen, where it divides into the main leg arteries. Some aneurysms occur at the turn of the aorta in the chest, but most develop in the abdominal area.

At first an aneurysm may be small, but in time it tends to increase in size until finally it may rupture, suddenly spilling blood and producing in an individual previously in apparent good health excruciating abdominal and low back pain, and requiring emergency surgery.

To avoid this, preventive surgery in advance of rupture is advisable. A still-intact aneurysm of the aorta may produce no symptoms. It may be felt, however, during a routine physical examination or noted on a routine abdominal X-ray.

To reach the aneurysm, a long abdominal incision from rib cage to pelvis is required. The aneurysm is cut out and the section of artery containing it is replaced with a properly shaped plastic substitute.

An aneurysm repair operation is serious. When an aneurysm has ruptured and emergency surgery must be performed, the operative death rate is about 33 percent. When performed in advance of rupture as an elective procedure before symptoms appear, the death rate is about 4 percent.

Following aneurysm repair, the patient usually spends several days in intensive care. Recent reports indicate that the life expectancy of patients with abdominal aortic aneurysm who are treated by elective surgery is about double that of those not surgically treated.

SEE ALSO PART II for pertinent information about choice of surgeon, preoperative and postoperative care, anesthesia, tests, costs, and other aspects of your operation.

Stroke

Stroke, also known as apoplexy and cerebrovascular accident (CVA), involves injury to the brain. It may be followed by such serious consequences as paralysis of one side of the body, loss of speech, memory impairment, and even death.

Until recently, strokes were looked upon with such fatalism that little was done to prevent them or their end results. Now, fortunately, strokes are better understood and there has been progress in their prevention.

A stroke is the result of hardening of arteries either in the brain or leading to it. In some cases an artery may leak or burst, resulting in hemorrhage into the brain substance. In most cases, as many as 80 percent, an artery becomes obstructed.

Since a stroke may result from an accident to a large or small artery anywhere in the brain or leading to the brain, the consequences can be quite varied. A stroke may block out a tiny area of the memory center or it may deprive a large section of brain of oxygen, producing unconsciousness, paralysis, labored breathing, and death.

Significant developments in stroke

One major development has been the discovery in recent years that a fairly substantial number of strokes arise from damage to arteries outside the brain itself—arteries in the neck leading to the brain and even in main arteries in the chest that supply the neck vessels and eventually the brain. These vessels are accessible to surgical repair.

Another important development is the recognition that although a major stroke may seem to come on suddenly, the stroke process is not necessarily sudden and may provide early warning signals. In fact, three stages of stroke are now recognized: impending, developing, and completed.

An impending stroke is brief, over in a few minutes. It

may involve fainting, stumbling, numbness or paralysis of fingers of one hand, blurring of vision, or loss of speech or memory—all brief indications that part of the brain has imparied blood oxygen supply. Any one or a combination of such symptoms should be reason for an immediate trip to the doctor or to a hospital. There may be another reason for such an incident, such as insulin overdosage in a diabetic. But if the incident seems to be a minor stroke, special X-rays of the arteries leading to the brain may be taken and if obstruction is found in an artery in the neck or other accessible location, surgery may be considered or anticoagulent medication may be tried to prevent the clot from causing a major stroke.

A developing stroke—a stroke-in-progress—is recognized when symptoms progress. For example, headache and clouding of the mind may be followed by blurring of speech; numbness in an arm may be followed by paralysis. This is an emergency situation, requiring hospitalization for confirmation of diagnosis and start of treatment. Anticoagulants may be used and oxygen may be administered. At this stage, it may still be possible to operate.

When major stroke has occurred, all is not necessarily lost. It has been learned that vigorous rehabilitation efforts can do much to overcome paralysis and speech impairment and achieve self-care.

Surgery for stroke

Operations for stroke are mostly in the neck where the carotid and vertebral arteries are most often affected. Either under general or local anesthesia, an incision several inches long is made along the side of the neck. Usually, the blocked area is an inch or even less in length. Commonly, the endarterectomy procedure is used: the affected section of artery is opened and the clogging deposits along with the artery lining are removed, thus opening up the channel for increased blood flow. In some cases, a bypass may be used, as in artery surgery elsewhere in the body, and blood is provided with a new channel to flow through around the obstructed area.

After such surgery, pain is moderate, easily relieved, and the patient may be moving about the following day or even later the same day of operation. Recovery is fast, often within a few days.

If surgery is performed to clean out or bypass a blocked artery in the upper part of the chest, the operation is more serious since the chest must be opened; there is more pain for several days afterward and recovery is slower. (See Chest Surgery, page 104, for special measures used.)

The sympathectomy operation

For some artery problems, operation not on the arteries but on sympathetic nerves may be used.

Through the electric impulses they feed to muscles in artery walls, sympathetic nerves automatically control artery size. Their impulses cause artery wall muscles to contract and the contraction squeezes the artery, diminishing its diameter.

In some cases, excessive sympathetic nerve impulses may keep arteries too constricted, impeding normal blood flow. It's possible to deaden sympathetic nerves temporarily by injection of a local anesthetic solution. This can be used as a test to determine whether once nerve stimulation is stopped, the arteries will open enough to provide significantly improved blood flow.

If so, sympathectomy is performed. Sympathetic nerve fibers are cut. The operation is most commonly used to try to help leg artery circulation. The sympathetic nerves acting on leg arteries are found at the sides of the spinal column in the flanks. Through an incision across the flank between ribs and hip bones, the nerves are divided.

The operation, in a different location, may be used when a circulatory problem lies with arteries in the arms and hands. These arteries are under control of sympathetic nerves in the neck area, and the incision and snipping are done in the neck.

Sympathectomy is carried out under general anesthesia; the patient is usually out of bed the next day; pain is moderate for a few days and can be readily controlled, and the patient is usually home within a week.

Since the sympathetic nerves that are cut have no connection with the muscles of movement in thighs, legs, arms or hands, there is no interference with normal activities of these muscles.

SEE ALSO PART II for pertinent information about choice of surgeon, preoperative and postoperative care, anesthesia, tests, costs, and other aspects of your operation.

Genitourinary Surgery

Every body cell must build its substance and obtain energy from nutrients supplied in food. It must get rid of wastes. All cells deliver their waste products continuously to the blood which in turn carries them to various centers for excretion. In the lungs, some water vapor and all carbon dioxide are removed from the blood. Additional water and salts pour out through the sweat glands in the skin. Other wastes—including water, salt, urea, and uric acid—leave the blood in the kidneys.

Blood enters the kidneys through the renal or kidney arteries and leaves through the renal veins, and while in the kidneys goes through a remarkable filtering system. Located deep in the abdomen at about the level of the lowest ("floating") ribs, the kidneys—each about 4½" long, 2½" wide and 1½" thick and weighing about 5 ounces—are basically filters containing an intricate system of tiny plumbing tubes called nephrons, whose combined length in each kidney is about 140 miles.

Every twenty-four hours, the kidneys filter about 200 quarts of fluid and salts, sending back to the body its needs of water, amino acids, proteins, glucose, and minerals but removing for elimination in the urine the blood's content of wastes. Actually, the kidneys have tremendous reserve capacity and could clean nine times more fluid than they are called upon to do, which is why one healthy kidney can serve body needs. Each day one or two quarts of waste go from the kidneys to the bladder to be flushed out of the body.

A tube, or ureter, leads from each kidney to the urinary bladder. The bladder empties into the urethra, a tube leading to an external opening called the meatus. Serving as collecting and temporary storage point for urine, the bladder expands to accommodate increasing amounts and, with accumulation of about half a pint, a desire to urinate develops.

Genitourinary problems and diagnostic aids

Problems may arise at various places in the urinary tract and may call for surgery. The problems include stones, benign and malignant tumors, or an obstruction that may lead to infection.

X-rays, catheterization, and cystoscopy are often important aids to diagnosis of urinary tract problems. In catheterization, a flexible catheter or tube is introduced into the bladder for drainage or injecting of solutions (in the case of men, this is done through the penis). A still longer catheter can be moved through the bladder up into the ureters which connect bladder to kidneys.

In cystoscopy, an instrument called the cystoscope, a metal tube containing lighting system and viewing lenses, is introduced into the bladder to view its interior. With the cystoscope, too, catheters can be moved into the ureters. Long-handled instruments tipped with scissors, pincers, or teeth for removing small specimens of the bladder can be introduced through the cystoscope. And it can accommodate an electric needle that may be used when necessary to stop bleeding.

X-ray techniques, including use of X-ray-visible materials, today permit study of the kidney in detail—the kidney substance, its blood supply, its excretory channels.

Stones

Kidney Stones

Stones are a fairly common problem. They are deposits of mineral or organic substances which may vary in size from tiny "pebbles" to a staghorn stone which may be large enough to fill the entire pelvis of a kidney.

There are several types of stones. Most common are those made up of calcium phosphate or oxalate or uric acid. Some disorders—such as gout and overactivity of the parathyroid glands—may encourage stone formation.

Kidney stone symptoms

Not all kidney stones produce symptoms. Some may remain silent for years and may in fact never cause symptoms or trouble. Others start to pass out of the kidneys and in doing so can cause alarming symptoms: severe pain and tenderness over the kidney area, frequent and painful urination, blood in the urine, fever, chills, and prostration.

Small kidney stones may get through and be eliminated in the urine. Larger ones, however, may become impacted in the kidney, ureter, or bladder and may have to be removed surgically. A kidney stone, if it blocks passage of urine, can cause back-pressure and infection and may eventually lead to kidney destruction.

Kidney stone surgery

Stones sometimes may be removed from the lower end of the ureter with the aid of the cystoscope. The instrument is passed into the bladder and through the scope, a long, thin, loop-tipped catheter is moved up the ureter. With the loop it may be possible to move the stone into the bladder where it can be removed through the cystoscope. Sometimes, when the loop can't grab the stone, catheters may be passed to try to stretch the ureter enough for the stone to move into the bladder for removal.

Stones too firmly lodged to be removed by such methods require open operation. An incision several inches long is made in the abdomen over the stone area, and through a small cut in the ureter the stone is removed. The operation is safe, usually done under general or spinal anesthesia; there is moderate pain after operation; the patient is usually out of bed in two or three days and recovered and home within a week or ten days. A drain may be passed from the ureter to the outside to take care of any temporary leakage of urine for a week or a little more.

In a minority of cases, kidney stone formation may recur. To help prevent such recurrence, a large fluid intake (eight or more glasses of water daily) is advisable. Depending upon the composition of the stone, diet modification and acidifying or alkalinizing medication may be prescribed for prevention.

When a stone develops in a kidney and becomes too big to move into the ureter, it may remain in the kidney for years without producing apparent symptoms since it does not obstruct the flow of urine. It may in time, however, produce infection and bleeding, requiring surgery.

Through an incision beginning in the loin and carried eight inches or more toward the front of the body, the kidney is reached. General anesthesia is used. The kidney pelvis may be slit open for stone removal or the kidney may be sliced in halves to get the stone out. The cuts into the kidney are sutured closed and drains inserted and brought out through the skin, remaining in place for about a week. In some cases, when the kidney has been damaged extensively by the stone, it may be necessary to remove the kidney (nephrectomy).

The patient is usually out of bed within two or three days; postoperative pain is moderate, and it is usually possible to go home within ten days to two weeks.

Some people who are repeated stone formers are found to have an excess of calcium in the blood and urine. This may be the result of excessive activity in one or more of the parathyroids, four little glands that lie alongside the thyroid gland in the neck. In such cases, further stone formation may be prevented by removal of the abnormal parathyroid tissue.

Bladder Stones

Bladder stones are relatively rare and occur for the most part in middle-aged and older men in whom stone formation may be encouraged when prostate enlargement prevents complete emptying of the bladder.

Bladder stone symptoms

Bladder stones may cause frequent, painful, bloody urination. Diagnosis is confirmed when the stones are seen on X-ray examination or under direct vision through the cystoscope inserted into the bladder.

Bladder stone surgery

Small bladder stones can be removed through the cystoscope. Larger stones often can be crushed with an instrument passed into the bladder through the cystoscope and the tiny pieces than can be washed out through the cystoscope.

Some larger stones cannot be crushed and are removed through an incision in the lower abdomen and another incision in the bladder. The relatively simple operation, which takes about half an hour, may be performed under spinal, general, or local anesthesia. It is well tolerated even by the elderly, and the patient may be home in two weeks.

Tumors

Kidney Tumors

Tumors, either benign or cancerous, may arise in any part of the kidney at any age. The benign growths often are filled with fluid and in reality are cysts rather than tumors.

They vary in size and are usually harmless, but since the cysts cannot always be distinguished on examination from tumors, surgery may be required. The fact that they are nonmalignant is quickly apparent on operation.

Cancerous kidney tumors tend to be found more often in older people except for one kidney malignancy, Wilms's tumor, which occurs mostly in children under six years of age.

Symptoms

Kidney tumors may produce blood in the urine and pain over the kidney area; sometimes a lump may be felt in the kidney area. There may also be fever for which no usual cause can be found. A child with Wilms's tumor may experience pain, fever, loss of weight and appetite, nausea and vomiting.

Diagnosis

A major diagnostic aid is pyelography, in which X-rays of the kidney are taken after a contrast medium is injected by vein or sometimes by way of catheters inserted in ureters. Study of the urine may show malignant cells.

Kidney tumor surgery

For a kidney cyst, surgical treatment is removal of the cyst. For a malignant tumor in child or adult, surgical treatment is removal of the kidney (nephrectomy), which may be combined with radiation treatment and use of anticancer drugs (chemotherapy) with the hope of eliminating the last vestiges of cancer.

The nephrectomy operation, which may be carried out under general anesthesia, involves an incision from the loin carried around toward the front of the body, and removal of the entire kidney and associated tissues and veins. While kidney removal is a major procedure which may require up to three hours to perform, 95 percent of patients come through it, may be out of bed within two or three days, and in uncomplicated cases may be home within two to three weeks and able to return to normal activities within two months.

One healthy kidney is sufficient for normal living. When kidney cancer is treated before malignancy has spread, cure can be expected. Overall five-year cure rates have been increasing and now apply to the majority of children with Wilms's tumor and to almost half of adults with kidney cancer. It has also been noted that removal of the primary kidney cancer occasionally has led to spontaneous regression of cancer lesions which had spread from the primary site.

Bladder Tumors

Bladder tumors may be benign or malignant but most often are malignant and affect men about twice as often as women.

Symptoms

Bloody urine, pus in the urine, burning and frequency of urination are the most frequent symptoms.

Diagnosis

Diagnosis may be established through examination with the cystoscope and through the appearance of cancer cells in the urine.

Bladder tumor surgery

Many bladder tumors are superficial. They have grown, wartlike, from the lining membrane of the bladder and have not penetrated deeply into the bladder wall. They often can be removed through the cystoscope without an abdominal incision. In the procedure, called transurethral resection, the growth may be cut away or burned out with instruments passed through the cystoscope. The likelihood of cure for superficial tumors may be as great as 90 percent.

There may be recurrences but the recurrent tumors often can be treated effectively.

When a tumor penetrates through the bladder wall muscle layer, an incision must be made in the lower abdomen and the bladder opened. In some cases the entire growth can be removed; in other cases, part of the bladder containing the growth must be removed.

When the tumor is deeply penetrating or extensive, it is necessary in some cases to remove the entire bladder. A substitute bladder may then be formed from a short isolated length of the small intestine (ileum). The ureters are connected to the substitute bladder, which is then fixed so that it opens to the outside on the abdomen, and a plastic container to receive urine is glued to the skin about the opening. Such surgery is required only for very malignant bladder cancer, and most patients recover from the operation and can expect longer survival than without the operation.

SEE ALSO PART II for pertinent information about choice of surgeon, preoperative and postoperative care, anesthesia, tests, costs, and other aspects of your operation.

The Prostate

The prostate gland adds a lubricating and nourishing fluid for the transport of sperm cells, which pass through it on their way from the testicles to the urethra, the tube leading from the bladder through the penis to the outside. The gland, which normally weighs about two-thirds of an ounce and is chestnut-size, is located at the neck of the urinary bladder and surrounds the urethra. Thus, an enlargement of the prostate can constrict the urethra and, in so doing, can impede the flow of urine.

At about age fifty, the gland often begins to enlarge. The enlargement puts a strain on the bladder, which has the added burden of forcing urine past the partial obstruction. This leads to bladder enlargement and, with some lessening of urine flow, the stage may be set for urinary infection triggered by stagnant urine. Because of obstruction, there may also be back-pressure of urine in the bladder sufficiently high to force urine into the ureters leading from the kidneys. The kidneys then may be damaged by stretching and may also be infected by the stagnant urine. An end result may be loss of so much kidney function that uremia, or poisoning from waste products, may develop or blood pressure may become elevated because of the kidney disease.

Symptoms

Often one of the first symptoms of enlargement is need to urinate one or more times during the night. There may also be difficulty in starting or stopping the urinary stream. Another symptom may be frequency of urination, with the patient noticing that he feels the urge to urinate again almost as soon as he thought he had finished urinating.

Diagnosis

The physician's gloved finger inserted into the rectum can examine the prostate and detect enlargement. An enlargement of a portion of the gland which cannot be felt through the rectum may also occur. The extent of enlargement also can be determined by passing a rubber catheter into the bladder after the patient has voided to determine what residual urine may be present. The amount of residual urine is a measure of obstruction. Additional information can be obtained by examination of the urethra from within through a cystoscope.

Cause

The cause of benign enlargement of the prostate is unknown. After age sixty, most men may have some enlargement and many of them some degree of obstruction.

Medical treatment

As many as three-fourths or more of men do not need surgery. When symptoms are mild and there is no serious degree of back-pressure, conservative treatment may be used. Medication to control any infection that may be present, prostate massages through the rectum to minimize congestion of the gland, and mild, warm tub baths with water circulating around the buttocks and lower abdomen may be helpful.

When surgery is needed

When medical treatment fails to ease symptoms, or when there is uncontrolled infection, marked obstructive pressure, formation of bladder stones, and evidence of danger to the kidneys, surgery becomes essential.

Types of operation

Four types of operations are available, each approaching the prostate in a different way.

Transurethral prostatectomy. This is a closed operation, requiring no incision. It is the most commonly performed and does not remove the entire gland. Under spinal or general anesthesia, a special instrument, the resectoscope, is inserted through the penis and with an electrically charged wire loop prostatic tissue is removed piece by piece until the obstructing portion of the prostate gland has been cleared away. The pieces of tissue are washed out through the resectoscope; bleeding points are sealed with the electric loop; and a catheter is left in the urethra for several days. The patient is out of bed within several days and usually home within ten days, able to void normally and with complete control in a short time.

Suprapubic prostatectomy. This is performed under spinal or general anesthesia through an incision in the abdomen below the navel. The bladder is opened and, by inserting his finger through the opening and into the bladder outlet forward into the urethra to where the urethra is surrounded by the prostate, the surgeon can work through the urethral lining and, with his fingertip, remove prostate tissue from its capsule.

This operation is often preferred when the prostate is very large and when there is a problem in the bladder such as stones. Catheters and drains are left in place for about ten days until there has been sufficient healing to allow normal urination. The operation takes about an hour. Only moderate pain which can be relieved by medication is felt afterward. The hospital stay is about two weeks and about a month of convalescence is needed.

Retropubic prostatectomy. This, too, is done through an abdominal incision under spinal or general anesthesia, but the bladder is not opened. The thick fibrous capsule of the prostate is opened so prostate tissue can be cut out with scissors or removed with a finger. A catheter to the bladder is left in place for about ten days during healing. Pain after operation is moderate and after removal of the catheter, the patient may go home from hospital and, after about a month of convalescence, resume normal activities.

Perineal prostatectomy. In this procedure, the incision is between the legs in the perineal area forward of the rectum and close to the gland. Except for the incision, the operation is carried out in the same way as in retropubic prostatectomy.

Success rate

In the great majority of cases, prostatectomy is curative. With advances both in surgery and anesthesia, even sick, weak and very old patients do well.

A complication which may develop, sometimes several weeks after surgery, is bleeding, which the patient quickly notices and which may require rehospitalization for about a week while irrigation through a catheter is used to stop the bleeding.

Once removed, the chances that a prostate will grow back are less than 5 out of 100.

With successful prostate surgery, length of life is not affected nor is there usually any interference with sexual activity which, in fact, may improve because of improvement in general health.

Prostate Cancer

Prostate cancer may occur in men in their forties and fifties but is more common after age sixty. It is the most frequent malignancy in American men.

Symptoms

Cancer of the prostate is generally slowly progressive and may cause no symptoms in early stages. Later it may lead to urinary obstruction, blood and pus in the urine and, when it spreads to pelvis and spine, may produce bone pain.

Diagnosis

Cancer may be suspected in relatively early stages when a firm, hard nodule in the gland is felt during rectal examination. The presence of cancer can be confirmed by snipping off a small piece of prostate tissue for microscopic examination.

Surgical treatment

In some men, prostate cancer remains locally confined for a long period. When the malignancy is confined within the capsule of the prostate, the gland can be removed by an operation of the type used for benign prostatic enlargement. The entire gland is removed.

When the cancer is too advanced and has spread too widely for prostate removal to provide a chance for cure, its growth may be controlled by treatment with female hormones, which act as antagonists to the male hormone which furthers growth of the cancer. Although hormone treatment is not curative, it may stabilize the disease, relieve pain, and have a long-lasting effect. In other men, castration—removal of both testicles—eliminates the main source of male hormone and adds to results with female hormone treatment. Castration does not necessarily end sexual intercourse.

Radiation therapy as a supplement to surgery is helpful in some cases, and occasionally triple anticancer drug treatment may cause dramatic regression of some seeding of prostate cancer in other organs.

Success rate

When prostatic cancer is detected and treated early, the chance for cure is excellent. When the cancer has spread, there is still considerable hope. Although some prostatic cancers are highly malignant and the five-year survival rate is virtually nil, others are of lesser degrees of malignancy: five-year survival rates approaching 80 percent are seen with some less malignant types even after spread has begun.

SEE ALSO PART II for pertinent information about choice of surgeon, preoperative and postoperative care, anesthesia, tests, costs, and other aspects of your operation.

Hypospadias

In this birth defect in a male baby, the urethral urinary channel, instead of running the full length of the penis, is short and opens to the exterior on the underside an inch or more from the penis tip. In some cases, the opening is far enough forward so that surgical correction is not needed. But in other cases, directing the urinary stream is a problem. Also, there may be a fibrous band which curves the penis so that sexual intercourse later in life will be difficult and may prevent proper sperm deposition.

When surgery is indicated, it should be performed between one and two years of age. Usually two surgical procedures are required. In the initial procedure, the fibrous tissue band is removed to eliminate the bend in the penis. Some months or a year later, the urethra is reconstructed. Many techniques are available for this. One employs a rolled strip of skin placed on the underside of the penis. The likelihood of success is excellent in about 90 percent of cases. In the other 10 percent of cases, reoperation may be needed, and it usually leads to good results.

Hydrocele

In this defect, a sac or bag of watery fluid surrounds a testicle. It may be small or large, may cause little or no discomfort, may occur at any time from infancy to old age. It may result from excessive accumulation of fluid as a consequence of overproduction or diminished resorption of fluid.

Diagnosis can be made—and a hydrocele can be distinguished from a tumor—by shining a light through the scrotum or by inserting a needle into the scrotum and withdrawing some fluid.

Although nonoperative treatment may be used—and consists of removing fluid through needle and syringe followed by injection of an irritating (sclerosing) liquid which cases scar tissue to form and obliterate the sac—recurrences are frequent, and surgery is preferred.

The operation is simple and may be done under spinal or general anesthesia. Through an incision in the scrotum, the sac is emptied and its wall is removed. The patient is out of bed in a day, home within a week.

Varicocele

In varicocele, veins of the spermatic cord are dilated and varicosed. The condition is not serious. There may be no symptoms or only a somewhat vague dragging sensation in the lower abdomen or groin.

Unless discomfort is considerable, surgery may be unnecessary. The operation, which may be done under spinal anesthesia, is relatively simple, involving an incision in the scrotum and tying off and removal of the varicose veins.

The operation relieves symptoms and does not impair normal function of the testes.

SEE ALSO PART II for pertinent information about choice of surgeon, preoperative and postoperative care, anesthesia, tests, costs, and other aspects of your operation.

Special Operations for Women

The reproductive system anatomy in the female takes the form of the letter "Y." At the ends of the two top arms are the ovaries. The arms themselves are the fallopian tubes, also called oviducts, through which eggs or ova released from the ovaries travel. At the center of the Y is the uterus, or womb, which houses and nourishes a fertilized egg through all phases of fetal development, enlarging greatly in the process. The neck of the uterus, the cervix, seals off the uterine cavity until just prior to birth of a baby, when it changes shape. The cervix leads into the vagina, the receiver of sperm and the exit passage at childbirth.

The ovaries produce female hormones as well as eggs. The hormones control menstrual periods. A single normal ovary is enough for all normal functions. Each ovary is about 1½" long, 1" wide, and 1" thick, shaped somewhat like an almond.

Released into a fallopian tube, which is about 4" long and connected to the uterus, a mature egg passes down to the uterus, taking about seven days to do so. If it has been fertilized by a male sperm in the tube, it becomes implanted in the wall of the uterus on arrival there.

The muscular uterus, about three inches long, two inches wide, and one inch thick, has an interior lining, or endometrium, which takes part in menstrual flow. It is this lining which is shed unless an egg has been fertilized. The purpose of the uterus is to nourish the fertilized egg. It has nothing to do with sexual desire or sexual activity, and removal of the uterus interferes with neither.

The vulva and the vagina are the external genitals. The vulva has two major and two minor lips (labia majora and labia minora). It is also composed of the hymen and vaginal opening; the small, firm clitoris above the urinary opening; and, near the vaginal opening, two small Bartholin's glands that secrete mucus.

The vagina, which receives the penis in coitus, is a canal extending from the vulva to the cervix. The adult vagina is normally about three inches long and slopes upward and backward. In front of the vagina is the bladder; in back of it, the rectum.

Some disorders and upsets of the reproductive system are mild and fleeting, others of more serious nature. Medical treatment is very often effective. Sometimes surgical treatment is required.

Dilation and Curettage (D and C)

D and C—dilation of the cervix and curettage or cleaning out of the lining of the uterus—is a very common minor operation. It accounts for nearly one of every seven surgical procedures among women, about the same as the next two most common procedures combined. At ages twenty-five to forty-four, it makes up 20 percent of all operations among women.

Thousands of lives have been saved by D and C and, in addition, the procedure has eliminated discomfort, doubt, and anxiety for millions of women.

One important purpose of a D and C is diagnostic, to determine what is causing abnormal functioning of female organs—bleeding or pain or illness. Another is therapeutic, to cure or correct the condition. Sometimes a D and C does both at the same time. A D and C also is often used for abortion, but only in the first ten to twelve weeks of pregnancy.

Indications for D and C

When there is excessive bleeding during or between periods, dilation and curettage is helpful in determining the presence of some of the most common causes. These include inflammation of the uterus; tumors; small fleshy growths called polyps which are no more dangerous than warts but often bleed; and cancer of the uterus.

D and C also may indicate hormonal disturbances that need correction. It is also an essential part of the evaluation of postmenopausal bleeding. It is used, too, to remove remnants of tissue that are not shed naturally after a miscarriage.

Most often, excessive bleeding is due to a benign condition. The D and C not only is diagnostic, but in well over one-half of patients is curative as well. Many others can be helped by hormone therapy.

D and C may also be used to determine the cause of infertility and of failure to menstruate.

The operation

D and C takes only a few minutes. It may be done under light general anesthesia.

After the canal leading through the cervix to the uterus is stretched or dilated with an instrument called a dilator sufficiently so a long, thin, scoop-shaped instrument called a curette can be inserted into the uterus, the uterine lining, called the endometrium, is scraped out. The curette at the same time removes any polyps that may be present. A specimen of the lining can be examined under a microscope.

A hospital stay of one or two days may be required. There is virtually no pain after the operation. Slight vaginal bleeding may occur for a short time and usually stops within two weeks or so. Sexual relations can be resumed when the staining ceases. In most cases the patient is back to work in less than a week. There is no interference with ability to become pregnant.

Although most surgeons prefer to perform D and C in hospital because of the long-established safety of the procedure when done there, some investigational trials suggest that it may be performed in the doctor's office under local anesthesia.

Hysterectomy

In women aged twenty-five and over, hysterectomy—the surgical removal of the uterus—is the second most frequent operation after dilation and curettage. More than one-quarter million hysterectomies are performed yearly in the United States.

There are a number of indications or reasons why hysterectomy may be considered. In some cases, the operation may be essential; in others, advisable; in still others, not at all inevitable.

Fibroids

The uterus has two layers. The inner layer or lining undergoes monthly changes. If no pregnancy occurs, it is shed. If conception takes place, the lining receives the egg and eventually forms the placenta and other membrances that surround and nourish the fetus.

The outer layer of the uterus, making up the bulk of the organ, is muscle. The muscle contracts rhythmically for childbirth; it may also contract irregularly during menstruation, accounting for cramps sometimes associated with menstrual flow.

Tumors that develop from the muscular layer are very common and are known as "fibroids" or myomas. Myomas are usually multiple and almost always benign. They may grow within the muscle layer or on stalks. Most myomas cause no symptoms or problems and may be detectable only on pelvic examination. When there is any doubt about their nature, Pap smears, X-ray films taken after instillation of a dye into the uterus to outline it clearly, or dilation and curettage can make the diagnosis certain.

In some cases, when myomas become large enough to press on the lining of the uterus or on nearby structures, they may lead to varied menstrual disorders. Sometimes they may so distort the normal shape of the uterus that implantation of the fertilized egg is difficult, and there may be infertility or miscarriage.

When myomas are found, regular pelvic examinations may then be performed to assess their rate of growth and detect any new ones, as a guide to determining if and when surgical removal may be adivsable. Many women who develop myomas are in their thirties and forties. Often, the growths tend to enlarge under the influence of estrogen and when estrogen secretion diminishes after menopause, they may get smaller and sometimes may disappear. For this reason, it may be advisable in some cases to delay decision about surgery until after menopause.

Surgical removal is the cure for myomas. But occasionally a D and C may correct menstrual abnormalities caused by myomas, and removal may be delayed or avoided. There are many reasons, however, to remove myomas—for example, if they cause pain by pressure on adjacent bowel or bladder; if they will interfere with pregnancy; if they enlarge rapidly; if they produce persistent menstrual irregularities or uncontrolled bleeding.

If surgery is required, *myomectomy* may be used. This is a procedure, carried out through an abdominal incision, in which the fibroid tumors are cut out but the uterus is left intact. Myomectomy may be used for younger women who wish to have children.

Most women past childbearing age who need surgery for myomas may be advised to have the uterus removed at the same time. While myomectomy is often helpful, new myomas may develop afterward in about 10 percent of patients and may require further operation. The removal of the uterus is curative and does not add much to the surgical procedure or to postoperative discomfort. Since the ovaries can be left intact, there is little if any interference with sexual desire and enjoyment. Some surgeons favor removal of ovaries along with uterus as a preventive measure against development of ovarian tumors in the future. After ovary removal, female hormones can be prescribed to make up for the deficits.

Any decision to operate should usually be confirmed by a specialist in gynecology.

Uncontrolled Excessive Bleeding

Sometimes when severe menopausal bleeding due to hormonal imbalance or other persistent uterine bleeding fails to yield to other measures, including dilation and curettage, hysterectomy may be required.

Premalignant Conditions

If microscopic examination of uterine lining removed during dilation and curettage reveals a condition known to be precancerous in nature, hysterectomy can avoid cancer. Cells of a type that foreshadow malignancy can be seen during a pathologist's viewing of the lining sample under a microscope.

Uterine Cancer

Uterine cancer occurs most often in the cervix. The disease is called *carcinoma in situ* when only the surface cervical lining is cancerous. In some cases, treatment may involve surgical removal of a cone-shaped piece of the cervix (*conization*), followed by checkups to guard against recurrence. More often, hysterectomy is performed.

The most serious form of cervical cancer, *invasive carcinoma,* means that the malignancy has broken through the cervical lining into deeper tissues. Treatment may consist of external radiation with X-ray or cobalt and internal use of radium. In some early cases, removal of the uterus and pelvic lumph glands is preferred.

Malignancy of the inner uterine lining, *carcinoma of the endometrium,* is most common after menopause and usually causes bleeding. If a D and C, performed to establish the reason for bleeding, reveals endometrical cancer, radium is frequently placed in the uterus to be followed in a month by removal of the uterus, cervix, and both tubes and ovaries. In some cases, the operation alone may be considered adequate treatment.

In both cervical and endometrial cancer, the disease appears to follow a progressive course. The more advanced the disease when treated, the more extensive treatment becomes and the less the chance for cure. Complete cure is possible for a very great percentage of patients treated for early malignancies.

Post-childbirth

Rarely, hysterectomy may be needed following childbirth because of life-threatening bleeding cause by large uterine tears.

Sterilization

Recent reports indicate use of hysterectomies solely for sterilization purposes in some areas. Such use of hysterectomy in place of tubal ligation or other methods of contraception is controversial. While risks of complications after hysterectomy are not great, they are higher than for tubal ligation, and many authorities consider that a case for routine elective hysterectomy for sterilization has not been made.

The Hysterectomy Operation

Two methods are available for removal of the uterus. In one, vaginal hysterectomy, the operation is performed through the vagina. In the other, abdominal hysterectomy, an incision in the abdomen is made to reach the uterus.

The abdominal approach is usually required when the uterus is large because of a tumor or if the uterus is not freely movable because of adhesions to other organs.

In vaginal hysterectomy, an incision is made deep in the

vagina. Through the incision, the supports for the uterus can be severed, and the uterus is then removed. Because there is less need for moving the intestine, gas pains afterward are less bothersome. In older women who may have sagging of muscles supporting vagina, bladder, and rectum, repairs of these can be made through the same incision.

In abdominal hysterectomy, an incision about six inches long or a little less is made low in the abdomen.

With either type of hysterectomy, the entire uterus, including the cervix, can be removed. The fallopian tubes and ovaries may be left in place—or they may be removed in whole or in part if there is evidence of disease or abnormality in these structures. As a precaution against the possibility of development of disease later in the tubes or ovaries, it may be considered advisable in a woman past menopause to remove these structures as well.

Anesthesia

Hysterectomy is usually done under general anesthesia, but spinal anesthesia may be used instead.

Length of operation

The operation may require from an hour or a little less to ninety minutes.

Postoperative care

Discomfort after vaginal hysterectomy may be relatively mild; after abdominal hysterectomy pain may be severe, especially if there is gas bloating, but can be relieved with medicine by mouth or injection. After either type of operation, a catheter may be required for several days to empty the bladder. When stretched bladder and rectal muscles have been tightened during the operation, the catheter may have to remain in place for about a week.

Often patients are out of bed the day after surgery, but this may be delayed a few days if considerable internal repair work was done. In all cases, bowel function returns but may not do so for several days.

The hospital stay may range from about eight days to two weeks. For two to three weeks while healing is taking place, there may be vaginal discharge and bleeding; these are no cause for alarm. Showers may be taken almost immediately after vaginal hysterectomy and after healing of the incision in abdominal hysterectomy. Usually tub bathing can be resumed about a month after operation. It is usually safe to resume intercourse within six to eight weeks.

Success rate

The overall success rate for hysterectomies for most of the indications previously discussed is high, including hysterectomy for precancerous conditions. It is also high for early cancer and some possibility of cure exists for later stages of cancer.

Like any major operation, hysterectomy has risks. The death rate from the operation is relatively low, averaging overall 16.4 per 10,000 patients, less than 0.2 percent.

Are you left with any limitations?

With successful hysterectomy, any symptoms previously present and related to the uterus will be eliminated. There is no interference with sex life, which may in fact be improved because of elimination of symptoms or because of freedom from need for contraceptive measures. No breast changes result from hysterectomy. Menstruation, of course, ceases. With removal of ovaries, manifestations of abrupt menopause, which may include hot flashes and other distressing symptoms, can be controlled by medication.

Deciding on a hysterectomy

Except in cancerous and precancerous states, the decision to perform hysterectomy warrants careful consideration. It is sometimes possible for symptoms to arise from areas other than the uterus, and these must be considered. When pain and bleeding arise from the uterus, conservative treatment, including rest, medication, and sometimes D and C may warrant trial before hysterectomy.

There is no question that some unnecessary hysterectomies are performed. The question is how many, what proportion? Nobody knows the precise answer, but there have been charges that in some areas as many as one out of three or even more hysterectomies are not really necessary.

When cancerous and precancerous conditions are present, the need for surgery is very clear. For other conditions, a patient may best be served by having a second independent consultation, which most conscientious doctors welcome. The fee of the consultant is well worthwhile because of the confirmation he may provide that surgery is needed or because of suggestions he may have for conservative measures which, in his experience, may solve the problem without recourse to surgery. A competent gynecologist may provide such consultation.

SEE ALSO PART II for pertinent information about choice of surgeon, preoperative and postoperative care, anesthesia, tests, costs, and other aspects of your operation.

Ovary Operations

Several conditions may require ovary surgery.

Cysts

A variety of cysts or fluid-filled cavities may develop in an ovary. Each month a cyst is formed around the egg to be released at ovulation and subsequently disappears. In some cases for unknown reasons, such a follicle cyst may not vanish for a time although it eventually does disappear. Occasionally, however, a follicle cyst persists, enlarges, produces pain and menstrual disturbance and may then require surgical removal.

Occasionally, mucous cysts develop and may enlarge to great size, filling much of the abdomen and damaging the ovary. Surgery then is required for removal of the cyst and very often the damaged ovary.

Some ovarian cysts twist and in so doing may cause severe pain in the lower abdomen, nausea, vomiting, and muscle spasm. Such cysts, which may need to be distinguished from appendicitis or abdominal obstruction (which may produce similar symptoms) by pelvic examination, require surgery for their removal.

Not infrequently, multiple cysts of the ovaries may produce menstrual and ovulation disturbances and may be responsible for infertility. When the cysts persist or increase in size, surgery—partial removal of the ovaries—may be needed for cure.

Tumors

Benign tumors of the ovary may range from walnut to grapefruit size. Some, even when massive, may produce no symptoms; others may lead to menstrual disturbances or lower abdominal or groin pain. Malignant tumors often develop silently in early stages, that is, producing no symptoms.

Enlargements of the ovary can be discovered during regular yearly pelvic examinations. They call for exploratory surgery to establish definitely the presence of a tumor. The affected ovary is then removed and tissue from it is immediately examined under the microscope. If the growth is benign, no further surgery may be required. If malignant, the other ovary may also be removed along with tubes and uterus.

Some ovarian tumors produce sex hormones, occasionally male sex hormones, which may be responsible for excessive hair on the face, deep voice and other male characteristics. Surgery is required for their removal.

The operation

The removal of an ovary, oophorectomy, is a relatively simple procedure. Under spinal or general anesthseia, an incision about four inches long or a little longer is made in the lower abdomen, and the ovary can be lifted into the wound, its base tied, and the ovary snipped off. The operation takes an hour or less. This applies to benign tumors and cysts. When the problem is a cyst and especially when the patient is a young woman, only the cyst-containing section of the ovary is removed when possible. When ovarian cancer is the problem, the operation is more extensive, with both ovaries removed and often the uterus and tubes.

Postoperative care

Pain after oophorectomy is relatively mild. No special postoperative measures are needed and the patient may be out of bed within a day or two, home from the hospital in seven or eight days, able to bathe in two weeks, able to resume household duties or work in about a month, and sexual relations about then or a week or two later.

Success rate

Almost invariably, cysts and benign tumors are curable by surgery. Ovarian cancer also is curable if treated before it has reached advanced stages and spread widely.

Are you left with any limitations?

The removal of part or all of one ovary produces no noticeable effects. If the remaining ovary is normal, as it usually is, menstrual periods are unaffected and pregnancy can take place. The onset of menopause is not hastened.

When both ovaries must be removed, menstruation stops and the symptoms of menopause develop. These may be treated effectively with synthetic hormone medication.

SEE ALSO PART II for pertinent information about choice of surgeon, preoperative and postoperative care, anesthesia, tests, costs, and other aspects of your operation.

Cervix Operations

Biopsy

This is a minor surgical procedure for removal of a small amount of tissue from the cervix for microscopic study. It is commonly done when a cancer detection test (Pap smear) indicates possibility, but not certainty, that malignancy may be present. It may also be done at other times when there is some doubt about the complete health of the cervix.

A cervical biopsy may be performed in office or hospital under light general anesthesia. There is almost no discomfort afterward but slight bleeding may be expected for a few days.

Cauterization

The mucuous membrane lining of the cervix may become inflamed (endocervicitis) and the condition, although not dangerous, may lead to vaginal discharge, and may become chronic. Electrical or chemical cauterization, a burning-off process, may be used to treat the condition. Often the procedure can be done without anesthesia in a gynecologist's office. When there is considerable inflammation, brief hospitalization and light anesthesia may be used. Even then, the procedure produces no great discomfort afterward, but for a time slight bleeding and vaginal discharge may be expected.

Cervical Polyp Removal

Polyps—benign, fleshy growths—sometimes grow from the lining of the cervix, protruding into the vagina. Often they produce no symptoms but occasionally may bleed after intercourse. When small, they can often be removed as an office procedure; larger ones sometimes may be removed under light general anesthesia in a hospital. There is virtually no discomfort after their removal but some staining may be expected for a few days.

Cancer of the Cervix

This form of cancer is the second most common among women—and one which has been becoming much less deadly. Thanks to the use of the Pap test, a greater number of cervical malignancies are discovered at the highly curable *in situ* stage before spread.

When a routine Pap smear test suggests the possibility of early cervical cancer, a biopsy is needed to make the diagnosis.

If early cancer is present, radiation treatment is usually used. In a hospital procedure, under general anesthesia, radium is implanted in the cervix. Later, radium treatment can be followed by supervoltage X-rays or cobalt 60.

In more advanced cancer, surgery may be required for removal of the cervix, part of the upper vagina, uterus, fallopian tubes and ovaries, and nearby lymph glands. The procedure is a radical hysterectomy.

In the last twenty years, there has been a marked increase in the number of early *in situ* cancers—cancers that are more or less resting and inactive—while the incidence rate for invasive or advanced cancers has declined. Overall, including all stages of cervical cancer, the five-year survival rate, which is used as a measure of cancer cure, has been 60 percent. For women with localized disease, the five-year survival rate has come close to 80 percent, and more widespread use of the Pap test could further increase the chances of survival.

SEE ALSO PART II for pertinent information about choice of surgeon, preoperative and postoperative care, anesthesia, tests, costs, and other aspects of your operation.

Vaginal Plastic Operations
(Prolapse, Cystocele, and Rectocele)

Muscles that support the uterus, the bladder, and the rectum are sturdy. But they may be stretched during childbearing and they may lose their tone and become flabby with lack of adequate physical exertion.

When the uterus has lost firm muscular support, it may *prolapse,* descending in the vagina and sometimes protruding from the opening. There may be some degree of lower abdominal discomfort and sometimes lower back pain and easy fatigue.

With loss of firm muscular support, the bladder may become loose and bulging. This is a *cystocele.* It may cause stress incontinence, or loss of urine with sneezing, coughing, laughing or straining. But a cystocele may be present without interfering with urinary control.

With loss of support, the rectum may sag. This is a *rectocele* and may cause difficulty with bowel movement, although a rectocele may be present without producing symptoms.

When is surgery necessary?

It isn't needed when there are no symptoms.

Even when there are symptoms, many surgeons believe it isn't usually advisable until a woman has had all the children she wishes. Until childbearing is completed, relief may be obtained by use of a pessary, or plastic ring, which is inserted into the vagina to prevent protrusion of uterus, bladder, and rectum. While use of a pessary may require frequent vaginal irrigations and may sometimes be accompanied by irritation and vaginal discharge, it may be advisable until a time suitable for surgery arrives.

Types of operations

Various operations—known as plastic repair operations—are available to tighten supporting muscles, remove bulging membranes, and draw separated muscles together. If one defect is present, a single repair in needed. When several are present, they can be repaired at the same time.

To repair a rectocele, for example, some of the membrane extending from the vaginal opening for several inches inside the vagina is removed, separated muscles at the sides of the vagina are brought together and tied, and the membrane's cut edges are fitted together. Similarly, to repair a cystocele, excess membrane is trimmed, muscles from the sides of the vagina are drawn together and tied beneath the urethra, or urinary channel, thus tightening urethra and weak bladder-outlet muscle.

The incisions are made within the vagina and are not visible.

Vaginal plastic operations may be carried out under general or spinal anesthesia.

Postoperative care

Usually the patient is out of bed the day after surgery. For a few days, because urination may be difficult, a catheter is used to drain the bladder. The period of hospitalization is about a week; convalescence thereafter is rapid. Light work may be resumed after three to four weeks, heavy work after two months, and marital relations after about eight to ten weeks.

Success rate

Vaginal plastic repair operations are considered major surgery but the risk is minimal and the success rate high. Symptoms are overcome in the vast majority of women.

SEE ALSO PART II for pertinent information about choice of surgeon, preoperative and postoperative care, anesthesia, tests, costs, and other aspects of your operation.

Caesarean Section

The delivery of a child through an incision in the lower abdominal wall and lower portion of the uterus is known as Caesarean section and is used for 4 to 5 percent of all deliveries. There have been various theories about the origin of the term. A common idea that Julius Ceasar was delivered this way is not true. The term may have derived from a Roman law during the time of the Caesars requiring that in the case of a pregnant woman who died before the birth of her child, the delivery must be accomplished surgically immediately following her death. But it could also have derived from the Latin word, *caedere,* to cut.

Indications for Caesarean section

A frequent reason for surgical delivery is a disproportion between baby head size and the mother's pelvis. This is determined by calipers and X-ray. Frequently in such situations, labor may be allowed to proceed under close watch for a few hours after onset of labor pains to see whether, if the disproportion is minor, good labor may overcome it and allow safe vaginal delivery. If not, Caesarean delivery can be used then.

Caesarean section may also be called for under certain other specific circumstances: when labor is prolonged or ineffective; when the placenta, or afterbirth, is very low in the uterus or separates (abruptio placenta) before birth, producing internal bleeding that may threaten both baby and mother; when, in some, but not necessarily all cases, the baby is in an abnormal position, with shoulder, arm, buttocks, or feet coming first; and also in some but not all cases when a woman has very high blood pressure, diabetes, or kidney disease; when a tumor may block the birth canal; or when a previous cervical or vaginal operation may make normal delivery difficult.

It is not invariably true that "Once a Caesarean, always a Caesarean." Commonly this is the case, since pelvic disproportion, if it was the original reason, does not change and also because the uterine wall may be somewhat weakened by earlier Caesareans and may give way during violent labor contractions. Although there are records of eight and ten Caesareans for the same woman, often it is suggested that three or four such deliveries be the limit.

The operation

A Caesarean may be performed under general or spinal anesthesia, sometimes under local anesthesia. An incision about five inches long is made in the center of the abdomen below the navel, after which the wall of the uterus is opened. Once the incision was always high in the uterus; now commonly it is low since a low incision leaves a stronger scar less likely to give way in future pregnancies. With hand inserted in the uterus, the surgeon can readily withdraw the baby, clamp and cut the cord, and hand the child to a waiting nurse, all in a few minutes. The placenta, or afterbirth, is removed and the uterus and the abdominal wall are sutured.

Postoperative care

The patient can usually be out of bed the day after Caesarean section and home from the hospital in seven to ten days. If she so desires, a woman can breast-feed her baby after Caesarean. Bathing, driving a car, and light household duties can be resumed within four weeks, marital relations within six weeks, and all activities a few weeks later.

Success rate

Caesarean section is successful, for both mother and child, in the overwhelming majority of cases. Performed by a qualified obstetrician in an approved hospital, the operation is very safe, carrying about the same risk as an appendectomy.

Getting a second opinion

Although a Caesarean is safe, a first Caesarean should be used only when really needed in the judgment of a competent specialist in obstetrics, since the same type of delivery is likely to be needed thereafter for subsequent pregnancies. Sometimes the decision must be made in an emergency, but usually there is time for consultation; accredited hospitals are required by the Joint Commission on Accreditation of Hospitals to make it a rule that a second surgical opinion be obtained before proceeding with a Caesarean.

Breast Surgery

The breast is made up of glandular tissue arranged in a complicated pattern of lobes, with milk ducts leading into the nipple at the approximate center of the lobes. It is subject to a number of disorders that can be difficult to differentiate by physical examination alone since they most commonly take the form of a lump or mass.

A lump may be a benign growth, a cyst, or a cancer. Of all lumps, the majority are not cancerous. About half are cysts. Another 10 percent or so are nonmalignant tumors.

Although the chances are thus greater that a lump is nonmalignant rather than malignant, any lump may be cancerous, and it is essential to try to make certain of its nature. In some cases, it is possible for a physician to arrive at a more or less certain diagnosis by feeling a lump, noting its consistency and whether it is well demarcated.

Special X-ray study—mammography—can be helpful in diagnosis. In the technique, which is painless, without risk, and may require as long as an hour, X-rays are taken of the breasts in various positions. Mammography often helps when a physician feels that a lump is not cancerous but wishes additional supportive evidence. It is also used when many cysts are present in a breast, making it difficult to detect a new mass. It often is helpful when a lump is difficult to feel and outline clearly or when there is persistent pain in one breast. It is often used routinely for women who have a strong family history of breast cancer or who have had a malignancy removed from one breast, since they may have a higher-than-average risk of developing cancer in the other breast.

Mammography is not always conclusive. For 100 percent certainty, it is often necessary to remove a piece of tissue for microscopic examination. The surgery is minor even though it is usually done in an operating room under general anesthesia. The lump tissue is removed, frozen, cut into extremely thin slices, stained, and analyzed under the microscope by a pathologist. In about ten minutes, the surgeon has a report.

If no cancer is found, the small incision is closed and the patient is usually home next day, free of the lump, assured there is no malignancy, with a small scar that is red at first but often becomes almost imperceptible after a few months. If cancer is found, the breast must be removed and this is done as soon as the report arrives in the operating room. Early detection and prompt treatment are vital for winning the battle of breast cancer. If cancer is removed before it has spread, the five-year cure rate is 75 to 90 percent; that is, 75 to 90 percent of patients are alive and well at the end of five years. If removed after such spread, the cure rate is in the 50 percent range.

Cysts

The glands which make up much of breast tissue enlarge and contract in response to hormones secreted by the ovaries. Sometimes some glands fill more rapidly than others or gland openings become plugged, causing localized swellings, or cysts. Cystic disease—chronic cystic mastitis—is a benign condition and the most common disease of the female breast, occurring in about 5 percent of middle-aged women, less often in others. There may be pain or premenstrual breast discomfort but often there are no symptoms and a woman usually seeks medical advice because of feeling a cyst.

A cyst may enlarge, gradually or suddenly, to half an inch or an inch in diameter. Sometimes, if a physician is certain that a lump is a cyst and nothing more, needling may be used to remove the fluid in it. In some women, following aspiration, as the needling is called, a cyst never reappears. Aspiration must be used cautiously, never when there is the slightest doubt about the nature of a lump. If a cyst recurs after aspiration, it is best removed or at least biopsied.

Removal of a cyst, performed under local or general anesthesia, is a minor operation and requires only one or two days of hospitalization.

Nipple Discharge

Bleeding or discharge of a yellow, red, green or dark brown fluid from a nipple often is the result of an intraductal papilloma, a small fleshy growth within one or several of the ducts leading to the nipple.

Papillomas may occur from adolescence to old age. Most are benign, especially at younger ages. But 12 to 25 percent are malignant, and the incidence of bleeding in breast cancer increases with age.

Some papillomas are large enough to be detected with the finger and when such a growth can be precisely located, it can be removed through a small incision. When precise location is not possible and surgery should be done without delay, an incision can be made to elevate the nipple, ducts can be removed, and the nipple then restored to original position, and thereafter secretions will be absorbed into the bloodstream.

Benign Tumors

A common tumor of the breast is the benign fibroadenoma, or adenofibroma. It occurs most often in young women and is the most common lump in the breast of women under age thirty. It is usually readily recognized. It has a firm, rubbery consistency, is well circumscribed, and may be easily "popped" about within the breast tissue. Sometimes a fibroadenoma may grow to large size and cause pain.

The usual treatment is surgical removal. The removal of a benign breast tumor is simple and ranks among the least risky of all operations. The lump can usually be removed through a small incision in from fifteen to thirty minutes, and the patient may be home in one to three days. Healing is rapid and the small scar often becomes hardly visible in a few months.

Cancer

Cancer of the breast is the most common malignant condition among women. It is rare before age thirty. Its incidence increases rapidly after menopause. The cause is unknown.

Those at risk of breast cancer

Although no woman may be completely immune to breast cancer, some women may have higher risk than others. Recent efforts to draw up risk profiles may be helpful in identifying those more susceptible to the disease so that they may be checked more intensively for earliest signs of the malignancy.

One such profile, for example, suggests that, as compared to the general population of women, the daughter of a mother who had breast cancer has twice the risk, the sister of a patient with cancer 2½ times the risk. An infertile woman may have 1½ times the risk of a fertile woman; a woman whose first pregnancy came after age twenty-five has twice the risk of one pregnant before that age; and one who had her first child after age thirty-one may have three times the risk of one who had her first child before twenty-one. A woman with cystic breasts may have twice the risk of one with normal breasts; so may a woman who began to menstruate early and has had a prolonged menstrual history. Also at somewhat greater risk than other women may be those who eat large amounts of fat, have wet rather than dry earwax, have underfunctioning of the thyroid gland, live in cold rather than warm climates, and have high rather than low socioeconomic status.

Symptoms

Cancer of the breast is generally not painful. The great majority of breast malignancies manifest themselves by the appearance of a slowly growing painless mass.

Diagnosis

A patient's clinical and family history, her physical examination, and mammography may strongly suggest breast cancer, but the diagnosis can be made definitively only by microscopic examination of excised breast tissue.

Treatment

The choice of treatment for breast cancer depends to a great extent upon the extensiveness of the disease.

Breast cancer begins in a small area and for a time is confined to that area. It can spread in two ways—through the bloodstream or through the lymphatics.

If cancer cells get into the bloodstream, they may be carried and seeded anywhere in the body—in bone, lung, or brain. Ordinarily, breast cancer does not get into the bloodstream early. Once it does and has spread to distant sites, surgery may be used to remove the primary or original cancer but usually cannot extirpate the metastases or distantly spread cancer growths.

More commonly, when breast cancer spreads, it does so by way of the lymphatics, thin-walled vessels that drain fluids from body tissues, including the breasts. When cancer cells get into tissue fluid, they may be filtered out by lymph glands, most of them in the armpit and some behind the breastbone inside the chest.

A cancer confined to the breast, with no evidence of spread to the armpit lymph glands, is ideal for surgery, and the chance for cure is 75 to 90 percent. When the cancer has spread to the armpit glands, the likelihood of cure is reduced to less than 50 percent.

With further spread, the possibility of cure by surgery is drastically reduced. With such spread, radiotherapy with or without surgery often slows advance of the disease and controls bone pain due to metastases.

Hormone treatment, in itself or combined with radiotherapy, can be palliative, delaying advance of the disease and helping to relieve bone pain. Estrogen may be used first and has been helpful principally in postmenopausal patients. If results are disappointing, male sex hormone may be tried and may help. In some cases, corticosteroids—or cortisone-like drugs—are useful in slowing progress of the disease and in increasing a sense of well-being. In women before menopause, castration may be helpful and in some cases may be achieved by radiation, but more often removal of both ovaries may be more effective.

In advanced disease, when hormone and other forms of treatment are not helpful, anticancer agents such as fluorouracil or thiotepa sometimes are useful for palliation.

Still-early studies of various agents designed to help increase natural body defense activities against cancer suggest that this form of treatment may eventually prove useful.

Surgical treatments

Several types of operation, most of them involving breast removal and some of them involving more than breast removal alone, are available.

Lumpectomy. In this procedure, only the tumor is removed, leaving the remainder of the breast intact. It may sometimes be used, when enlarged lymph glands cannot be felt in the armpit, for women over seventy or for women whose general health is poor.

Simple mastectomy. In this procedure all breast tissue is removed, but not the lymph nodes nor the underlying muscle on the chest wall. The operation takes about half an hour, involves very little risk to life, and only remote possibility of complication.

Modified radical mastectomy. This is a simple mastectomy carried a step further to include removal of easily reached glands in the armpit. The time required for it is a little longer and the possibility that there may be some swelling of the arm afterward due to edema is slightly greater.

The standard radical mastectomy. This procedure, which has been the one advised in most medical centers, involves removal of the breast, the underlying muscles of the chest wall, all glands in the armpit, and all glands beneath the chest wall muscles. The operation may take two to four hours and about one in five women afterward may have swelling of the arm due to edema.

Supraradical mastectomy. Some surgeons believe it necessary to go beyond the standard radical mastectomy and in addition to open the chest and remove glands on the underside of the breastbone.

There is controversy, not over the need for and value of surgery for breast cancer, but over how extensive surgery must be. Very much aware of the spreading capabilities of breast malignancy, most surgeons for over half a century have lived by a rule of "find a breast cancer, do a radical mastectomy." Occasionally, some have tried other operations, either lesser or more extensive, and have come back to the radical mastectomy as the seemingly best means of removing all of the cancer and preventing spread. But there have been no hard data to allow comparisons of the effectiveness of the various operations.

Currently, comparative studies are under way at more than twenty major hospitals and university medical centers across the country, but it will be years before survival-rate figures will be available.

Meanwhile, competent surgeons must weigh many factors, including a patient's age, general health, and apparent extent of the cancer, in arriving at a decision. Women are demanding the right to participate in the decision. If you are told you have a suspicious lump, you can discuss with family physician and surgeon what is likely to be the approach if the lump should prove malignant. If you dislike the approach, you can get a second opinion.

After the operation

Commonly there is pain in the wound area and shoulder and arm on the involved side. The pain may last up to a week. Swelling of the arm sometimes develops, but not inevitably. The swelling comes from accumulation of fluid because of interference with drainage. Patients are usually encouraged to be out of bed the day after operation and to use the arm on the involved side. Movement is helpful in minimizing swelling. Physical therapy is, too. When necessary, a special tube around the arm through which pumping pressure can be gently exerted to help move fluid out of the arm into the body is useful, and an elastic sleeve helps keep the swelling from returning.

Exercises may be used for strengthening shoulder and arm. The exercises, shown in literature published by the American Cancer Society and available through the Society or your surgeon, make it possible for normal activities, including swimming, tennis, golf, and other sports, to be resumed.

Help from those who have been there

About 69,000 women each year now have mastectomies. A great help to many of them is Reach to Recovery, organized by Terese Lasser (herself a breast-cancer victim), and now part of the American Cancer Society program. Reach to Recovery has 2,000 volunteers who themselves have had a breast removed and who visit women in 1,000 hospitals in almost every state. Recently, many husbands of these volunteers have become volunteers as well, visiting husbands of mastectomy patients.

A Reach to Recovery volunteer usually visits a patient in the hospital about four days after surgery, when the patient needs consolation and comforting. The volunteer brings with her a kit containing a ball on a plastic string and a length of rope, both for use in arm exercises; a temporary breast substitute for the patient to wear home from the hospital; a special manual to answer common questions, including: How should I act around family and friends? How do I do the arm exercises? How should I dress? Also in the kit is a list of manufacturers of artificial breasts and a letter to husbands.

If the patient wishes it, the volunteer visits again about six weeks later, when the patient is ready to be fitted for an artificial breast. If the patient desires it, the volunteer continues contact. Breast forms now are remarkably realistic; they come in foam rubber, air-filled plastic, liquid-filled plastic, and silicone; some even have nipples; prices range from 75¢ to $500.

The recovery time after mastectomy is usually six weeks or less. Normal sex relations can be resumed after the wound has healed. Although some women have had babies successfully after mastectomies, some doctors feel that pregnancy is inadvisable because hormonal processes during childbearing may increase the chance of recurrence of cancer.

SEE ALSO PART II for pertinent information about choice of surgeon, preoperative and postoperative care, anesthesia, tests, costs, and other aspects of your operation.

Breast Plastic Surgery

Effective methods for reshaping the breasts have been developed. Plastic surgery may be considered for marked enlargement of the breasts, hanging or pendulous breasts, marked disparity in the size of the breasts, and for marked underdevelopment.

Plastic surgery on the breasts is performed in hospital under general anesthesia and is usually advocated only when there is more than a minimal problem, not as a whimsical exercise. As much as two hours or a little more may be required for each breast.

Breast Reduction

The operation, called reduction mamoplasty, involves removal of breast tissue, somewhat like removal of tissue for biopsy, but with consideration for breast contouring. It goes beyond, of course. An incision is made around the nipple but the nipple is left attached to breast tissue. Excess breast tissue is excised. Remaining breast tissue, with nipple, is moved upward, a hole is made for the nipple in the upper skin, lower excess skin is removed, and suturing is done.

The patient is out of bed in many cases the following day, and within two or three days drains left in the wound to remove fluid that may form are removed. A few days after surgery, a bra is fitted and a few days later the patient is ready to go home. Hospitalization may total about a week or a little less. Usually breasts that have been excessive in size do not regrow unless much weight is gained, and pendulous breasts that have been elevated remain so for many years unless there is great weight gain.

The incision mark about the nipple usually becomes virtually invisible and incision marks under the breast fade away. Within a month, virtually all activities—housework, exercise, marital relations—can be resumed.

Breast Enlargement

Breast enlargement, or augmentation mamoplasty, is more difficult than breast reduction. A plastic implant must be used. Through an incision below each breast in the breast tissue on the chest wall, a properly shaped plastic implant is inserted. The skin incision is then sutured. The scar is not noticeable afterward.

Complications may occur but do not very often. If fluid accumulation is evidenced by swelling, firmness, or discomfort, a needle may be inserted through the skin to drain it. Sometimes as healing progresses, the breast may become firmer than desired as the result of formation of a thick fibrous capsule pressing against the implant. This may relax after several months; if not, the capsule may be loosened. Occasionally, infection is a complication; it may respond to antibiotic treatment; if not, removal of the implant may be required.

The results of breast enlargement surgery are rated excellent by some surgeons when there is natural softness, good contour, and no margins between implant and breast tissue that can be felt. They consider results good when there is slightly less softness but good contour and a slightly detectable margin; fair, when the breast is slightly hard and a margin can be felt. Breast implants have not been shown to cause cancer.

Silicone fluid, injection of which was once tried as a means of breast enlargement, is not approved for such use by the Food and Drug Administration at the present time, although a few unscrupulous operators may be using it surreptitiously. Silicone fluid sometimes may shift and drift after injection, even reaching other parts of the body, and it cannot be removed. Its use also makes early detection of cancer of the breast almost impossible.

SEE ALSO PART II for pertinent information about choice of surgeon, preoperative and postoperative care, anesthesia, tests, costs, and other aspects of your operation.

Enlargement of the MALE Breast

Gynecomastia, or enlargement of the male breast, most often occurs either in adolescence or after forty. In adolescents, the enlargement may be due to the increase in hormone secretions at that point and may later disappear. When it occurs later in life, it may involve one or both breasts. When it involves one, it may lead to some worry about the possibility of cancer of the breast.

Enlargement should, of course, receive medical attention. Rarely, the enlargment may be associated with liver disease or a tumor of the testicle. Some drugs may produce gynecomastia as a side effect which disappears when the drugs are stopped. Often gynecomastia occurs for unknown reasons in men who are normal in every other respect.

If the enlargement should be marked, persistent, and a cause of much embarrassment, surgery can be used. The operation is relatively minor, and simple. Under general anesthesia, breast tissue is removed through an incision about three inches long or a little longer. The patient is home from the hospital within two or three days.

Cancer of the MALE Breast

Such cancer is infrequent. When biopsy shows that a male breast growth is malignant and confined to the breast and the lymph glands under the arm, the operation—for removal of the malignancy, surrounding breast tissue, and glands under the arm—is the same as for such cancer in women.

SEE ALSO PART II for pertinent information about choice of surgeon, preoperative and postoperative care, anesthesia, tests, costs, and other aspects of your operation.

Nose, Throat and Neck Surgery

Tonsillectomy and Adenoidectomy

In the side of the throat, behind and above the tongue, are two masses of lymph tissue known as the tonsils. The adenoids, similar but smaller masses of the same kind of tissue, are located close to the opening of the eustachian tubes which drain the ears.

The tonsils and adenoids serve useful purposes, acting to filter and remove inpurities, especially bacteria, from air. Sometimes the tonsils become overloaded by a heavy invasion of germs and, instead of destroying the germs, themselves are overwhelmed and infected. When acutely infected, they become swollen. There may be sore throat and high fever. If the tonsils become chronically infected, they may act as a focus from which infection spreads to other sites in the body.

Chronically enlarged and infected adenoids may also act as a focus for the spread of infection. When they are chronically enlarged, they may interfere with nasal breathing so a child breathes chiefly through the mouth. They may also block the eustachian tubes and in so doing may cause pain or a sense of pressure in the ears and sometimes, middle ear infections and interference with hearing.

Is surgery necessary?

Once tonsil removal—almost invariably accompanied by adenoid removal—was routine, virtually a childhood ritual. Many hospitals set aside regular "tonsil days" for children. The theory was that without tonsils and adenoids, children would be less susceptible to repeated sore throats and colds.

The operation is still the most common surgical procedure in the United States but no longer is accepted as one to be done routinely. For several decades, the operation has been under increasingly critical review. For example, an investigation reported in 1957 covered 5,000 children for ten years, about half of whom had tonsils removed, the other half not. No significant difference was found between the two groups in the number of colds, sore throats, and other upper respiratory infections. Other studies in New York City, Cleveland, and England have confirmed these findings.

While routine operations are no longer advocated, there remains much controversy over when removal of tonsils or adenoids or both is essential. Some authorities maintain that even now the majority of "T and A's" being done are unnecessary; others believe that that is not the case and some children who might benefit by surgery are being denied it mistakenly.

One pediatric authority believes surgery can help in (1) children under five and not older than eight who have persistent nasal obstruction not caused by allergy, with evidence of large adenoids or very large tonsils that interfere with swallowing and (2) children under eight who have had four or more proven attacks of bacterial tonsillitis within a year. When a child suffers from middle ear infections, he suggests, treatment with decongestants, allergy therapy, antibiotics and drainage through eardrum puncture should be tried before operation—and even then, if operation is necessary, sometimes adenoid removal alone is effective. Few children under two, he believes, should have the operation and rarely should both adenoids and tonsils be removed before four years, while in older children, it may be wise to wait a year even when the operation seems indicated.

Usually tonsil and adenoid tissues tend to shrink with maturity. This is particularly the case with adenoid tissue. Sometimes surgery is required for adults; when it is, usually only the tonsils need removal.

If you have any doubts about whether tonsillectomy or adenoidectomy or both may be needed for your child, or possibly for yourself, you can get a second opinion from a qualified ear, nose, and throat specialist.

The surgery

For children, general anesthesia is used. For adults, local anesthesia may be employed. A tonsil can be grasped and pulled with forceps so the edge of the tonsil capsule can be cut with a knife, allowing the tonsil to be separated from its bed. A wire snare is placed around the stalk of the tonsil and is tightened until the stalk is cut through and the tonsil is free.

Adenoid tissue is removed with a delicate instrument that can be moved into the throat behind the nose to snip off the tissue and collect it in a basket.

Either operation is brief, and tonsillectomy and adenoidectomy can be completed, after the induction of anesthesia, within about half an hour. Immediately afterward, when a general anesthetic has been used, the patient is taken to the recovery room with face down so blood and mucus in the throat drain out readily. There are no stitches to be removed later.

The throat is sore for five to seven days. Sometimes pain referred from the operative site may appear in the ears. Discomfort can be minimized with medication and use of an ice collar. Liquids may be swallowed when the patient wakes and later the same day small quantities of milk, ice cream, and sherbet may be taken at frequent intervals. Many surgeons start patients on at least a soft diet the day after operation.

In less than 5 percent of cases, bleeding may occur within a few hours after surgery or as long as two weeks later, but usually between the fifth and tenth days. Sometimes a scab falls off and there will be some bleeding. If there is very much, the doctor should be informed and can stop it.

Recovery is usually complete within ten days to two weeks when all activities, including the most vigorous, can be resumed. Usually a child can return to school sooner, about a week after operation. Sometimes a child may have a peculiar nasal type of speech after adenoid removal but the voice returns to normal after a month or two.

Preparing a child for surgery

While no special diet is required before tonsil and adenoid operations, your doctor may prescribe a laxative and, possibly, vitamin K as an aid in minimizing the likelihood of bleeding after surgery.

Psychological preparation is important. There should be no concealing of the truth from a child. He should know that he is to have his tonsils or adenoids or both removed; that this is likely to make him feel better and healthier; that he will feel nothing at all while the operation is going on and will actually be asleep during that time; that he will have some discomfort afterward but that it will be relieved as much as possible and will stop after a few days. He should also be told that he will wake up in the recovery room. In many hospitals it is possible for him to visit the recovery room in advance of surgery so he is familiar with it.

SEE ALSO PART II for pertinent information about choice of surgeon, preoperative and postoperative care, anesthesia, tests, costs, and other aspects of the operation.

Thyroid Surgery

The thyroid gland, in front of the throat below the Adam's apple and just above the breastbone, is roughly U-shaped, with each end of the U flaring out to a lobe about the size of a big toe. The gland is very important. It determines the rate at which the body utilizes oxygen and controls the rate at which various organs function and the speed with which the body utilizes food.

In effect, the thyroid functions as a thermostat. Each body cell can be looked upon as a tiny power plant, burning food and releasing energy, with some of the energy coming off as heat. Thyroid hormone regulates metabolism: how hot the fires get in the cells and the speed of activity in the cells.

When the thyroid gland is underactive, producing and releasing inadequate amounts of hormone, the effects may include feelings of sluggishness, excessive weight gain, puffiness and slowed mental pace. The hormone deficiency is counteracted by use of thyroid pills.

When the gland is overactive, producing excessive amounts of hormone (hyperthyroidism), the effects may include weight loss, large appetite, heart pounding and skipping of beats, nervousness, muscle quivering, feelings of warmth and, occasionally, conspicuous bulging and protrusion of the eyes (exophthalmic goiter).

Goiter is a term popularly but not accurately used for any enlargement of the thyroid gland. Goiter indicates overgrowth of the thyroid but does not include all enlargements.

Colloid goiter, a swelling of the gland without obvious change in body functioning, stems from insufficient iodine in drinking water and food. Once common, colloid goiter is no longer, because it was discovered that thyroid hormone consists of about 65 percent iodine, and iodine has been added to drinking water and table salt.

Nodular goiter is relatively common and of concern. In this condition, the thyroid has one or more nodules or lumps which may be seen or felt in the neck. In some cases, these eventually lead to overactivity of the thyroid, or hyperthyroidism; in other cases, they may sometimes grow and press against the windpipe or press against the larynx and lead to hoarseness; in up to 10 percent of cases, they may develop into cancer.

Enlargement of the thyroid also may be produced by *thyroiditis,* inflammation of the gland. The swelling may be painful and accompanied by fever. In many cases, thyroiditis subsides within a few weeks; in other cases, steroid, or cortisonelike medication, may be used to bring it under control.

Enlargement may be the result of benign thyroid gland tumors called adenomas, or malignant tumors. Fortunately most thyroid malignancies remain localized within the gland for long periods before spreading, and their removal has a high cure rate.

Diagnosis

Various blood tests are now available to determine at what rate a gland is functioning. They provide accurate measurements of thyroid function.

A valuable procedure for helping to determine the nature of a lump in the thyroid is the thyroid scan (scintiscan). A small dose of radioactive iodine is swallowed. The iodine is attracted to the thyroid. When a Geiger counter is placed over the neck, its sensitivity to the radioactive iodine allows mapping of the gland. If there is an area of nonactivity in the gland, a "cold" area, it indicates a change in the gland and may suggest the diagnosis. So may a "hot" area of great activity. Generally, cold nodules are more apt to be cancerous; hot areas may be indicative of benign growths.

Medical treatment

In some cases of goiter, when the gland is not large enough to warrant removal, medical treatment may suffice. If the goiter is due to insufficient iodine, it may be treated with iodine, which may prevent further enlargement. In some cases, thyroid hormone may be used and will have the effect of stopping the stimulation that leads to goiter formation.

For hyperthyroidism, medical methods are available now to suppress the production of excess thyroid hormone. Antithyroid drugs such as propylthiouracil may ameliorate the disease by blocking production of thyroid hormone, and after several months of treatment a normal thyroid function may be achieved. Radioactive iodine treatment, with larger doses than used for diagnosis, may also control hyperthyroidism by destroying enough of the gland to reduce excess hormone production. These medical methods are not always effective. Antithyroid drugs may fail to control hyperthyroidism or in about 9 percent of patients may produce toxic reactions such as drug fever, skin outbreaks, and blood disturbances. Because of the possibility that there may be long-delayed effects from radiation not yet apparent, radioactive iodine is usually limited to patients over forty.

When surgery may be needed

Surgery may be required under several circumstances: when there is the possibility of cancer; when medical treatment proves inadequate; when the gland enlargement in itself is a hazard because of pressure on the windpipe.

Thyroid operations

Surgery is performed, usually under general anesthesia, through a 3½ to 4-inch incision in the neck above the collarbone. The muscles in the neck can be readily separated to allow the gland to be brought into view.

According to the amount of thyroid tissue that must be removed, the operation is called subtotal thyroidectomy, hemithyroidectomy, or total thyroidectomy.

Subtotal thyroidectomy refers to removal of parts of both lobes of the gland lying along the windpipe and of the connecting strip (isthmus) of thyroid tissue over the windpipe, or removal of a whole lobe and part of the other.

Hemithyroidectomy refers to removal of one whole lobe and usually the isthmus.

Total thyroidectomy refers to removal of all thyroid tissue.

The amount of thyroid tissue that must be removed depends upon the nature of the problem and the individual circumstances. If surgery is required for thyroiditis because of pressure on the windpipe, only the isthmus over the windpipe may require removal. A nonmalignant tumor may be removed with little loss of thyroid tissue. In some cases of thyroid cancer, hemithyroidectomy can be adequate; in other cases, more extensive surgery is essential and may include removal of lymph nodes and some neck muscles.

Length of operation

Thyroid surgery may require three or four hours because the thyroid touches or has connections with nerves, veins, windpipe, esophagus, and parathyroid glands, and great care must be used.

Recovery

Usually, recovery is rapid; patients may be out of bed in a day or two, home from hospital within a week. There is some discomfort but much less than from an abdominal or chest wound, and healing is rapid. For a few days there may be soreness of the throat and some hoarseness. A drain is left in place temporarily but is removed with virtually no discomfort within twenty-four to seventy-two hours. A thin scar left by thyroid surgery may remain red for six months or longer; usually, after a year it has faded and become less conspicuous. The shirt collar in men usually covers it; women may use a necklace.

Corrective surgery usually can be expected to relieve many or all symptoms previously arising from the thyroid problem, including hand tremor, heart palpitation, nervousness, excessive appetite, neck pressure, hoarseness, breathing difficulty.

Sometimes after surgery, a previously overactive gland may become underactive, leading to weight gain and other symptoms of thyroid deficiency, in which case thyroid medication can be used to correct the deficiency and eliminate the symptoms. Thyroid medication also can be used as needed after total thyroidectomy.

In most cases, a patient after thyroid surgery is back at

work within two or three weeks, a little longer if the work is of the heavy manual type.

SEE ALSO PART II for pertinent information about choice of surgeon, preoperative and postoperative care, anesthesia, tests, costs, and other aspects of your operation.

Parathyroid Surgery

Four small glands, the parathyroids, are attached to the thyroid gland. The hormone parathormone, secreted by the parathyroids, has much to do with the balance in the body and the excretion in the urine of calcium and phosphorus derived from milk and other foods and necessary for bone growth and maintenance. If the parathyroids are underactive, the calcium level in the blood falls and muscles go into painful spasms, called tetany; in severe cases, convulsion and death may result. Administration of parathyroid hormone, or certain synthetic compounds with similar actions, or a potent vitamin D preparation, will usually keep calcium output normal and stop the spasms. Feeding calcium is helpful in such cases.

If the parathyroids secrete too much hormone, calcium leaks out of the bones and phosphorus out of body cells. Calcium stones may form in the kidneys and tumors or cysts may develop in and soften bones.

Tests showing excessive parathyroid activity may indicate need for surgery to remove excess functioning tissue or a tumor which often is confined to a single parathyroid gland. The incision is similar to that made for thyroid surgery; as much tissue as necessary is removed to reduce parathyroid functioning or eliminate the tumor, and recovery is rapid. If a large amount of tissue has to be removed because of widespread involvement, tetany with its muscular twitching and spasm can be prevented by administration of synthetic parathyroid hormone and other medication.

SEE ALSO PART II for pertinent information about choice of surgeon, preoperative and postoperative care, anesthesia, tests, costs, and other aspects of your operation.

Salivary Glands

A pair of salivary glands, known as the parotid glands, lie in the sides of the face in front of and slightly below the ears. Saliva from these glands reaches the mouth through parotid ducts, which open on the inner surfaces of the cheeks opposite the second molar teeth. There are also a pair of submaxillary glands in the angles of the lower jaws and a pair of sublingual glands under the tongue. Ducts from these glands open into the floor of the mouth beneath the tongue. Saliva from the six glands mixes with food in the mouth and softens and lubricates it. Saliva, too, contains a digestive enzyme, ptyalin, which acts to convert cooked starch to sugar. There is enough saliva so that, if necessary, one or two glands may be removed without causing any deficiency.

Several salivary gland problems may require surgery.

Salivary Stones

Stones, or calculi, may form in any of the salivary glands but most commonly occur in the submaxillary. When the duct or tube from gland into mouth is blocked by a stone, the gland swells. Sometimes the stone can be felt in the duct inside the mouth under the tongue. If not, it may be located by X-ray examination after injection of a material into the duct opening to help visualize the stone.

Often the stone can be removed by a minor operation under local anesthesia in which an incision is made into the duct directly over the stone. If the gland remains swollen persistently, it may be removed through an incision under the jaw. The incision follows the jawbone conformation so the scar will not be conspicuous. A hospital stay of only a few days may be required.

In rare cases a sublingual gland may become blocked and swollen with saliva. The swelling is usually visible as a ranula, or fluid-containing bag, under the tongue behind the front teeth. Under local or general anesthesia, the top of the bag is removed and the gland duct's entrance into the mouth is reconstructed. No more than a day or two of hospitalization is needed.

Salivary Tumors

Tumors of the salivary glands, most often the parotid glands, are frequent. Most are not cancerous. Painless and slow-growing, they are most likely to start on the outer surface of a parotid gland near the ear, protruding outward from the cheek. In that case, if the tumor is benign, only the outer half of the gland may have to be removed. When the tumor is in the inner half bulging into the mouth, the entire parotid gland is removed.

Removal is through an incision in the skin running from in front of the ear to the neck, long enough to allow careful separation of the gland from the facial nerve so that the nerve is not cut. Cutting the nerve causes distortion and paralysis of that side of the face. If the tumor is malignant, the nerve may have to be cut.

For a few days after surgery, a drain will remain in place. The patient may be out of bed the following day, home in a week or less. A fluid diet may be used for several days because of pain caused by chewing, but thereafter diet can be unrestricted. Usually the wound is healed in about ten days. Often a fine, thin scar can be expected.

SEE ALSO PART II for pertinent information about choice of surgeon, preoperative and postoperative care, anesthesia, tests, costs, and other aspects of your operation.

Larynx Surgery

The larynx, or voice box, which forms the Adam's apple in the neck, is at the top of the windpipe or trachea which takes air to the lungs. While incoming air passes through the larynx, it is air expelled from the lungs that makes voice sounds.

In the front of the larynx, two folds of membranes, the vocal cords, are attached and held by tiny cartilages. Muscles attached to the cartilages move the vocal cords, which are made to vibrate by air exhaled from the lungs. The vibrations are carried through the air upward into the throat, mouth, nasal cavities, and sinuses, which serve as resonating chambers.

Growths that affect the larynx and require surgery may be benign or malignant. With either, the prime warning symptom is hoarseness that persists for more than a few weeks. While cancer of the larynx is fairly common, it can be removed by surgery when detected early and the voice may be saved. Nonmalignant growths also can be removed and the voice can be restored to normal.

Nonmalignant Growths

Most tumors of the larynx are benign and in fact are not so much tumors as overgrowths of the mucous membrane lining the larynx and vocal cords. In addition to hoarseness, they may make for difficulty in breathing when they become large enough to obstruct the airway and sometimes may cause coughing and difficulty in swallowing.

A growth can be seen by reflecting light from a physician's head mirror onto a small mirror held against the back of the throat.

To determine the nature of the growth—and benign growths may be caused by allergy, irritation, infection, or overuse of the voice (singer's nodes, for example)—a laryngoscope is used. In the hospital, under general anesthesia or after painting or spraying the throat with a local anesthetic, the tubular instrument is inserted through mouth and throat to the larynx and allows a direct look at the larynx.

The benign growths are removed through the laryngoscope with special instruments that can simultaneously cut away and catch pieces of overgrowth tissue. There is little pain or discomfort afterward; a liquid diet may be used for a day; and the patient is home in two or three days. For healing purposes, the voice cannot be used for about a week.

Cancer of the Larynx

Mainly a disease of smokers over fifty, cancer of the larynx occurs most often on the vocal cords. When it does, it gives its warning of persistent hoarseness and in nine of every ten cases can be cured when treated early. Cancer on a vocal cord tends to be confined there for a relatively long time, spreading only after hoarseness has persisted for several months or longer.

Some cancers of the larynx occur elsewhere in the larynx, in cartilage, muscles, passage from throat, or passage to windpipe. These may not cause hoarseness in early stages and may spread sooner than vocal cord cancer.

Treatment

Either surgery alone, radiation alone, or a combination of both may be used. In some cases, when the cancer is only superficial, radiation alone is enough.

Surgery may involve complete removal of the voice box (total laryngectomy) or partial laryngectomy, which preserves the voice.

Partial laryngectomy

Under general or local anesthesia, an incision is made in the neck, starting at the top of the Adam's apple and extending about 2½ inches. The cartilage of the larynx is split and the growth on a cord can be then cut away.

When a considerable amount of tissue must be removed, a tracheostomy may be performed to make certain that there is an adequate airway. This involves making a hole in the windpipe and inserting a metal tube which can be removed without difficulty a few days later; the opening closes on its own without suturing.

There is only minimal, easily relieved pain after the operation. In order to help with swallowing, the patient may sit part-way up in bed for a few days. Sutures are remove within a week, and the patient goes home within ten days.

When the cancer is confined to the epiglottis, the leaflike flap of cartilage between the back of the tongue and the entrance to the larynx and windpipe, all of the larynx above the vocal cords may be removed. The voice is preserved but there may be some difficulty in swallowing, and a temporary feeding tube, through nose to stomach, may be used for a week or a little longer until swallowing becomes easier.

Variations of partial laryngectomy may be used when growths are located away from the vocal cords in other areas of the larynx or when they occupy much of the larynx. The voice is still preserved. In some cases, the extent of the cancer may require that radical neck node dissection (see page 216) also be done.

Total laryngectomy

Carried out under general anesthesia, total laryngectomy is a much more extensive operation. A longer incision along the center of the neck is made. The windpipe is cut across just above the collarbone, and a tube is inserted so the anesthetic gas goes directly to the windpipe. The entire larynx is removed. Because one wall of the larynx forms part of the throat and esophagus, this area is reconstructed. Sometimes a plastic feeding tube through the nose to the stomach may be used temporarily to give the area time to heal, but frequently this is not necessary and swallowing of soft foods is possible within a day or two.

After total laryngectomy, a patient must breathe through a permanent opening in the neck which is provided for by suturing the end of the windpipe to the skin.

For a few days after operation, the neck feels weak, movement is uncomfortable, help may be needed to raise the head, and after total laryngectomy a patient may be cared for in a special care section or have a special nurse for a day or two. He may be home from hospital within two weeks.

Adjusting to life after total laryngectomy

Total laryngectomy is radical but very often often life-saving. Adjustments have to be made afterward and require effort; many thousands of well-motivated patients have successfully made the adjustments.

In addition to having to learn a new method of speaking, the patient must be careful about not sucking water into his lungs when bathing or showering. Although a dressing is not absolutely essential for covering the tracheal opening in the neck, the patient may wish to cover it with a small square of gauze or cotton material or wear a collar or scarf of porous material to conceal the opening. Such coverings are also useful in that they serve as filters and remove dust and other irritants from the air being inhaled through the opening.

Until he has learned a new way of speaking, he should have a pencil and notebook to write messages to those caring for him. His family can do him great service by anticipating his needs and wishes whenever possible to minimize frustration and tension for him.

Instruction is a new method of speaking can begin as soon as the operative site has healed. Esophageal speech, the simplest, is usually the first one the patient learns. He is taught to belch and form simple sounds and words while burping. With practice, he can make sustained belches that cause a column of air to vibrate in his throat and the walls and roof of his pharynx, and the air column substitutes for the vocal cords as he forms words with his mouth. Esophageal speech is not smooth and after mastering it the patient can begin to learn the more advanced and smoother pharyngeal method.

Pharyngeal speech uses the limited amount of air that enters the nose and mouth during breathing through the tracheostomy tube. Sounds can be produced by blocking this air with tongue actions, making it vibrate against the roof of the pharynx at the back of the mouth. With practice, it becomes possible to so control and slowly expel the air that almost normal, fluent speech is achieved, and the voice sounds ordinary but slightly hoarse.

For those who cannot master esophageal or pharyngeal speech, various electronic speaking devices are available. An electric vibrator can be held against the side of the neck while words are formed with tongue, teeth, and palate and the result is communicative speech even though with artificial tone.

A source of valuable information for patients who have had total laryngectomies is the International Association of Laryngectomees, 521 West 57 St., New York, N. Y. 10019. Information may also be obtained from telephone company offices' special equipment services.

SEE ALSO PART II for pertinent information about choice of surgeon, preoperative and postoperative care, anesthesia, tests, costs, and other aspects of your operation.

Lip and Mouth Surgery

Lip Tumors

The lips, the fleshy margins of the mouth composed of skin and mucous membrane, are commonly sites for benign tumors. These are usually warty in nature or made up of blood vessels that cluster together (hemangioma). Such benign growths almost invariably can be cured. They may be removed with good cosmetic results in one of several ways most suitable for the individual patient: by freezing, electric needle, radiation, or excision and suturing.

Cancer of the lip, many times more common in men than in women, most often occurs on the lower lip, usually in middle age or later. Usually it is curable because it is visible, discovered often in early stages, and tends to be slow-growing, often requiring months to spread to the lymph nodes in the neck.

For some early cancers of the lip, radiation alone is sufficient to cure. When surgery is advisable, the operation, which may be performed under general or local anesthesia, is relatively minor. A V-shaped area containing the tumor and enough healthy tissue on each side to provide a margin of safety, is removed, and the remaining healthy lip is then sutured. As much as half of a lip can be removed and the remaining healthy lip tissue can stretch and adapt well enough so that within six months, the lip is flexible and virtually normal in appearance.

Usually the patient is out of bed when he recovers from the anesthesia, uses a liquid diet for a few days, and is home from hospital well within a week.

When a lip cancer is very large, or when lymph nodes in the neck are enlarged and the malignancy may have spread, cure is often possible with radical dissection of the neck nodes and removal of all the glands (see page 216).

Leukoplakia

Thickened white patches that sometimes form on the lips, gums, tongue, or other mucous membranes tend to grow into larger patches or may take the form of ulcers. They may in time cause pain during swallowing or speaking and have a pronounced tendency to become cancerous.

Leukoplakia affects mostly middle-aged and elderly men, apparently as the result of prolonged irritation from such factors as smoking or badly fitting dentures.

Treatment is aimed at removing any possible cause of irritation—tobacco, possibly alcohol, and extremely hot food.

Dental attention may be required if teeth are uneven or dentures fit improperly. The white patches may be removed with an electric needle under local anesthesia. Many systematic treatments may be required to remove them all. The patches also may be removed surgically under local or general anesthesia with an overnight stay in hospital.

Torus Palatinus

This is a benign bony overgrowth of the hard palate in the roof of the mouth. The tumor sometimes grows to an inch or more in diameter but so slowly that it may not be noticed. Unless there is some difficulty, as in fitting dentures, it may be left alone without danger.

When necessary, the growth can be removed in a minor operation under local anesthesia. The membrane of the palate is opened, the excess bone is chiseled away, and the membrane is then sutured.

Tongue Cancer

Tongue cancer appears mostly in men of middle or older ages and in the majority of cases it is situated at the tip or along the sides of the tongue, where it can be discovered early. Many tongue cancers remain confined for months to their original site before spreading to the lymph nodes of the neck. Cancer towards the back of the tongue tends to spread to lumph nodes on both sides of the neck, requiring extensive surgery.

Smaller cancers, up to about 3/8″, often can be removed by excising a wedge of the tongue. With suturing and healing, the deformity is not great. Larger cancers, when located along the side of the tongue, may require removal of as much as a third of the tongue from the tip back. Speech is changed but remains understandable. Swallowing becomes awkward but still functional.

With increases in the amount of tongue that must be removed, disability increases. After removal of as much as

75 percent of the tongue, chewing may be impossible, requiring that the diet be confined to finely blended or puréed foods.

Surgery for tongue cancer is carried out under general anesthesia, and an operation for cancer at the back of the tongue may be supplemented, before or after, by radiation.

When tongue cancer has spread to the lymph nodes, radical neck node dissection (see below) will be needed to remove the nodes in the neck. When it has spread to the floor of the mouth, the affected areas under the tongue will be removed along with the cancer of the tongue. When part of the jawbone must be sacrificed, it may be replaced with a bone graft or metal splint.

In some cases, the treatment of extensive tongue cancer has to be extreme and there is extreme disability to be adjusted to. Yet, with the saving of life, life can be worth living, and many patients make excellent adjustments, much as do those who require total laryngectomies.

SEE ALSO PART II for pertinent information about choice of surgeon, preoperative and postoperative care, anesthesia, tests, costs, and other aspects of your operation.

Radical Neck Surgery

Cancers such as those of the lips, tongue, and larynx sometimes require removal of the lymph nodes in the neck. The nodes act as filters. In addition to destroying any invading bacteria they trap migrant cancer cells and may hold them for months to prevent their spread throughout the body.

If the cancer is small and the lymph nodes are not enlarged, their removal may not be needed. But if a cancer is sizable, hope for cure may rest with removal of the nodes even if they are not enlarged.

Radical neck node dissection is done under general anesthesia and may require up to five or six hours when done together with removal of the primary cancer. An incision may run from below the ear to the collarbone. Everything in the front of the neck on one side or both sides is removed. In addition to the lymph nodes this may include blood vessels, nerves, and the salivary gland under the jawbone.

Extensive as the operation is, the patient is usually out of bed within a day or two and home from hospital in about ten days. The neck, of course, is thinned, but deformity is much less than might be expected.

SEE ALSO PART II for pertinent information about choice of surgeon, preoperative and postoperative care, anesthesia, tests, costs, and other aspects of your operation.

Sinus Operations

The sinuses are cavities in the skull which help both to reduce the weight of the head and to make the voice more resonant. The sinuses connect through small openings (ostia) into the nasal passages, and the soft, moist mucous lining which coats the inside of the nose extends into the sinuses.

Sinustis, an inflammation of the mucous membrane lining of one or more sinuses, may be caused by almost anything that can irritate, infect, or obstruct the interior of the nose. The sinuses may be affected by colds and other respiratory infections, allergies, sometimes by tooth infection.

In the vast majority of cases, sinusitis can be controlled by antibiotics, moist heat, drugs that act to shrink the mucous membrane lining of nose and sinuses so that pus or secretions can drain from the sinuses.

The modern tendency is to try to avoid direct surgical penetration of the sinuses to establish drainage or remove diseased lining membranes. Such operations are held in abeyance until more conservative measures have been tried. If there are allergic sensitivities, they may need treatment. Pus from sinuses can be cultured and the offending germ identified so an antibiotic specific for that germ can be used. Infected teeth are treated.

On both sides of the septum, the cartilage partition that separates the nostrils, are rounded ridges called turbinates, which are outgrowths of thin bone covered with mucous membrane. Sometimes cauterization of boggy turbinates helps to establish drainage. Sometimes minor surgery to remove polyps or correct a deviated septum may be called for.

In the minority of patients who do not respond well to conservative treatment, sinus surgery may be used.

Sinus procedures

The sinuses most often affected are the maxillary sinuses in the cheekbones. An infected maxillary sinus can be opened through an incision beneath the upper lip. An opening is cut through the bony front wall of the sinus; membrane within the sinus is removed; another opening or "window" is made in the inner sinus wall into the nose through which drainage can occur; and the incision beneath the lip is closed. The operation may be done in hospital under local or general anesthesia and the patient is usually recovered in four or five days. In some cases, the window opening alone may be enough and can be made under local anesthesia from within the nose.

The frontal sinuses are above the bony orbit of the eyes. The ethmoid sinuses are between the eye sockets and the nose. The sphenoid sinus is at the back of the nose. These sinuses can be reached through an incision that begins in the inner half of the eyebrow and extends along the side of the nose. It is also possible to reach the frontal sinuses through a scalp incision at the hairline and the ethmoids from within the nose.

The operations are performed under local or general anesthesia; there is postoperative discomfort but it may be less than the original sinus pain; there may be some facial swelling and eye discoloration for some time after operation. Usually the patient is out of bed the next day and home after several days during which antibiotics may be administered along with pain-relieving agents. The scar, which follows a natural crease, usually in inconspicuous and will not be visible at all when glasses are worn.

When sinus surgery is required, it is usually best performed by a specialist in such operations. If you have any doubts about the need for or help to be expected from an operation, it is advisable to have a second opinion.

SEE ALSO PART II for pertinent information about choice of surgeon, preoperative and postoperative care, anesthesia, tests, costs, and other aspects of your operation.

Nasal Polyps

Nasal polyps—growths extending outward from the mucous membrane—grow in the nasal cavity or in the sinuses. They are produced by local irritation or may be the result of allergy. They are not dangerous, but if they grow large enough, they may cause stuffiness and headaches and obstruct nasal breathing.

It is necessary to treat the allergy or any other source of irritation responsible for the growth of polyps. If the polyps continue to be troublesome, surgery may be necessary, but unless the cause is treated and brought under control, the polyps often recur.

In most cases, polyp removal can be carried out under local anesthesia in the surgeon's office, using snares and forceps that permit them to be snipped or twisted off. In some cases of large and extensive polyps, hospitalization may be needed to allow cutting through the wall between the sinus and the nasal cavity or, sometimes, to allow opening of the sinuses from the outside, in order to permit removal of all polyps.

Deviated Septum

The septum, the cartilage structure separating the nostrils, sometimes is bent or deviated. Airflow on one side then may be reduced. Many people with deviated septum have no difficulty.

When there is trouble, it is important to determine that the deviated septum is the cause or a major contributing factor. It is possible for the septum to be a factor when it obstructs sinus openings or in some people whose membranes swell as the result of allergy, dust, or excessive humidity.

The corrective operation, called submucous resection, may be done under local anesthesia in hospital. An incision is made in the membrane lining the septum on one side of the nose and deflected portions of the septum are removed. The septum is intact afterward. At the completion of the operation, lubricated gauze is packed into both nostrils to prevent bleeding and to hold the lining membrane against the septum. The packing is uncomfortable and pain medication may be required for a day or two. The packing may be removed after several days.

The results of correction of a deviated septum are excellent when the septum was responsible for trouble.

Broken Nose

Fractures of the nose, common injuries, are best treated very soon after the event. After ten days, treatment can be difficult and possibly unsuccessful.

Often the diagnosis of fracture is obvious from the shape of the nose and feeling of the broken bones. X-rays are used to determine the precise extent of the fracture and to make certain no skull fracture may have occurred.

While a nose fracture sometimes may be set without anesthetic in the office, often local or general anesthesia and an overnight stay in the hospital are required.

To manipulate the broken bones back into proper alignment, pressure is applied from the outside and also with special instruments that go inside and can push out bone fragments. A lubricated gauze packing may be kept in the nose for several days, with a mild sedative used to help relieve discomfort. There may be swelling which will persist for a few weeks beyond the three or four required for complete healing of an average fracture.

Brain and Nerve Surgery

In recent years, major advances have been made in understanding the functioning of the brain and nervous system and in neurosurgical techniques for operative treatment of disorders of the system. Those techniques now are often lifesaving.

The Brain

One measure of the intricacy of the human brain is that it weighs only about twelve ounces at birth and about three pounds in an adult, yet it can store, it is estimated, more facts, impressions, and total information than is contained in the nine million volumes of the Library of Congress.

Another is that when necessary we can get along with only half the brain. After removal of much of one side of the brain because of tumor, physicians, lawyers, and others have been able to carry on their regular work. Studies of servicemen who suffered penetrating head wounds during World War II showed that upon retesting for intelligence their scores remained largely the same as upon first entering service. The evidence is that if the brain is compartmentalized, with specific areas for specific functions, another area can, when necessary, take over the functions of a damaged area.

The brain has some 15 billion nerve units which permit

221

storage of memory images and learning. In addition, it has great numbers of connections which control the more than 600 muscles in the body. Other connections into the brain from eyes, ears, and nerves in the skin allow us to record and remember what we see, hear, feel, smell, and taste.

The brain is composed of several parts. The cerebrum takes the form of two hemispheres divided by a groove. The surface, or cortex, of the cerebrum is gray matter formed by the cell bodies of nerve cells. Fibers from these bodies lead inward to form the white matter of the cerebrum. The fibers cross over so that those entering the brain from the left side of the body cross to the right side of the brain, which is why the right lobe of the cerebrum controls most of the left side of the body while the left lobe controls the right side.

At the base of the cerebrum are three structures: pons, medulla, and cerebellum. The pons connects the medulla with higher brain centers. The medulla, just below the pons and at the upper end of the spinal cord, is a switching center for nerve impulses to and from higher brain centers. It also has centers which act through the autonomic nervous system to control heart activity, breathing, and other functions that go on without our conscious effort.

The cerebellum, or little brain, has areas that control muscle tone, equilibrium, and coordinate voluntary movements.

The skull, a tough bony cage, surrounds the brain and protects it. The skull itself is protected by the scalp, which is made up of five layers: skin and hair, cutaneous tissue, a tough layer of fibrous tissue, loose tissue, and periosteum, which covers the bone of the skull.

Additional protection is provided. Within the brain are four reservoirs, the ventricles, containing cerebrospinal fluid. The fluid circulates around the brain so that in effect the brain floats on and in fluid, an excellent shock absorber system. Finally, within the bone of the skull the brain is wrapped in layers of tissue, one of which, the dura mater, is especially tough and protective.

The Nervous System

The brain can be considered a control center; the nervous system is like a two-way communications network for informational messages to flow to the control center and command messages to be transmitted from the center. The informational or sensory messages come from the eyes, ears, and other sense organs and also from many billions of receptors within the body itself concerned with various body functions.

Actually, we have two nervous systems: central and autonomic. The central nervous system includes the brain and spinal cord. The spinal cord is suspended within a cylinder formed by the spinal bones. From the spinal cord emerge forty-three pairs of nerves that connect to every part of the body. Twelve, the cranial nerves, go to the eyes and other sense organs, the heart and other internal organs. The thirty-one other nerve pairs go to skeletal muscles throughout the body. They come off the spinal cord between the bones of the spine, one of a pair going to the right side of the body and the other to the left.

The central nervous system works in more than one way. When, for example, you touch a hot object, pain stimulates a sensory nerve; the nerve shoots informational impulses to the spinal cord; there the impulses are transferred quickly to a motor nerve to muscles which jerk your hand away. All this takes place in a fraction of a second; it's a reflex action requiring no thought.

But while it is going on, something else is taking place. Impulses from the sensory nerve also are transferred to another sensory nerve traveling up the spinal cord to the cerebrum and, as you feel pain, you look at your finger and at the hot object and associate the two—and, because of knowledge stored in memory centers in the cerebrum, you quickly put your fingers under cold water.

The other nervous system, the autonomic, provides for automatic control of internal organ functioning. It has two parts—the sympathetic and parasympathetic—which oppose each other and permit a precise balance.

The sympathetic begins at the base of the brain and runs along both sides of the spinal column. Nerves from the system go to glands, muscles, heart, stomach, intestines, and bladder. The parasympathetic system has two major nerves. One, the vagus, comes from the medulla and sends branches through chest and abdomen. The other, the pelvic, comes off the spinal cord in the hip area and sends branches to organs in the lower part of the body.

The sympathetic system dilates the pupil of the eye, speeds the heartbeat, raises blood pressure; the parasympathetic constricts the pupil, slows the heartbeat, and lowers blood pressure.

Emotions strongly influence the autonomic system.

Brain Surgery

To reach brain structures, entry can be gained readily through the skull.

In some cases, for example, when a blood clot is sought, a burr hole may suffice. A ½″ to 1¼″ diameter plug of bone is cut out with a circular saw.

In other cases, when surgery must be more extensive, a craniotomy may be performed under general or local anesthesia. A number of holes are cut in the skull and a wire saw or an air or electrically driven saw may be used to connect the holes to make a bone flap.

After operation, plugs or flap may be replaced or a metal or fabric mesh may be used to cover the opening.

When brain tissue is exposed, a salt solution is repeatedly sprayed and suctioned off to keep the tissue moist. The handling of brain tissue is very gentle; forceps are tipped with cotton pads. An electric needle is used to seal tiny severed blood vessels supplying the scalp. Bleeding from the brain itself can be reduced with a drug that lowers blood pressure and with a cooled blanket under the patient that lowers brain temperature and reduces the amount of oxygen-carrying blood it needs during operation.

Aids to diagnosis

To help in the diagnosis of brain conditions, one or more procedures may be used.

Ordinary X-rays of the skull yield information which in some cases may be sufficient.

A special X-ray study—a ventriculogram or a pneumoencephalogram—may be needed. A *ventriculogram* makes the brain's ventricles visible. For this, a burr hole is made in the skull and through a needle placed in one of the ventricles, a small amount of fluid is withdrawn. The fluid is replaced with air. With X-rays taken as the patient's head is turned to various positions, all aspects of all four ventricles, which connect with each other, can be viewed and any abnormal structure such as a tumor can be detected.

For a *pneumoencephalogram,* a needle is inserted into the spinal canal between two vertebrae at the point just above the hip bones. A little spinal fluid is removed and air is injected. Since the brain ventricles connect with the fluid around the spinal cord, they can be viewed in similar fashion to a ventriculogram.

An *angiogram,* an X-ray study to view the arteries, veins, and other blood vessels of the brain and covering membranes, is made by injecting a small amount of a radioopaque substance into arteries of the neck leading to the brain. A local anesthetic is used. Although briefly uncomfortable, an angiogram is helpful in revealing the presence of new blood vessels in a tumor or displacement of brain blood vessels indicative of a growth. An angiogram can also reveal an aneurysm, or ballooning out, of a brain blood vessel.

An *electroencephalogram,* or brain wave tracing, obtained by taping wires to the skull, does not directly reveal tumors or clots but can indicate abnormal brain functioning, which may help in diagnosis.

For a *brain scan,* a radioactive chemical solution is taken by mouth or is injected. About a day later, a radio counter moved back and forth over the head reveals how much of the chemical has concentrated in the brain and where. The scan may show the position, size, and shape of a tumor.

Brain Tumors

However frightening the thought of a growth within the brain, a brain tumor is not invariably hopeless.

More than a third of brain tumors are benign, and about 30 percent more are moderately malignant, growing and spreading slowly.

Several kinds of tumors develop within the brain. As many as one of every five are *meningiomas,* or growths arising from the brain coverings, or *neurofibromas,* which are growths arising from brain nerves. Often such tumors are accessible to surgery and can be removed completely for cure.

About 10 percent of brain tumors are *pituitary gland adenomas,* growths arising from the gland which descends from the brain and is located in a niche of the skull between the optic or eye nerves. Usually these tumors grow slowly and do not spread to other parts of the body. Many may be treated successfully by X-ray therapy alone without surgery or by implantation of radioactive isoptopes in the tumor via a needle under X-ray guidance. Patients not helped by radiation may benefit from surgery. One approach to a pituitary tumor is through a craniotomy, with the incision made above the forehead. Another is through the nose, upward through the sphenoid sinus.

An *acoustic neuroma,* a tumor of the hearing nerve, is not malignant but can be dangerous because of its pressure on brain structures. An early sign is impaired hearing, sometimes with head noise, and acoustic neuromas are often discovered early. With early enough discovery, a neuroma can be removed completely through an opening in the back part of the skull and sometimes, at the very earliest stages, through the ear.

A little more than half of brain tumors are *gliomas* developing within the brain substance. When a glioma is superficial, in an outer or frontal area of brain, it is possible to remove it and effect a cure. A deeply located glioma, however, usually cannot be removed without the destruction of dangerous amounts of normal brain tissue.

For some tumors, radiation therapy to retard further growth may be used in combination with surgery to get out as much as possible of the tumor.

In a little less than half of brain tumors, the results of surgery are excellent. In about three out of ten cases, surgery fails completely. But in some cases when only palliation, not cure, is possible, patients may live fairly comfortably for extended periods, sometimes as long as ten or fifteen years.

When a tumor is successfully removed after having caused disturbances—of speech, vision, hearing, motion—the disturbances often may improve considerably or disappear after a period of time. But this is not invariably the case.

Surgery for brain tumor varies in length from an hour or so to as much as three or four hours. There is usually not much pain afterward. The hospital stay may be about two weeks.

SEE ALSO PART II for pertinent information about choice of surgeon, preoperative and postoperative care, anesthesia, tests, costs, and other aspects of your operation.

Parkinson's Disease (Shaking Palsy)

Parkinsonism, also known as Parkinson's disease and shaking palsy, is a disorder of unknown cause that produces tremor or shaking, stiffness, weakness. Until recently, medical treatment often produced less than satisfactory results and surgical attempts were made to help parkinsonism patients.

Certain areas deep within the brain, such as the thalamus and the globus pallidus, are involved in producing parkinsonism symptoms. While cutting directly through to these areas is not feasible because vital brain tissue would be severed in the process, a needle can be maneuvered to them under X-ray guidance, and it has become possible to destroy the small guilty areas by freezing, cautery (burning) radioactive chemicals, or ultrasonics.

The operation does not cure but it often relieves shaking and trembling and to some extent rigidity.

More recently, there have been major advances in drug therapy for parkinsonism. One drug in particular, levodopa, introduced in 1967, has proved helpful in relieving symptoms for many patients. While the long-term value is not yet known, it may make surgery unnecessary in some patients.

Other movement disorders

Surgery has been showing promise in the treatment of other movement disorders, including dystonia musculorum deformans, previously considered a progressive, incurable disease. In dystonia, the first symptom is appearance of an involuntary motion or posture which may come and go at first, then become constant. The second most common symptom at the beginning is involuntary bending of the wrist. Later, abnormal muscle contractions, spasm, and deformed postures of the neck and trunk appear.

Surgery, performed under local anesthesia in the thalamus area of the brain, has relieved symptoms in more than three-fourths of patients, and relief has continued for up to ten years thus far.

SEE ALSO PART II for pertinent information about choice of surgeon, preoperative and postoperative care, anesthesia, tests, costs, and other aspects of your operation.

Hydrocephalus

Hydrocephalus—often referred to as "water on the brain"—begins in most cases in infancy. Cerebrospinal fluid forms in the ventricles of the brain and circulates, flowing out into the protective cushion surrounding the nervous system, there to be absorbed by veins in the membrane coverings of the brain.

When there is interference with the cerebrospinal fluid circulation, a large volume of fluid accumulates in and distends the ventricles, spreading the child's skull bones. The head may expand to huge proportions. If allowed to continue, hydrocephalus may lead to mental and physical deterioration.

Various surgical procedures have been devised to overcome hydrocephalus by routing cerebrospinal fluid around an obstruction into the blood circulation. A frequently used procedure is called ventriculo-atrial shunt. Through a small scalp incision and burr hole in the skull, a fine plastic tube is moved into one of the ventricles and then carried under scalp and skin of the neck to the jugular vein and through the vein to the atrium or entrance chamber of the heart. Through such a shunt or bypass, the cerebrospinal fluid can flow for absorption.

Adult hydrocephalus

In recent years, there has been the discovery that in some older adults, what seems to be senile deterioration related to hardening of brain arteries may in fact be the result of a form of hydrocephalus which is not obvious, as it is in children. In occult hydrocephalus, as it is called, there is no head enlargement, But symptoms may include memory defects, disorientation, confusion, incontinence, gait disturbances.

With increasingly refined diagnostic techniques to reveal occult hydrocephalus, such symptoms traceable to the condition often can be eliminated by shunt surgery that creates a new passage for cerebrospinal fluid through the jugular vein.

SEE ALSO PART II for pertinent information about choice of surgeon, preoperative and postoperative care, anesthesia, tests, costs, and other aspects of your operation.

Cerebral Aneurysm

When an area of wall in an artery becomes weakened, it may, like a weak spot on the wall of an automobile tire, become distended, ballooning out. This is an aneurysm, and the condition may sometimes occur in a brain artery. Usually an aneurysm produces no symptoms until it becomes so weakened that it bursts. As blood from the ruptured artery accumulates in the brain, it may press upon vital structures, causing stroke indications or coma.

To stop the bleeding, the carotid artery in the neck may be tied shut. Since this is a major carrier of blood for the brain circulation, there is a reduction in the flow of blood.

When the patient's condition permits, an operation to place a metallic clip on the ruptured artery in the brain may be successful.

Surgery for Head Injuries

Head injuries, even seemingly severe ones, may not require surgery. Sometimes, however, surgery is needed for a skull fracture, hemorrhage, penetration of a foreign body into the brain, or collection of blood.

If a blow on the head fractures part of the skull, some of the bone may be depressed into the brain. Usually surgery is performed under local anesthesia. After burr holes are made around the affected skull area, bone fragments can be manipulated back into position or in some cases may have to be discarded. If much bone has to be removed, some months later a second operation may be performed to implant bone from the hospital bone bank or a plastic or metal plate.

When there has been penetration of brain substance by fragments of bone or metal or other material, these may be carefully picked out or flushed out with salt solution.

Extradural hemorrhage occurs when a blood vessel outside the outermost brain covering, the dura, bleeds. Often, the patient, after a brief episode of unconsciousness, seems to be recovering, when some hours later he experiences head ache. Surgery consists of making an inch or 2-inch opening in the skull, removing any blood clot present, then sewing or clipping the bleeding vessel. In most cases, recovery is rapid.

Subdural hemorrhage, involving bleeding underneath the dura covering, calls for the same type of surgery.

Trigeminal Neuralgia

Also known as tic douloureux, trigeminal neuralgia produces brief attacks of stabbing or lightninglike facial pain. Although the trigeminal (fifth cranial) nerve is involved, usually there is no evidence of organic change in the nerve.

In up to two-thirds of patients,. treatment with a drug, carbamazepine, may satisfactorily reduce the frequency of attacks. Other medications, including diphenylhydantoin, may be helpful.

Medical measures have sharply reduced the number of surgical procedures needed in trigeminal neuralgia, but when medical measures fail, surgery may be considered.

It is possible to free a patient of the pain attacks for a period that may last as long as a year or more by injecting an alcohol solution into the nerve. With the injection, as with cutting the nerve, there is numbness of the face. If the patient is satisfied with the numbness in exchange for the freedom from pain, the operation to sever the nerve permanently can be performed under a general anesthetic through a burr hole made in the skull at the temple area. The procedure is relatively safe.

SEE ALSO PART II for pertinent information about choice of surgeon, preoperative and postoperative care, anesthesia, tests, costs, and other aspects of your operation.

Psychosurgery

Psychosurgery is the surgical modification of the brain for the relief of mental and psychic symptoms.

An early procedure for such purposes was lobotomy, which involved cutting the brain's frontal lobe. While the operation was in some cases helpful in ameliorating mental symptoms, its destruction of a considerable amount of brain tissue could produce deficits. With the advent of modern drugs for the treatment of mental and emotional illness, lobotomy was largely abandoned.

Because even with drugs there remain some patients who do not respond adequately, surgeons have been investigating many other operative procedures.

In one procedure, known as cingulumotomy, minute holes are bored in the skull under a local anesthetic and an electric current is then used to cauterize and destroy bundles of nerve cells connecting various parts of what is known as the brain's limbic system. Patients usually recover the same day. There have been reports that cingulumotomy may be helpful in relieving otherwise unyielding severe neuroses and other serious disorders.

The amygdala is a small almond-shaped body in the brain. Some reports indicate promising results in operating on the amygdala to relieve behavioral abnormalities, depression, and periodic attacks of violent, even homicidal rage.

Investigational work by other surgeons indicates some promise in surgery of the hypothalamic brain area as a means of controlling violent patients.

Psychosurgery generally is considered a promising investigational area; its possible use is indicated only in patients with extreme disorders who cannot be helped by any other means.

SEE ALSO PART II for pertinent information about choice of surgeon, preoperative and postoperative care, anesthesia, tests, costs, and other aspects of your operation.

Spinal Cord Surgery

The spinal cord can be reached anywhere along its length from base of the skull to lower back. It occupies the canal within the column of vertebrae. Forming the back wall of the canal are two bony plates called laminae.

To reach the cord, the laminae of two or three vertebrae are removed. The procedure is called laminectomy. Because the laminae play a relatively minor role in supporting the vertebrae, several can be removed without interference with spine motion.

Aids to diagnosis

A spinal puncture may be done for diagnostic purposes. Under local anesthesia, a hollow needle is inserted between vertebrae in the lower back and introduced into the spinal canal. Pressure measurements can be made to determine if spinal fluid flow may be obstructed as would happen with a tumor. Some of the spinal fluid can be withdrawn for laboratory analysis.

In addition, a small amount of radioopaque material can be introduced through the needle. In this procedure, called myelography, the patient is placed on an X-ray flouroscopic table which can be tilted. As the table is tilted, the movement of the radioopaque material can be followed, any obstruction to its flow can be noted, and tumors and disks can be detected by the distortion they produce in the shape of the canal.

Another valuable diagnostic aid is electromyography. Very fine, coated needles are inserted into various muscles of the back. The needles carry wires and can pick up electric potentials from localized areas of muscle fibers. Electromyography can help in detecting muscle and spinal cord diseases.

Knowing which nerves innervate which muscles, the physician can suspect from any abnormalities of potential in specific muscles whether, for example, a herniated spinal disc is pressing on a specific nerve root.

Myelography is sometimes followed by headache. Electromyography has no adverse side effects.

Spinal Cord Tumors

As many as half or more spinal cord tumors start outside the cord itself in a membrane around the cord or in a spinal nerve. Most of these are nonmalignant, cause pressure on the cord and nerve pathways within it, and can be removed completely by surgery, with cure or marked relief of symptoms, such as pain and burning and tingling sensations.

Tumors growing within the cord tend to be cancerous more often, but usually grow slowly. They are extremely difficult to remove completely without destruction of a section of the spinal cord. Often such tumors can be arrested by radiotherapy.

Tumors that originate in the spinal vertebrae may compress the cord, and sometimes surgical removal of the section of bone pressing on the cord may bring relief.

When a cancer originating elsewhere in the body spreads to the spinal cord, radiotherapy may be helpful in shrinking the growth.

Spinal Cord Injuries

When a spinal cord is injured, it is usually in connection with a fracture of the spinal column. There may be paralysis or abnormal sensations in the feet and legs or in some cases in the upper extremities as well.

With damage to the spinal column, pieces of broken vertebrae or projections of disks may press upon the cord. If these should cut the cord, it will not regrow and the damage is permanent. Thus far, despite many efforts to find ways to stimulate cord regeneration, there has been no success.

Fortunately, the spinal cord is quite strong and resistant. It may remain intact despite considerable pressure. If, below the level of a fracture, movement is completely lost and no sensation at all can be felt, it is likely that the cord has been severed and no improvement can be expected. If there is the slightest movement or smallest degree of sensation, there is a good chance that pressure is involved and surgery may be helpful.

In the operation, which may be performed under local or general anesthesia, the spine is opened and bone fragments are removed to ease pressure. If supporting areas of vertebrae have been cracked, small pieces of bone from a bone bank may be used to fuse the vertebrae. The fusion of bone grafting eliminates motion in that area of the spine but not to an incapacitating extent, and routine bending movements can be accomplished.

After fusion, a period of some months, sometimes as long as a year, in a brace or body cast may be needed, but during this time the patient can be up and around and walking.

Surgery for Pain

When pain is extremely severe and unyielding, relief may be provided by cutting the nerve carrying pain impulses.

The nerve may be cut within the spinal cord. Its precise location is known. Under local or general anesthesia, a laminectomy is performed, removing enough bone to allow entrance into the spinal canal, and the pain nerve is clipped without affecting other nerves controlling movement. The operation is called chordotomy. In perhaps 5 percent of cases, an initial chordotomy may fail because of an unusual arrangement of nerves, and a second chordotomy may be needed.

In another method, called percutaneous chordotomy, a needle is inserted through the skin and carefully guided under X-ray to the pain nerve, which is then destroyed by means of an electric current transmitted through the needle.

The site usually is high in the neck, and local anesthesia is used.

Intervertebral Disk Surgery

The herniated or "slipped" intervertebral disk has received much blame, often wrongly, for back pain.

Between each vertebra and the next is a spinal disk, a circular cushion of connective tissue and cartilage, which serves to absorb the impact of body weight and movement. If the tough outer covering of a disk is severely injured, suddenly or over a period of time, gelatinous material within the disk may pour out much like toothpaste from a tube when the tube develops a small hole. If the material is extruded at a site where it presses upon a nerve root, there will be pain. If the material later breaks off so the pressure on the nerve root is relieved, the pain will disappear.

Depending upon the location of a damaged disk and the nerve root involved, one or more areas of the body may become painful. Most often, however, because it is the disk between the fifth lumbar and first sacral vertebra low in the back that herniates, pain is felt along the course of the sciatic nerve, down the back of the thigh and usually into the side of the foot.

Usually the leg pain comes first; it may be followed by "pins and needles" sensations, numbness and weakness of the leg; then may come low back pain and spasm of back muscles.

There are many possible causes of back pain, including sprains, strains, arthritic changes, radiation of pain to the back from diseases elsewhere including peptic ulcer, colitis, gallbladder diseases, menstrual disturbances. It is now generally agreed that by far the majority of backaches, however, are the result of weak musculature, most often weak muscles of the abdominal wall which, unable to carry their share of the load of supporting the spinal column, put an extra burden on muscles in the back, which are then more subject to sprain, sudden strain, and spasm.

Generally, disk operations do not cure backaches. Often pain in the leg from nerve root compression from a herniated disk is not intractable, provided proper measures such as bed rest, traction, and spasm relief are used. But there are some cases in which pain cannot be relieved within a reasonable period of time without surgery.

Operation

Surgery may be carried out under spinal or general anesthesia through a 4 or 5-inch-long incision in the back, over the herniated disk area. The disk material may sometimes be removed without removing any part of the vertebra bone, but in other cases a laminectomy, with removal of part of the bony ring, may be used to get at and remove the material. During the procedure, the intervertebral foramen, the hole through which the nerve passes, may be enlarged so as to make it unlikely that there can ever again be pressure on the nerve root.

Generally, the hospital stay is ten days or less. The patient is out of bed within a day or two, and usually light work can be resumed about three weeks after surgery, heavy manual work after several months.

Sometimes surgical fusion is required. In fusion, two separate bones are united so as to eliminate motion at the joint between them. Fusion may be needed when motion causes pain at a joint—as the result, for example, of arthritis which has affected joint surfaces or of disk degeneration which, with or without compression of a nerve root, has narrowed the space between vertebral bodies so they rub painfully against each other. Sometimes, with extrusion of disk material, the cushioning effect of the disk is lost, and pain may arise from motion as well as pressure on a nerve root. In such a case, both laminectomy and fusion may be advisable.

For fusion, bone surfaces are first denuded. Bone chips, taken from part of the vertebra itself, or from the hip bone, or from a bone bank, are placed on the denuded surfaces of the two adjacent vertebrae. The chips eventually die; their purpose is to act as a framework over and through which bone cells in the remaining portions of the two vertebrae can grow. When such growth is completed, the two bones have become one. The bone growth is similar to that involved in the healing of a fracture and, as with fracture healing, the growth may be slow and require three to six months for completion, during which time excessive back motion must be avoided and a cast may be used.

Success rate

Disk surgery is safe.

As many as 90 percent of patients, who have been carefully diagnosed and for whom surgery is definitely indicated, benefit. In the past, success rates ranged down to 30 percent or less when disk herniation tended to be regarded as *the* major cause of back trouble and surgery was mistakenly resorted to when it could not possibly help.

Today the approach is conservative as a rule. Time is taken to determine whether conservative measures can eliminate need for surgery. Diagnostic tests, including electromyography and myelography, are more helpful now. More and more patients are, in fact, willing and eager to try other measures before undergoing surgery. There is increasing use of consultation, often between neurosurgeon and orthopedic surgeon.

There have been preliminary reports recently that in some cases injection of an enzyme may help patients with herniated intervertebral disks sufficiently to avoid need for surgery. The enzyme, chymopapain, is injected into the disk space and appears to digest extruded disk material. In so doing, it may relieve pressure on a nerve root. The effectiveness of the technique over a prolonged period is yet to be determined.

SEE ALSO PART II for pertinent information about choice of surgeon, preoperative and postoperative care, anesthesia, tests, costs, and other aspects of your operation.

Nerve Injuries

Unlike nerves in the spinal cord and brain, which cannot regrow when destroyed, peripheral nerves—nerves throughout the body which transmit messages to and from the spinal cord and brain—can regenerate.

When a nerve has been cut in an accident, the ends may be trimmed and sutured together—immediately if the wound is not contaminated and there is no danger of infection, or several weeks later after infection has been overcome with antibiotics.

Peripheral nerves grow slowly, at a rate of about an inch a month. Under some circumstances, restoration of function must depend upon such growth. Sometimes, to aid the growth, a section of nerve that can be spared from elsewhere in the body may be transplanted, not to serve as a transmitting nerve but to guide the regrowth of the damaged nerve. In some cases, the time needed for a damaged nerve to regenerate sufficiently to reach a muscle it is meant to serve may be so long that the muscle may atrophy or waste away if left to itself, but it may be kept active and functioning through physical therapy measures, including electrical stimulation.

Orthopedic Surgery

Two hundred and six bones form the basic framework, the skeleton or chassis, of the body, providing support for the rest of the body, able through strength to resist pressure and through flexibility to absorb some shock without shattering. But bones may be fractured, joints where bones connect to each other may be dislocated, and other conditions including wear and tear and disease, may call for orthopedic surgery.

Fractures

A fracture is a break in a bone—any break, small or large. A simple fracture is one that has not involved any break through the skin; a compound fracture is one in which there has been skin penetration.

Far from being inert, bone is living material, containing living cells and blood vessels. Among the cells are osteoblasts, which function in the construction of new bone material and repair of broken bones.

In order to assure proper healing and restoration of useful function, a fractured bone can be "reduced" or set, often by pulling or manipulation so that the fractured bits are aligned properly, followed by application of a splint or cast to hold them properly aligned until healing has been completed. This is called "closed reduction" since the area does not have to be opened up for proper placement of the bone ends.

When, however, X-rays reveal that the bone is broken or splintered in many places or the break is at such an angle that closed reduction will not work because proper positioning can't be achieved and maintained through closed reduction, surgery is required to bring the fracture into view and to allow the bone ends to be properly aligned and held in place with some mechanical internal fixation device. This is called open reduction.

For a compound fracture, surgical attention is needed because with bone marrow exposed to contamination from bacteria and dirt that may enter through torn skin and muscle, the wound must be cleaned out and in some cases some tissue may have to be removed if dirt has been ground into it. After such cleaning out, the fracture may be reduced, but if the contamination seems to be too severe, gauze packs may be placed in the wound and a cast applied for up to a week or so, permitting drainage of organisms, after which the fracture can be reduced.

Internal fixation devices

Many types of metal plates, nails, screws, pins, wires, and rods made of special alloys that usually do not bother body tissues and can remain in place permanently are available for use in securing fractured bones. Occasionally wiring around a break may be adequate. Nails or pins inserted through the bone marrow may hold a break together effectively. A metal plate may be placed alongside a reduced fracture and held in place with screws. A long rod sometimes may be inserted so that it extends the length of the bone through the marrow canal, holding the bone ends aligned.

When necessary, under X-ray guidance pins can be inserted through the skin into bone to achieve internal fixation without need for an incision.

While internal fixation alone may be enough in some cases to help a fracture heal properly, additional support may be provided by a cast on the outside.

Anesthesia

For the setting of small bone fractures, local anesthesia may be adequate. For major fractures, general anesthesia may be used.

Healing time

The time needed for healing depends, of course, upon the extent of the fracture and the size of the bone—and whether, too, the bone is a weight-bearing one or not. Up to six months may be needed for solid enough healing of long weight-bearing bones before they are strong enough to carry body weight. Most bone requires a minimum of six weeks to heal.

Occasionally, a fracture may not heal. It may not have been reduced properly or may not have been kept properly aligned. The broken ends may have hardened without knitting to each other. Infection may have interfered with healing.

In such cases, healing may be achieved by resetting, draining off pus and treating infection, or by removing hardened bone end areas and placing chips of bones (obtained from the hospital bone bank) to stimulate new bone growth and knitting.

Arm Fractures

While a patient with a broken arm may be inconvenienced to the extent of having to carry the arm in splint or cast, he can be out of bed and walking about.

Spine Fractures

Usually it is a single vertebra that is fractured in an accident. To assure proper healing, the spine must be kept from bending forward. This can be done with a brace extending from shoulders to below the hips or a body plaster cast; unless the fracture is extremely severe, walking can usually be resumed within a week.

When a vertebra has been so badly fractured that satisfactory healing cannot be achieved, or when several vertebrae have been broken, spinal fusion surgery may be used, with bone grafts placed to unite two vertebrae thus stiffening the spine in this area. After such surgery, a brace or cast may be required for up to six months or more, although many patients with brace or cast can be walking a few weeks after operation.

Leg Fractures

Patients with leg fractures can be mobile through use of a cast with a walking heel. The cast serves to keep the leg bones aligned so they can carry some of the body weight and the cast itself carries part of the weight.

Thighbone Fractures

The femur, or thighbone, of course carries body weight. When the bone has been broken, a long nail may be introduced, under general anesthesia, into the upper end of the thighbone through a small incision at the hip, and through another incision in the thigh about the site of the break, the nail can be maneuvered through into the lower end of the femur. Although weight cannot be born on the femur until bone knitting can be seen on X-rays and this may require a few months, many patients can get about on crutches within a few days after the nail placement.

Pelvic Bone Fractures

Pelvic bones bear body weight, and yet it is sometimes possible that a fracture may be so minor and so situated that little weight is borne in that area and walking may be possible in a few weeks. With severe fractures, because no means is available to take weight off the pelvis, several months of bed confinement may be required.

Hip Fractures

Usually what is called a broken hip does not involve a fracture of the pelvic bone, which is one part of the hip joint, but rather of the upper end of the femur, or thighbone, which is another part of the joint.

Such fractures are most common among the elderly. Some hip fractures will heal if nothing is done surgically and the patient is immobilized in bed for three to six months. But keeping an elderly patient bedfast and immobilized with cast or weights for that long may lead to serious complications, including pneumonia, bladder infection, and pressure sores, and may end in death.

Usually an operation is needed as quickly as possible after the patient is restored to the best possible general health. Under general or spinal anesthesia, the fractured bone ends can be set and secured by nails, screws, or plate. Once this is done, it is possible to move the patient in bed and not long afterward to get him into a chair or walker until bone knitting occurs. When X-ray films show that bone knitting has occurred, weight can be placed on the bone.

If the fracture should occur very high up in the femur, the head of the bone, which is ball-like in shape, may die and in that case may have to be replaced by a metal socket secured to the bone shaft (see page 256).

Total hip replacement (see page 257) may sometimes be used when a fracture is so bad that nothing else will do, or if the first hip operation does not produce a painless, effective hip joint.

Results

In most cases, the results of necessary surgical treatment for fractures are excellent. With healing there may be some shortening of bone, but this is usually only a small fraction of an inch and matters little if at all.

Although a fractured bone must be immobilized to heal properly, muscles that normally move the immobilized part must be kept limber and strong. Special exercises achieve this, and it is vital for the patient to carry them out faithfully. If function should not return to normal, intensive physiotherapy with exercises, massage, heat, and other treatments can be used and often leads to marked improvement.

Other than simple fractures, which often can be treated by a general practitioner, most fractures should be evaluated and treated by an orthopedist.

SEE ALSO PART II for pertinent information about choice of surgeon, preoperative and postoperative care, anesthesia, tests, costs, and other aspects of your operation.

Dislocations

A dislocation is the displacement of a bone from a joint. It is usually caused by a blow or a fall, although unusual physical effort may produce it. Symptoms include loss of motion, temporary paralysis of the joint, pain, and swelling.

As soon as possible, a dislocation should be reduced—the bone replaced in normal position—by a surgeon. No incision may be needed. Often, traction and expert manipulation can get the bone back where it belongs, and the joint then can be immobilized for a time to allow for healing of torn ligaments, tendons, and capsule. The joint then may become stable again.

In some cases, however, surgery may be needed to stabilize the joint. In these cases, dislocation tends to recur when there is any strain on the joint or even with relatively moderate movements.

Shoulder

A common site for dislocation is the shoulder, which is a ball joint with a relatively shallow socket, out of which the smooth round head of the humerus, the bone of the upper arm, may slip. In surgery to overcome recurrent dislocation, a tunnel may be made in the humerus and the tendon which attaches the biceps mucle to bone can be used to stabilize the joint. When it is rerouted through the tunnel, it allows the humerus to move freely but prevents it from moving out of the socket.

The operation, which may sometimes include taking a tuck in the capsule to tighten it, is usually successful. A cast is used for up to six weeks after surgery. When it is removed, physical therapy is employed to restore normal motion.

Elbow

Recurrent dislocation of the elbow is much less common. In surgery to overcome the problem, the biceps muscle tendon attachment to the forearm bone is moved from its normal position at the outer side to the inner side of the elbow where, by preventing the elbow from straightening completely, it can prevent dislocation. A cast is used during healing, and physical therapy is employed afterward.

Knee

The knee, one of the largest joints of the body and one that sustains great pressure, is formed by the head of the tibia, the inner and larger bone of the leg below the knee, the lower end of the femur, and the patella, or kneecap. The bones are joined by ligaments, and the patella is secured to the adjacent bones by powerful tendons.

For recurrent dislocation of the kneecap, a tuck may be taken in the heavy patella tendon, or the tendon may be detached and then attached at a new position where it can provide for increased stability. In some cases, a bone graft may be used to keep the kneecap from sliding. Following surgery, a cast is used for as long as eight weeks, and sometimes longer, and after its removal physical therapy is employed.

Spine

Dislocations of the spine may occur. In most cases, even when a dislocation may produce paralysis, the dislocation can be corrected and the paralysis eliminated by traction or stretching of the spine with weights and pulleys to allow the dislocation to be reduced. In some cases, manipulation may be used for reduction. In the relatively few cases where stability cannot be achieved by such conservative measures, surgery may be needed and spinal fusion (see pages 235–38) may be performed.

SEE ALSO PART II for pertinent information about choice of surgeon, preoperative and postoperative care, anesthesia, tests, costs, and other aspects of your operation.

Torn Knee Cartilage

The knee is a frequently injured joint, particularly but not only in athletes. While it is basically a hinge joint, it is subjected to rotation, and it may be injured when there is much twisting and turning of the body, with excessive pivoting on the leg.

The two semilunar cartilages—gristlelike and crescent-shaped—in the knee joint are particularly likely to be injured. They serve to help guide movement and function as cushions. One is on the inner and one on the outer side of the knee.

In the usual injury, one of the cartilages is torn away from its attachment and may be caught between the bones. The result may be pain, swelling, inability to bear weight on the leg and locking of the joint with inability to straighten the knee.

After the first such injury, if the damage does not appear to be severe, a cast may be used for several weeks and symptoms may subside. Surgery, however, is often needed because symptoms persist or because there is a feeling of weakness in the joint and a tendency to recurrences.

In the operation, performed under general or spinal anesthesia, the joint is opened through a 3- or 4-inch incision, and the torn cartilage is removed. The operation is completed in half an hour or a little longer.

About the second or third day after surgery, an exercise is used in bed to strengthen the quadriceps, or front thigh muscle, which plays a part in keeping the knee stable. A day or two after operation, weight bearing can begin. There may be swelling of the knee from accumulation of fluid, and an elastic bandage may be applied to reduce it. In some cases, fluid may be withdrawn from the joint by needle after a local anesthetic numbs the skin surface.

While discomfort is not great after the operation, restriction of activity may be annoying. It may be a month or six weeks before normal activity can be resumed. Oddly enough, a knee from which a cartilage has been removed works virtually as well as before injury, and results of surgery are usually excellent.

SEE ALSO PART II for pertinent information about choice of surgeon, preoperative and postoperative care, anesthesia, tests, costs, and other aspects of your operation.

Bursitis

A bursa is a small fluid-filled sac that permits one part of a joint to move easily over another part or over other structures. Bursae act to facilitate the gliding of muscles or tendons over bony or ligamentous surfaces. They are found throughout the body.

In bursitis, a bursa becomes inflamed as the result of injury, gout, acute or chronic infection, arthritis, or other causes. Most commonly affected is the bursa of the shoulder.

Acute bursitis comes on suddenly; severe pain and limitation of motion of the affected joint are the principal symptoms. Resting the joint in a sling or splint and applications of moist heat often provide relief. Aspirin or another suitable analgesic may be used. Injection of a steroid drug, such as hydrocortisone, may be used to give relief.

Chronic bursitis may follow acute attacks. There is continued pain and limitation of motion. X-ray examination may show calcium deposits. Diathermy, hot packs or baths, and massage may be tried. Hydrocortisone or another steroid, prednisolone, and procaine may be injected into the bursa. At the same time the area containing calcium may be needled to break up the deposits. Cautious manipulation may be used to break up any disabling adhesions.

If satisfactory results are not obtained by such treatment, surgery may be utilized. An operation to remove a bursa is usually successful.

Surgery for a bursa on the elbow or kneecap is minor, requires only brief hospitalization. Because a shoulder bursa is deeper-lying and more closely involved with muscles, tendons, and other structures, physical therapy begun in the hospital is usually needed after the operation, requiring a longer stay. It may be four weeks or longer before normal activities can be resumed. Usually after a bursa operation at the knee or elbow, work can be resumed much more quickly even though there may be an annoying but expectable drainage from the wound for several weeks to a month or so.

SEE ALSO PART II for pertinent information about choice of surgeon, preoperative and postoperative care, anesthesia, tests, costs, and other aspects of your operation.

Frozen Shoulder

In addition to inflammation of a bursa in the shoulder, the capsule of the shoulder may become inflamed. Ligaments and tendons may be affected. Scar tissue may form. The end result may be a locking of the shoulder joint and pain accompanying any attempt at movement.

Sometimes gentle manipulation to stretch the capsule and tendons, performed under general anesthesia, may be successful in unlocking the joint and restoring pain-free motion. It often happens that a frozen shoulder, in effect, cures itself over a period of time, and normal motion may return after a year or even longer of locking.

Surgery is reserved for patients with prolonged severe pain and for those who must return to work without undue delay. The operation, performed under general anesthesia through an incision about three inches long across the shoulder cap, involves several procedures, including removal of some of the arch of the shoulder socket, splitting of several ligaments, and some transfer of muscle fibers. Afterwards a cast is worn for several weeks, and exercises are begun. Full recovery may require a month or even several months. Usually there is gratifying relief of pain and return of full motion.

SEE ALSO PART II for pertinent information about choice of surgeon, preoperative and postoperative care, anesthesia, tests, costs, and other aspects of your operation.

Osteomyelitis

With modern treatment, bone infection (osteomyelitis) no longer is the disabling disorder it so often was in the past. But it can sometimes be difficult to cure.

Infection may result from injury to a bone, such as a compound fracture, or entrance of a foreign body, or spread of infection from elsewhere in the body. Characteristically, osteomyelitis is ushered in with sudden pain in the affected bone and sharp rise in body temperature. The infection may be confused initially with rheumatic fever, sprain, or fracture.

With prompt antibiotic treatment, the chance of controlling acute osteomyelitis is excellent. Surgery may be needed, however, when symptoms do not disappear or in there is abscess formation. An incision is made over the affected area and the bone is opened to permit drainage of pus and infection. The operation is not dangerous. After the infected material has drained out, the wound may be sutured or allowed to close by itself.

Chronic osteomyelitis is now fortunately uncommon. It is characterized by the formation of draining tunnels or sinuses and repeated flare-ups of painful abscesses. Dead and dying bone tissue, which serve as the nidus for continuing infection, must be removed. It is sometimes difficult to remove all the infected or dead tissue at once and repeated relatively minor surgical procedures may be needed. In some very severe cases, more extensive procedures, involving the removal of fairly wide areas of skin, muscle tissue and bone, may be required, and extended hospitalization may be needed, but in almost all cases the infection can be cured with prompt institution of treatment.

SEE ALSO PART II for pertinent information about choice of surgeon, preoperative and postoperative care, anesthesia, tests, costs, and other aspects of your operation.

Dupuytren's Contracture

Of unknown cause, thought by some to be the result of injury and by others to be the result of an inherited tendency, Dupuytren's contracture involves a thickening and shortening of tissue under the palm. The fingers, most often the ring and little fingers, are pulled down into the palm, producing deformity.

Because neither tendons nor nerves are involved, only overgrown fibrous tissue, surgery to remove the affected tissue is relatively simple and does not affect feeling or movement.

Carpal Tunnel Syndrome

The median, a major nerve of the hand, passes through the wrist in a tunnel under the carpal ligament. When the nerve becomes compressed in the tunnel, there may be pain, numbness and tingling of the fingers. The disorder, which occurs most often in middle-aged women, may be produced by excessive wrist movement, arthritis, swelling of the wrist, and overgrowth of bone and connective tissue.

Conservative treatment, in which the wrist is splinted for several weeks until the irritation of the median nerve has had a chance to heal, may be effective. In severe cases, rapid cure can be achieved with surgery in which the tunnel is opened and the carpal ligament is divided, ending the nerve compression.

Clubfoot

Clubfoot is a deformity in which the foot is twisted out of normal position. The condition, known medically as talipes, is usually present at birth, but a few cases occur in older children as the result of injury or poliomyelitis. There are several types of clubfoot; the foot may be twisted inward, outward, upward, or downward. Sometimes a combination of defects may be present.

The treatment varies with severity of the deformity. Often milder cases may be corrected with casts, which are changed periodically. With each change, the foot is manipulated into position until it gradually achieves a normal position. A special splint also may be used. It consists of two plates attached to shoes with a crossbar between plates and set screws that allow the angulation of the foot to be changed as necessary.

More severe deformities may require surgery which may be performed under general anesthesia. Some fibrous tissue in the sole of the foot may be stripped away from the bones and with partial severing and lengthening of a tendon, the foot may be brought into normal position, after which a cast is applied to maintain the position.

It is sometimes necessary in older children or adults to remove portions of the bones of the foot and fuse joints in order to correct the deformity.

Bunion

A bunion is a deformity usually caused by tight shoes that push the great toe toward the little toe. As the result of the rubbing against the shoe of the inner side of the foot, particularly at the first joint of the great toe, a bony knob forms and overlying tissue becomes inflamed and swollen.

In mild cases, heat may relieve the pain and the condition may improve with the use of properly fitting shoes. In more severe cases, special corrective shoes may be used or an operation, bunionectomy, may be employed.

Through an incision from between first and second toes running backward to the ball of the foot, a muscle on the underside of the foot is transferred so that its pull can help straighten the inner foot border. Excess bone in the knob that makes up the bunion is chiseled or cut away. For a time after surgery, firm bandaging is used and, in some cases, a plaster cast with a rubber heel. Usually within a few days, sometimes within twenty-four hours, the patient can stand and even begin to walk with some assistance. Full motion is restored within several weeks. The operation is usually successful in eliminating pain, swelling, and soreness and, with the protruding bony knob gone, ordinary shoes fit well and walking is comfortable. About a week of hospitalization may be needed.

SEE ALSO PART II for pertinent information about choice of surgeon, preoperative and postoperative care, costs, and other aspects of your operation.

Arthritis

More than 18 million Americans suffer from arthritis. In recent years, physicians have become more skilled at treating arthritis with drugs, exercise, and rest. Particularly great strides have been made in the last decade in the treatment of arthritis with improved and new surgical techniques and newly developed synthetic materials which may be used when medical measures do not prove adequate.

Rheumatoid arthritis, one of the major forms of the disease, is really a systemic illness that manifests itself primarily by joint pain and inflammation, often leading to deformities. Usually it begins between the ages of twenty and forty, often starting with nonspecific symptoms such as fever, poor appetite, and general run-down feeling before producing joint stiffness, soreness, and pain. It most frequently affects the joints of fingers, wrists, knees, ankles, and toes, alone or in combination.

The cause is still not clear, although some recent findings suggest that an unusual type of bacterium or virus may be involved.

Osteoarthritis, sometimes referred to as degenerative joint disease, is arthritis associated with "wear and tear" in the joints. It does not usually become a problem before middle age except when a joint has been injured or subjected to much stress and overuse, as in the finger joints of some pianists, for example. Unlike rheumatoid arthritis, osteoarthritis produces no constitutional symptoms such as fever, but in some cases it may cause joint disability. The joints most commonly affected are the weight-bearing ones such as hips, spine, knees. Frequently, swelling of small finger joints occur (Heberden's nodes).

Surgery is not a cure for arthritis but it may relieve severe pain, restore joint function, improve appearance, and permit a patient to earn a living and care for himself. It may arrest or delay further joint destruction or save adjacent joints on which the patient is putting stress.

The following are the major procedures used in arthritis surgery.

Synovectomy

Synovectomy—the removal of diseased synovial membrane, the lining of tissue around an arthritic joint—is the most frequently used operation and may be employed for virtually any joint.

The synovium produces fluid to lubricate joint surfaces. In rheumatoid arthritis the membrane becomes inflamed and swollen. In severe cases the swelling may distend the joint. Then ligaments connecting bone ends in the joint may become stretched and damaged; and tendons that attach muscle to bone may drift out of normal position and shorten, with the shortening producing deformity. In the hand, for example, the tendon shortening may pull the fingers into useless positions.

Synovitis, or synovial inflammation, often responds to drug therapy. When this fails, the synovium may be removed surgically. Synovectomies are usually done after the disease has been in progress for some time. The results may be excellent, including relief of pain and control of inflammation for extended periods, as well as return to "normal" function.

Recently some surgeons have done synovectomies early in the course of rheumatoid arthritis hoping to prevent destruction of tissues. Early synovectomies do not cause any permanent damage since the synovium, like a fingernail or skin, grows back. At present, while early results of early synovectomy appear promising, definite conclusions about the value of the early procedure await completion of long-term studies comparing the state of health of snyovectomized joints with similarly affected joints not operated on.

Osteotomy

Rheumatoid arthritis may cause a joint to become fused, leaving it immobile, or may cause a joint to shift into abnormal position. An osteotomy, also called a resection, consists of separating a fused joint or shifting a joint back into normal position. For example, an arthritic hip ˙may be realigned to permit a patient to walk without a limp.

Arthrodesis

In this operation, a diseased joint is purposely fused or locked in a fixed position. Two bones forming a joint—for example, anklebone and leg bone at the ankle, or leg and thighbones at the knee—are fastened together so that movement between them is eliminated. In effect there is no longer a joint, since the two bones form a single continuous structure. This may be achieved by removing the cartilage surfaces from the bone ends, which is followed by new bone growth from the bared ends that knits the bones together over a period of four to six months or longer. During that time a cast or metal pins may be used to hold the bones together. In some cases, bone chips or grafts may be used to fill spaces between the bones.

Often, results of arthrodesis are gratifying. For example, in one series of patients, wrist fusion was used in twenty cases for pain alone and after surgery all were free of pain; in twenty other cases it was used for wrist deformities or instability, again successfully; in ten others who had no deformity but suffered losses in hand strength apparently because they had avoided gripping anything strongly to prevent pain it was likewise successful. Patients appear to make excellent adjustments to wrist fusion, developing new patterns of handwriting, making greater use of the elbow for such activities as combing hair or dealing cards. They often find that increased function resulting from alleviation of pain and increased strength more than compensate for loss of ability to bend the wrist.

Arthroplasty

This is the reconstruction of a diseased joint. The patient's own tissue or various materials may be used to help rebuild a crippled hip joint, for example. The operation may be performed under general or spinal anesthesia through a long incision, about eight or ten inches or more, over the front and side of the hip.

In the procedure, the hip socket of the pelvic bone may be reamed, made larger, and smoothed and the ball-shaped top of the thighbone may be shaped to fit the socket. A metal cap fitted over the thighbone top can be used to provide for smooth motion in the socket. In some cases, the upper end of the thighbone may be removed and a metal substitute fitted in place.

After such an operation, if healing proceeds well, the patient may start training to walk again in about three weeks, carrying weight at first only on the good hip. With physical therapy, hip muscles become able to control the new joint and full motion usually can be recovered.

Total Joint Replacement

Among recent surgical advances, those which have drawn most attention involve total joint replacement.

Hip replacement. Because the hip joint is a frequent target for both rheumatoid arthritis and osteoarthritis, there have been many efforts in the past to devise an artificial hip. But the material had to be strong enough to withstand the many millions of loading pounds placed on the hip over a period of years, compatible with and uncorroded by body fluids and tissues, and self-lubricating. A stainless steel ball had been tried as a replacement for the diseased femur head but the ball, screwed into the thighbone, sometimes worked loose. A socket of steel in which the ball could rotate had been tried, but a steel-to-steel joint had to be lubricated by body fluids and these were not always adequate.

Then, early in the 1960s, an English surgeon, John Charnley, used a plastic material, methyl methacrylate, commonly employed in dentistry, to hold ball and socket in place. He used a stainless steel ball and for the socket a high-density polyethylene plastic which proved to have excellent wearing qualities and requires no lubrication.

Hip replacement is, of course, a major operation but results have been excellent. Within ten years after its first use, more than 10,000 Americans were walking around with the man-made joints, according to the Arthritis Foundation, and reports from major institutions such as Mayo Clinic and Massachusetts General Hospital indicated that 96 percent of patients operated on had gained better motion and freedom from discomfort.

Typically, in the operating room, while the surgeon removes a diseased joint, nurses mix a liquid and a powder to form a paste. The surgeon pours the paste into place, molds it to shape, and it becomes cemented into the bones and provides a surface with much the same consistency as human bone. The metal and plastic artificial hip is implanted into the drying cement, and by the time the patient is off the operating table, the new joint is securely held. For the first four or five days, the operated leg is rested with traction in a light splint. Walking is attempted after between five and ten days, at first with a walker and then with crutches. On the average patients remain in the hospital about three weeks.

Knee replacement. Total knee-joint replacement now is becoming feasible. Bearing virtually all the body's weight, the knee is very susceptible to arthritis and may be the most frequently affected joint. Medical treatment is often helpful but in some cases fails.

Surgery has been used to fuse knees to stop motion and pain. There has been some use of partial prostheses, including metal disks, to separate the heads of thighbone and shinbone. For years there have been efforts to develop a total knee replacement. Recently two designs have been showing promise, and others are being studied.

One, the polycentric knee, consists of two crescent-shaped Vitallium half circles that are implanted into the thighbone so only their rounded edges protrude. The shinbone is fitted with two matching polyethylene tracks or grooves in which the upper part can rock back and forth each time the knee is bent and extended. Both parts are cemented in place with methyl methacrylate, the material used for hip replacement.

The geometric knee is a variant of the polycentric knee, in which the crescent-shaped tibial components are linked together. Both the tibial components and the two polyethylene tracks in which they rock back and forth are affixed to long stems, which are cemented into healthy bone.

In 1971, clinical trials started at five medical centers— Mayo Clinic, Johns Hopkins in Baltimore, Massachusetts General Hospital in Boston, Doctors' Hospital in Corpus Christi, Texas, and UCLA Medical Center in Los Angeles. Two hundred patients received the polycentric and one hundred the geometric knee. Early results have been excellent with both. Length of rehabilitation varies among patients: some use crutches for three months; some use a walker until they feel comfortable with a cane and are walking with a cane in 3½ weeks. After a year a follow-up study of sixty patients who had seventy-three knee replacements found that the operation relieved pain in 84 percent and provided normal stability in 93 percent. Seventy-eight percent of the patients needed no help in walking.

Finger joints. Arthritis may twist and gnarl the hands, producing pain and deformity. The use of synthetic finger joints made of silicone rubber has been proving helpful in many severe cases.

A typical finger-joint implant resembles a piece of taffy pulled out at both ends. After the removal of a deformed joint, the surgeon makes a channel in each bone entering the joint for the ends of the implant. The implant is positioned so its thickest part lies between the bones and keeps them properly aligned. For about three weeks, the patient wears a movable brace to help make certain that healing takes place in the right position.

In trials at more than 200 clinics throughout the world during which the synthetic joints were implanted in more than 4,000 hands, there were no adverse effects on surrounding tissues, no complications in more than 99 percent of patients. The synthetic joints appear able to provide as much as 75 percent of the efficiency of naturally healthy joints.

Other joints. Surgeons and biomedical engineers are now working to develop substitutes for elbow, wrist, and shoulder joints. The need for these is less because these joints often respond well to medical measures and other surgical procedures.

SEE ALSO PART II for pertinent information about choice of surgeon, preoperative and postoperative case, anesthesia, tests, costs, and other aspects of your operation.

Bone Tumors

While some tumors of bone are malignant, many are benign. Often pain is the first symptom. Often, too, a hard lump may be felt. While the X-ray appearance of many tumors is characteristic, final diagnosis depends on removal of a section of the tumor for microscopic study. When a malignant tumor is suspected, a chest film is usually made to search for any spread of the tumor to the lungs, and a skeletal radiologic survery is made to determine whether there are any additional bone lesions.

Benign tumors. There are several types of these, some of which may cause no pain or interference with joint action and may sometimes be left alone. When they do cause trouble, they may be removed by simple excision. Some, called giant-cell tumors, may destroy large areas of bone, leading to fracture. They often can be removed by curettage, which is scraping away of the diseased bone, or in some cases they may be cut out. Sometimes, when the tumors are difficult to get at, radiation treatment may be used.

Malignant tumors. There are also many types of these. Osteogenic sarcoma, one of the most common, occurs most often in young persons, many only in the teens. Amputation usually offers the best hope of cure. The tumor is not radiosensitive. Treatment with chemicals such as nitrogen mustard may be tried.

A less malignant form of sarcoma, parosteal, involves the surface but not interior of bone, and cure may be achieved by amputation or sometimes by local bone resection.

Ewing's sarcoma, occurring in children and young adults, is highly malignant. It is sensitive to radiotherapy. The primary tumor often responds well, with marked reduction in size and lessening of pain, but the disease tends to seed itself elsewhere and spread. Since the primary tumor can be well controlled by radiotherapy, amputation may or may not be justifiable.

Reticulum cell sarcoma, closely resembling Ewing's sarcoma, offers much greater chance for cure by either radiotherapy or amputation.

There are other types of malignant tumors, including giant-cell tumors which sometimes change from benign to malignant, and require removal of the entire portion of diseased bone and sometimes amputation.

SEE ALSO PART II for pertinent information about choice of surgeon, preoperative and postoperative care, anesthesia, tests, costs, and other aspects of your operation.

Amputations

The removal of a limb or other appendage or outgrowth of the body is sometimes vital in cases of cancer, infection, or gangrene. It may be needed after irreparable injury to a limb. Blood vessel disorders such as arteriosclerosis account for the greatest percentage of leg amputations.

More than 25,000 amputations a year are performed in the United States. Although an amputation is a means of saving life, the prospect seems grim. Yet more and more amputees now adjust well and quickly to the loss. There have been marked advances in prosthetic devices and their application and in rehabilitative techniques. With modern devices it is possible to thread needles, to stand for a full day's work, to dance.

Amputation may be performed under general or spinal anesthesia and in some cases may be done after use of ice to refrigerate the area to the point of insensitivity to pain.

The site or level of amputation is determined on the basis of several factors. One consideration is to save as much as possible of an extremity. Circulation at the site must be good, and it is also important to choose a site that will permit best results with a prosthesis. Thus, for example, amputation behind the toes and through the foot can allow use of a simple rubber shoe-filler. Amputation through ankle or heel bone is less practical than above the ankle; optimal fitting of a prosthesis may be obtained with amputation about six inches below the knee. When that amount of bone below the knee cannot be saved, an above-the-knee amputation may make possible use of a prosthesis and good functioning of the leg.

When forearm or arm amputation is required, it is sometimes possible to shape bones and cover them with skin so they work somewhat like fingers or to fashion a system in which muscle and tendons can be used to control mechanical devices in the prosthesis.

Before surgery, the affected limb may be shaved and thoroughly cleansed with an antiseptic. Afterward, the stump may be elevated on a pillow and special exercises ordered to prevent contractures of muscles leading to the stump. A clean amputation stump usually heals within two weeks. In the past, it was usual to apply an artificial limb about six to eight weeks after surgery, but more and more now, especially for lower limb amputations, a prosthesis is applied at the time of operation or soon afterward.

A sensation called phantom pain may sometimes be experienced after amputation. Pain is felt in the limb that has been amputated, as a result of irritation of nerve endings at the site of the stump. The pain can be quite disturbing to a patient unless he is told that the phenomenon occurs and he need not doubt his sanity or worry that surgeon and nursing staff doubt the existence of the pain. Drugs may be used to relieve the pain.

The length of surgery can vary from as little as ten minutes for a finger or toe amputation to as much as forty minutes for an arm or leg amputation. Similarly, length of hospitalization may range from one or two days for a finger amputation and up to a week for a toe amputation to up to ten days or two weeks for an arm or leg amputation.

If a patient is properly prepared for amputation, the chances of psychologic repercussions are greatly reduced. It is best that the patient learn as much as possible from the physician about the amputation itself, the treatment that follows, and the prosthesis. If at all possible, and often the surgeon may be able to arrange for this, the patient should talk to someone who has had a similar amputation. In almost every community, education, training, and financial assistance, if needed, are available through public rehabilitation agencies or private sources, and the surgeon may direct the patient to such sources.

SEE ALSO PART II for pertinent information about choice of surgeon, preoperative and postoperative care, anesthesia, tests, costs, and other aspects of your operation.

Eye Surgery

The Eye

The human eye, which contains in a single cubic inch of space more than 150 million light receptors, is commonly compared to a camera. The outermost layer of the eyeball forms the white of the eye, which becomes the transparent cornea at the front. The next layer is the iris, which has an adjustable aperture, the pupil, which becomes larger or smaller depending upon the amount of light entering.

Behind the iris and its pupillary opening is the oval-shaped elastic lens, which bulges out when its muscles contract, and flattens when they relax. The lens muscles, the fastest in the body, thus permit adjustment of the lens to bend and focus light rays properly on the retina.

The retina, which lines the back of the eye, contains the light receptors that react to incoming images. Responses of the receptors are transmitted along nerve fibers forming one outgoing cable, the optic nerve, at the back of each eye. The exit of the nerve leaves a "blind" spot, without receptors.

The brain, rather than the eye, does the actual seeing. The process is essentially this: Light rays striking an object and reflected to the eyes pass through the cornea, the clear front window, a watery liquid called the aqueous humor which is behind the cornea, the pupil, and the lens. The lens bends and focuses the rays on the retina. As rays impinge on light-sensitive pigments in the retina, chemical reactions occur that send impulses through the optic nerve to the brain. Because the lens inverts images, they are received upside down, but the brain interprets them realistically.

The eye is subject to some defects and diseases which may require surgery. A specialty, eye surgery, is performed by ophthalmologists. There have been marked advances in eye surgery. Pain control can be complete. Bed confinement is usually brief now, a day or so after major surgery.

Cataracts

Cataracts are opaque spots that form on the lens and impair vision of many elderly and some younger people. Spreading throughout the lens over a period of time, they keep light rays from getting through to the retina. Cataracts may result from injuries to the eyes, exposure to great heat or radiation, or inherited factors, but in most cases they are termed senile cararacts and appear to be part of the aging process.

Symptoms

Blurred and dimmed vision is often the first indication of cataract. You may find that you need a brighter reading light or must hold objects closer to the eyes. The continued clouding of the lens may cause double vision. Finally, a need for frequent changes of eyeglasses may be caused by cataract. These symptoms do not necessarily indicate cataract but if any are present, an ophthalmologist should be consulted.

Diagnosis

Upon examination with an ordinary light shined into the eyes, a cataract formation may be detected, and further examination with an ophthalmoscope reveals the extent of the opacity.

When surgery may be needed

The only known effective treatment for cataract is surgery. No ointments or drops can dissolve a cataract.

More than 250,000 cataract operations are performed yearly in the U.S. It used to be considered necessary to wait, sometimes for years, for a cataract to ripen, or spread throughout the lens and in the process loosen the lens from its capsule, before operation could be undertaken. With the ripening, it was easier for the surgeon to get out all of the lens, leaving none behind to cause possible vision interference later. Now, new techniques permit ready removal of the lens at any time without need for an extended period of partial blindness. Cataract removal is indicated when vision is impaired to the extent of interfering with work or other normal activities.

Cataract surgery

Cataract removal can be achieved under local anesthesia. Making an incision at the point where clear cornea and white of the eye meet, the surgeon can reach the lens. The lens then can be loosened by injecting an enzyme, chymotrypsin, that dissolves the lens ligaments without affecting other eye structures.

The lens can then be lifted out with forceps, or a freezing rod that can grip it securely, or an instrument with a suction cup. After lens extraction, fine sutures are used to close the incision (in some cases, the sutures are of the type that are absorbed and do not require later removal), and the eye is bandaged for several days. Many surgeons now allow the patient out of bed the first postoperative day.

Success rate

While removal of a cataract is a delicate operation, it is more than 95 percent successful in allowing vision restoration.

Since a lens is needed for focusing, glasses are required after surgery. They have thick, conspicuous lenses and tend to make objects appear larger, but most patients adapt to them quickly. Contact lenses, for those who can wear them, often make for better vision.

When both eyes are affected by cataracts, it has been usual to remove one cataract at a time, with an interval of from one to six months between. In some cases now, as the result of improved techniques, it is possible to remove both cataracts during the same hospitalization.

Experimental techniques

Under study are a number of new techniques which hopefully may further simplify cataract removal.

One new instrument is built around a hollow needle in which a tiny whirling blade, working like a blender, pulverizes the lens, which then is drawn off through a tube. In another new instrument, a needle vibrates at ultrasonic speed, 40,000 beats a second, to detach the cataract, and a sensitive system emits fluid to flush away the lens debris. With both devices, only a 110th-inch slit is needed to get at the lens, in contrast to an incision about ¾-inch-long used in conventional surgery. The smaller incision can be closed by a single suture and heals faster.

Also under investigation is the possibility that patients may not need a week to ten days of hospitalization but may be released safely in much less time, possibly even the same day as surgery.

SEE ALSO PART II for pertinent information about choice of surgeon, preoperative and postoperative care, anesthesia, tests, costs, and other aspects of your operation.

Glaucoma

Glaucoma has been called the "sneak thief of sight" because the common chronic type develops gradually, slowly, and painlessly. The less common acute form strikes suddenly, producing cloudy vision, severe eye pain, redness of the eye, nausea. Actually, there are dozens of different "glaucomas" but all have in common increased pressure within the eyeball because fluid cannot get out.

The hollow area inside the front of the eye is partly filled with a circulating fluid, aqueous humor, which continuously forms and drains off so it remains at the same pressure level. In glaucoma, drainage is impeded, and pressure begins to build up, inhibiting the blood supply and gradually damaging the nerve cells. The damage begins at the edges, slowly moving toward the center. The victim loses side sight (peripheral vision) and has "tunnel vision," which makes him seem to be viewing things through a telescope. He may also have blurring of vision and may see halos or rainbow-colored rings around lights.

Glaucoma rarely appears before age thirty-five; about two million Americans over forty have it; by age sixty-five, about 10 percent of the population is affected. Glaucoma causes 13.5 percent of all blindness. Each year about 4,000 people are needlessly blinded by it; glaucoma can be arrested and controlled when detected early enough.

The tonometer tests

A simple, painless one-minute test can detect glaucoma, and such testing is advocated for all people over 35. It involves only one act: placing the tip of a small, pressure-sensitive instrument against the front of each eye. The instrument registers any increase in pressure within the eyeball.

Medical treatment

When glaucoma is detected, eyedrops are prescribed. While the drops do not cure, they very often can control the disease, acting to control the production of aqueous humor or to facilitate its drainage so that pressure is brought down to normal.

When surgery is needed

Surgery is usually not undertaken until medicine has been given a trial and has been found inadequate.

Operative treatment

Iridectomy, the simplest operation, which may be used in early stages of glaucoma, involves cutting off a segment of the iris, the colored part of the eye around the pupil. The segment is snipped off through an incision in the white of the eye at the edge of the iris. A small, almost invisible opening remains and allows increased drainage. The operation may be done under either local or general anesthesia. The patient is out of bed within a day or two and home from the hospital a few days later.

Iridectomy is effective in about 95 percent of acute glaucoma cases. Usually, acute glaucoma will affect both eyes, one at a time. Surgery will usually be done for the affected eye and a preventive operation at a little later date may be advisable for the still unaffected eye. When acute glaucoma has not led to extensive eye damage, iridectomy will be followed by return of normal vision.

For chronic glaucoma, iridectomy may be used, or a filtering procedure may be done under local anesthesia. In one such procedure, *sclerectomy,* a tiny hole is made through the outer coat of the eye into the space under the sclera, the outer white eyeball sheath, opening a new fluid drainage channel. In some cases, a section of iris may be drawn into the new channel to serve as a wick for the fluid; the procedure is called *iridencleisis..* No scar is visible. Sutures of a type that can be absorbed may be used so no suture removal is necessary. If silk sutures are employed, they can be taken out later with little if any discomfort. A change of glasses may be needed after the operation and in some cases drops may be continued.

Surgery for glaucoma is not life-threatening, delicate as it is; the success rate for avoiding blindness is high and in many cases so is the rate for restoring good vision. Currently a daring new experimental treatment being tried in the Soviet Union involves firing up to a dozen bursts of high-powered Q-laser beams into the eyes to open clogged channels and restore drainage. It appears possible to complete the treatment in five minutes on an outpatient basis, without hospitalization.

SEE ALSO PART II for pertinent information about choice of surgeon, peoperative and postoperative care, anesthesia, tests, costs, and other aspects of your operation.

Crossed Eyes (Strabismus)

An infant's eyes often "float," momentarily turning in or out independently of each other. It may take several months for eyes to become coordinated. After three to six months of age, however, eye crossing warrants attention. Without attention, there may be loss of vision in an eye as well as marring of appearance.

When eyes cross, each views an object from a different angle. The brain then receives two different images. Since seeing double is disturbing, the cross-eyed child will squint and tilt his head in an effort to combine the images. Finally he may give up and resort to using just one eye. The sight in the other will deteriorate from lack of use. When a child is helped early, simple measures may be effective.

One cause of crossing is farsightedness, which may lead to such excessive use of the eye muscles that the eyes over-converge. Sometimes glasses alone, to correct the farsightedness, may be enough to straighten the eyes. A qualified or-toptic technician in an ophthalmologist's office can help many children by teaching them eye exercises and how to use them at home. Special devices allow each eye to see only half a scene; the eye muscles are strengthened while the child practices fusing the two images into a whole picture.

Restoration of vision in a crossing eye which, for lack of use, has become amblyopic—a "lazy eye"—can very often be achieved if treatment is begun early enough, preferably before age seven, although in some cases it may be achieved later. Eyeglasses and a patch over the good eye may be needed to force use of the weak eye so that, with increased work, its vision increases.

When surgery is needed

In some cases, when the eyes are badly crossed and exercises and other measures are inadequate, an operation to bring the eye muscles into proper balance is needed. It can be performed on a two-year-old, or even earlier if necessary. A muscle that does not pull enough may be shortened; or excessive pull may be reduced by reattaching the muscle at a different point on the eyeball.

Operations

Surgery for strabismus is safe. The eyeball does not have to be opened, since the muscles are on the outside of it. As a result there is virtually no risk of harming the eye or damaging vision.

For a child, general anesthesia is commonly used. For an adult, local anesthesia may be employed. An incision is made through the white part of the eye. The six eye muscles are attached in back to the socket and extend around the front of the eyeball.

After establishing which eye movements are not properly balanced, the surgeon adjusts the proper muscle or in some cases more than one. If the muscle is too taut, it can be removed from its position at the front of the eye and reattached further back. If a muscle is loose and weak, a tuck may be made in it to shorten it or a small piece may be removed and the cut ends sutured together. Often the problem lies in only one eye. If both eyes are involved, operation on both may be carried out at the same time, or correction may be made separately.

Postoperative care

Usually the operated eye is comfortable after surgery. Both eyes may be kept bandaged for a few days, and the patient may be kept in bed. Then, for several days in hospital, the eyes are unbandaged and the patient may get out of bed to sit in a chair. Children may be kept inactive at home for several weeks. Double vision may occur after surgery but usually disappears after several weeks.

Results

In as many as 90 percent of cases or even more, surgery is successful in straightening the eyes and, when performed early enough so that vision has not been permanently impaired in the "lazy eye," it is successful in producing normal vision. If farsightedness is present, glasses are needed to correct for it. If, in an older child or adult, vision in one eye has been permanently impaired, the operation cannot restore it but it can produce excellent cosmetic results.

SEE ALSO PART II for pertinent information about choice of surgeon, preoperative and postoperative care, anesthesia, costs, helping a child through surgery, and other aspects of the operation.

Detachment of the Retina

One in every 10,000 Americans each year suffers from a detached retina. The retina, which contains light receptors, lines the back of the eye and is held in place against the choroid, the middle coat of the eyeball, by the fluid filling the eyeball. When a tear or hole occurs in the retina, the fluid may seep in behind and lift the retina from the choroid. This is detachment of the retina which is partial at first. If untreated it becomes complete.

Symptoms

With detachment, flashes of light (stars) are seen, followed by a sensation of a curtain moving across the eye. The extent of loss of vision depends upon the location of the detachment

Diagnosis

The diagnosis of detachment can be made with an instrument, the ophthalmoscope, which discloses folds, tears,
or other irregularities in the retina.

Operations

Surgery is required for treatment of retinal detachment,
and the earlier the better.

With a local anesthetic dropped into the eye, an incision is made in the white of the eye. Through a needle,
fluid behind the separated portion of the retina is withdrawn.
The remaining fluid filling the eyeball then has a chance to
press the detached area back into place against the choroid.
When this is achieved, the retina is sealed in place by any
of several methods—an electric needle, freezing rod, or
laser light beam.

In another type of operation, a small plastic implant is
sutured to the eyeball over the area of detachment. It serves
to push and hold the choroid against the detached portion
of the retina.

Postoperative care

Surgery for retinal detachment is not painful. Afterward,
both eyes may be bandaged for up to a week, and the
operated eye may thereafter be kept bandaged for another
week or so. Complete rest may be advisable for ten days
to about two weeks to prevent bleeding within the eye and
to minimize the risk of jarring the retina loose. Thereafter,
it may be necessary to stay home from work for as long as
three or four months as a precaution against jarring.

Success rate

The smaller the detachment and the earlier surgery is
performed, the more likely a successful result. Overall, four
of every five patients can expect to benefit.

If, at the end of six weeks after surgery, the retina is holding firm, the likelihood of permanent success is great. Recurrences are not infrequent. Within a few weeks after surgery, the retina may be shaken loose again and resealing must be done. In people who do strenuous work, there is some risk that the retina may separate many months or years later, requiring reoperation.

SEE ALSO PART II for pertinent information about choice of surgeon, preoperative and postoperative care, anesthesia, costs, and other aspects of your operation.

Corneal Transplants

The transparent cornea, or window, at the front of the eye may be affected by physical injury or by infectious disease. If, as a result, the cornea becomes scarred, the blocking of light rays by the scar may produce partial or complete blindness in the eye. This is the cause of about 5 percent of all blindness.

Corneal transplantation is one of the oldest of transplant procedures. In most areas of the United States, eye banks store donated corneas from deceased people and fetuses. Synthetic corneas made of plastic are also available.

Operations

Keratoplasty, as corneal transplantation is known, is the most successful of all transplantation procedures, but there is risk of failure and usually the operation is reserved for eyes without useful vision.

Operation can be done under local anesthesia. Using an operating microscope or high-power lenses, the surgeon removes the scarred area of the cornea in one piece. With the same sharp coring type of instrument, he bores out an identical size plug from the donor cornea and sutures it in place in the living cornea. If the full depth of the cornea was not affected by scarring, only the affected outer layer may be removed and then replaced with a cornea graft of the same thickness.

Postoperative care

With present microsurgical procedures, the eye sometimes may be unpatched and the patient up within several days. The average period of hospitalization ranges from five to ten days, depending upon the individual case and ease of following a patient after hospital discharge.

For the first six months or so, the surgeon will usually check progress during office visits as often as once every one to three weeks.

Visual acuity can be expected to return rapidly enough so that final improvement occurs within a few months, although occasionally this may require up to a year. The operation does not produce any change in the appearance of the eye.

Success rate

Most corneal transplant operations today are successful. The likelihood of success has greatly improved in recent years as the result of use of operating microscopes, extremely fine suture material, better selection of donor tissue, and other advances. Currently, depending upon the type of condition which makes operation necessary, and the control of glaucoma or any other complicating factors, the success rate runs from 70 percent to 90 percent and even higher.

In most cases, an unsuccessful graft—one that is not transparent—does not worsen the original status of a patient's vision. Nor does an unsuccessful graft seriously limit the chance of success for reoperation later.

Not all ophthalmologists choose to do corneal surgery themselves, but specialists in this field are to be found in almost every state and most large cities.

SEE ALSO PART II for pertinent information about choice of surgeon, preoperative and postoperative care, anesthesia, costs, and other aspects of your operation.

Removal of an Eye

There are several situations, all of them serious, which call for removal of an eye. Immediate removal is required for a malignant eye tumor. The prompt removal, or enucleation, of the eye often can lead to cure. When all vision of an eye has been lost for any reason, enucleation is recommended by many surgeons because of a greater tendency for tumors to develop in a blind eye than in a normal one and because if a tumor should develop there will be no vision disturbance to provide warning.

Enucleation may also have to be considered because of a (rare) condition called sympathetic ophthalmia, which may follow eye injury involving the ciliary body, an organ connecting the iris and the choroid, one of the casts of the eye rich in blood vessels. Symptoms of irritability—sensitivity to light, tearing, transient blurring of vision, tenderness—may develop in the noninjured "sympathizing" eye after some weeks or months and may lead to blindness in that eye. Prompt and adequate treatment of an injured eye often can prevent sympathetic ophthalmia. But under some circumstances, enucleation of the injured eye—when it is sightless or when preservation of sight is unlikely—may be indicated to prevent sympathetic ophthalmia.

The operation

Enucleation is carried out under general anesthesia in children and under either local or general anesthesia in adults. While the operation is a major one, it is not dangerous and no pain is experienced during the procedure. With the good eye patched, the patient neither sees nor feels the eye being removed. In the procedure, the conjunctiva membrane covering the eyeball, the muscles attached to the eyeball's outer coat, and the optic nerve behind the eyeball are cut.

For a few days afterward, the patient stays in bed,

but he or she may go home in about a week. A patch is worn for three or four weeks, by which time the socket usually is healed.

An artificial eye, with iris colored to match the normal eye, usually is unnoticed by others. Tears form in front of it in the usual way. The artificial eye or prosthesis can move in unison with the normal eye because the capsule and muscles of the removed eye are sutured to form a base or stump that goes through the same motions as the good eye. The prosthesis can usually be placed in the eye after healing of the socket and virtually any child or adult can learn to insert, remove, and cleanse it.

Because two functioning eyes are needed for stereoscopic vision, there is some impairment of depth and distance perception when only one eye functions. Very often children quite readily, and adults with more effort, develop the ability to overcome the impairment to a considerable extent.

The need to lose an eye comes, of course, as a shock. Yet, there is comfort in knowing that, with vision in the eye lost or doomed, its removal can help to safeguard sight in the good eye, and that the cosmetic effect of a prosthesis of the type now available can be excellent.

SEE ALSO PART II for pertinent information about choice of surgeon, preoperative and postoperative care, anesthesia, costs, and other aspects of your operation.

Ear Surgery

In recent years there have been notable developments in ear, or otologic, surgery. To a large extent it has become microsurgery. With extremely precise and meticulous procedures performed with tiny instruments and with the aid of operating microscopes, it has become possible to help more of the hard-of-hearing than ever before. Other problems now often yield to microsurgical and other techniques, including stubborn infections within the ear, some head noises, and a form of dizziness.

The Ear

An organ of hearing and equilibrium, the ear is made up of the outer (external) ear, the middle ear, and the inner (internal) ear.

The outer ear collects sound waves. Separating the outer ear from the middle ear is the eardrum, or tympanic membrane. In the middle ear are three ossicles, or small bones: the malleus (hammer), incus (anvil), and stapes (stirrup), so called because they resemble these objects. The three bones form a chain across the middle ear from the eardrum to an oval window in a membrane that separates the middle ear from the inner ear. The middle ear is connected to the nose and throat area by the eustachian tube, through

278

which the air pressure on the inner side of the eardrum is equalized with the air pressure on its outside surface.

In the inner ear (or labyrinth) is the cochlea, a spiral cavity containing a structure, the organ of Corti, that translates sound vibrations into nerve impulses that go to the brain. Also in the inner ear are the semicircular canals, which are essential to the sense of balance.

When a sound strikes the ear, the eardrum vibrates. The ossicles in the middle ear, working like levers, amplify the motion of the eardrum and pass the vibrations on to the cochlea and from there the vibrations, having been translated into nerve impulses, are transmitted by the eighth cranial nerve to the auditory center in the brain.

Puncturing the Eardrum (Myringotomy)

Myringotomy, an incision in the eardrum, is sometimes necessary to relieve pressure behind the eardrum and allow for drainage from an infectious process in the middle ear. Middle ear infections may follow respiratory infections, particularly in children. Pain in the ear may indicate that infection is present and that pus or fluid is bulging the eardrum. Pus may build up to the point where it generates sufficient pressure to puncture or break the eardrum.

Surgical puncture of the eardrum for drainage of pus is a simple procedure carried out either under a local or a general anesthetic, involving an incision less than ¼-inch long. Pain is relieved almost at once. As the pus escapes, it is wiped from the ear canal. The drum heals quickly and smoothly.

Puncture of the eardrum may also be required for secretory otitis media, an inflammatory condition in which fluid collects in the middle ear. At first, pain, fullness, and decreased hearing are experienced in the affected ear. Pain may disappear after a few days but the fullness and hearing loss persist, and the patient may complain of a sensation of water in the ear, which varies with changes in position. The fluid may disappear in a week to ten days through absorption or drainage via the eustachian tube. But if it persists, surgery to establish drainage may be required.

In the procedure, an incision is made into the eardrum and fluid is sucked out with a needle. A small polyethylene tube is then placed in the incision to facilitate complete drainage. If necessary, the tube may be left in place for several months. During that time no dressing is needed but the ear should be kept dry, using a shower cap when bathing. At the appropriate time, the tube can be readily removed in the doctor's office, and the incision then usually heals within a week.

SEE ALSO PART II for pertinent information about choice of surgeon, preoperative and postoperative care, anesthesia, costs, helping a child through surgery, and other aspects of the operation.

Eardrum Repair (Myringoplasty)

Myringoplasty, or surgical repair of a hole in an eardrum, may be required when the hole refuses to heal. The healing failure may result from a mild but chronic middle ear infection that makes an ear "run," draining just enough to interfere with the healing process.

The repair procedure, carried out through the ear canal or through an incision behind the ear under local or general anesthesia, involves the placement of a small graft of skin, vein, or ligament to close the hole from the outside. This helps to prevent infection by microorganisms entering the middle ear from the ear canal and often improves hearing.

Several days of hospitalization may be needed, and while there is some discomfort after surgery, it is minimal and readily controlled with medication. Healing occurs within a month or a little more.

SEE ALSO PART II for pertinent information about choice of surgeon, preoperative and postoperative care, anesthesia, costs, helping a child through surgery, and other aspects of the operation.

Mastoidectomy

The middle ear is connected with cells in the mastoid bone just behind the outer ear. Because of the connection, it used to be, before the era of antibiotics, that mastoid bone infection was a common complication of middle ear infection. And one of the oldest of all ear operations is simple mastoidectomy in which through an incision behind the ear, the mastoid bone was exposed so a cavity could be made in it in order to allow drainage of pus.

Although acute infection of the mastoid bone is uncommon today, chronic mastoiditis may occur as a complication of chronic ear infections. With serious mastoid disease, a radical or modified radical mastoidectomy may be required to dry the ear and eradicate foci of chronic infection, and also to prevent spread of infection into the brain and major nerves and blood vessels nearby.

Mastoidectomy is usually done under general anesthesia. An incision may be made behind the ear lobe or inside the ear canal. In a radical mastoidectomy, all infected mastoid cells are removed and, because the middle ear structures—bones and eardrum—are diseased, these too are removed. In a modified radical mastoidectomy, infected mastoid cells are removed and as much as possible of ear bones and eardrum are saved in order to maintain as much hearing as possible.

Pain after a mastoidectomy can be controlled with medication and the patient may be out of bed within a day or so. Although the operation is a serious one because the mastoid bone is close to the brain and also to the nerve that moves facial muscles of expression, there is little danger with expert surgery, and mortality is almost nil.

Mastoidectomy sometimes may be combined with tympanoplasty in a double procedure in which the sound-conducting mechanism of the middle ear is reconstructed, using remnants of healthy bone along with skin or vein and substitute materials (see tympanoplasty).

Usually after mastoidectomy, the scar is not disfiguring. Only a small line may be visible in the ear canal or, if the incision was made behind the ear, only a thin white line may be apparent.

SEE ALSO PART II for pertinent information about choice of surgeon, preoperative and postoperative care, anesthesia, costs, helping a child through surgery, and other aspects of the operation.

Stapedectomy

Hearing impairment affects an estimated 17 to 20 million Americans. There are two types of impairment: nerve and conductive. When the nerve of hearing is diseased, the condition is usually irreversible. But in many cases of impairment, the problem lies with defective conduction—a physical interruption or resistance to the transmittal of sound waves to the inner ear. Often now in such cases surgery can be helpful.

One of the most common causes of defective conduction is otosclerosis of the stapes bone in the middle ear. As we have noted, the three small bones of the middle ear—the malleus, the incus, and the innermost, the stapes—act as a conducting mechanism to transmit sound through the middle ear space from the eardrum. The stirrup-shaped stapes fits into and closes the oval window in a membrane that separates the middle ear from the inner ear. When the stapes moves, it agitates fluid in the inner ear into vibratory waves and this physical motion of the fluid in the inner ear stimulates the auditory nerve endings in the organ of Corti, thus transforming mechanical energy into sensory energy that is relayed to the brain and interpreted as sound.

In otosclerosis, the stapes hardens and becomes rigid and fixed, unable to transmit the vibratory sound waves. Hearing is impaired, and there is ringing of the ear (tinnitus) in about seven out of ten cases.

The operation

Stapedectomy is performed under local anesthetic which may be supplemented by other measures to make the patient drowsy. The eardrum is lifted to expose the middle ear. The stapes bone is removed. The opening into the inner ear is then covered with a small piece of vein or other material. A tiny section of plastic or wire is then connected to the incus bone, forming a strut between the incus and the vein graft used to cover the inner ear window.

To test the integrity of the bone chain and new strut, the surgeon may gently lift the malleus handle. When this is done, there should be motion of the incus which is transmitted to the strut which in turn vibrates the inner ear fluid. The eardrum is then replaced and the procedure is completed.

Postoperative care

After the operation, the patient is returned to his bed and may be placed with operated ear down into a pillow so any drainage of blood will be away from the eardrum. The patient may be discharged from the hospital on the second postoperative day and may be asked to stay at home for about five days.

At the first postoperative visit to the surgeon, which may be about the twelfth day after surgery, any clots or crusts are removed from the external ear canal. By this time the patient is usually hearing. When the incision is fully healed, the patient can bathe and swim without worry about getting water into the ear.

Many surgeons report that over the next few months, there is often a vast change in the personalities of patients. An ease and a relaxed air replace the previous attitude of tension and strain.

Results

Stapedectomy is hugely successful but not foolproof. There is some possibility that the operation may be ineffective and may not improve hearing. About 92 percent of all otosclerotic patients undergoing the operation will benefit. About 8 percent will come away with no better hearing than before. However, one patient in every 150 will lose his hearing completely in the operated ear as a direct result of the operation, and the ear will no longer be able to use a hearing aid. Because of this calculated risk, most surgeons will not accept for surgery anyone who has only one usable hearing-aid ear.

Usually hearing loss from otosclerosis occurs in both ears and patients who have had successful surgery on one ear want similar surgery on the other. Many surgeons believe that no one should have a stapedectomy on the second ear for at least six months to a year.

If hearing is improved after stapes surgery, the ringing of the ear which may have been present before may subside or diminish.

Through tests before surgery which indicate the level of function of the auditory nerve, it is possible for surgeons to predict how much hearing can be restored through stapes surgery.

For patients with normal nerve function, it can be predicted that surgery is likely to lead to complete restoration of hearing, and if a hearing aid was required it can be discarded. If some degeneration of the auditory nerve with a loss of upper frequency sounds is present, successful surgery will allow normal hearing in most situations but will not eliminate some limitations in other situations. On the whole, hearing will be satisfactory without a hearing aid. With marked nerve degeneration, hearing will improve enough to justify surgery: it will be possible to hear close conversation and to hear comfortably on the telephone but for most social and business purposes, a hearing aid will be needed. For advanced nerve degeneration, where the hearing loss was so advanced that a hearing aid was ineffective, the aim of surgery is to permit use of a hearing aid effectively for the first time.

Age is not a factor in determining suitability for stapes surgery. The basic requirement is sufficient auditory nerve function. As a result, patients from seven to seventy-seven or beyond can be suitable candidates. Often, elderly patients have too great a degree of nerve degeneration to warrant surgery. But many elderly patients with good nerve function have had very satisfactory results.

SEE ALSO PART II for pertinent information about choice of surgeon, preoperative and postoperative care, anesthesia, costs, and other aspects of the operation.

Tympanoplasty

Tympanoplasty is an operation to overcome the serious consequences of chronic middle ear infection. It includes repair of a perforated, unhealing eardrum and reconstruction of the diseased bone chain within the middle ear. Such consequences of middle ear infection constitute a major cause of conductive hearing loss.

The operation may be performed through the ear canal under local anesthesia, but in some cases an incision behind the ear may be necessary and a general anesthetic will then be used.

Skin or vein grafts may be used to repair the eardrum. The extent of surgery within the middle ear will depend upon how much of the bone chain remains functional. Commonly, bone damage from infection takes the form of erosion of the long process of the incus, and in such cases the incus may be transposed to the head of the stapes. In other cases, it may be necessary to use substitute materials to take the place of damaged bones.

Usually the patient is out of bed the day after operation and may go home the same day. Improvement of hearing usually occurs within a period of two months.

Promising results are being achieved in some cases now with transplants from cadavers for patients who lack all or part of the bony chain. The operations vary according to need, and the transplants may consist of eardrum alone, eardrum with attached malleus, eardrum with all three middle ear bones, and the incus alone.

SEE ALSO PART II for pertinent information about choice of surgeon, preoperative and postoperative care, anesthesia, costs, and other aspects of the operation.

Surgery for Ménière's Disease

Ménière's disease is marked by attacks of severe true whirling dizziness or vertigo, with nausea, vomiting, sweating, and pallor. In addition there may be hearing impairment and ringing in the ears (tinnitus). Attacks last from a few minutes to several hours. Sometimes an attack develops so suddenly that the victim falls to the ground. Usually, however, the patient senses an oncoming attack and has time to sit or lie down.

Ménière's disease involves a little understood faulty functioning of the labyrinth of the inner ear. The course may vary. Sometimes the vertigo attacks stop but the hearing impairment and tinnitus continue. Or the vertigo may stop only when the deafness is complete.

There are theories that Ménière's disease may involve local disturbance of salt and water balance, local allergy, blood vessel disturbances in the inner ear, or anatomic changes in the cochlea.

Many measures may be tried with varying success. They include inhalation of oxygen and carbon dioxide to help promote circulation, low salt diet, use of a diuretic drug to promote fluid excretion, treatment for allergy and anxiety, use of vitamins B, B 12 and, most recently, E.

Operations

In severe, unyielding cases involving one ear, surgical treatment may be considered. If useful hearing in the ear is lacking, the inner ear labyrinth may be destroyed. The operative route may go through the ear canal, the eardrum, and the middle ear, or through the mastoid bone. Hearing is destroyed but other symptoms may be eliminated.

Although their success is not predictable, there are operations designed to eliminate attacks of vertigo and still maintain useful hearing. In one, performed through the mastoid bone, a tiny sac which functions to keep fluid pressure within normal limits around the hearing nerve and inside the ear canals is connected to the fluid space surrounding the brain.

Recently, ultrasound, or generation of high-frequency sound waves, has been used in an effort selectively to destroy nerve endings in the inner ear without harm to hearing or equilibrium.

SEE ALSO PART II for pertinent information about choice of surgeon, preoperative and postoperative care, anesthesia, costs, and other aspects of the operation.

Skin and Superficial Tissue Surgery

The Skin

The skin is the body's largest organ and in an average 150-pound person it has an area of seventeen to twenty square feet and weighs about six pounds, twice as much as brain or liver. It's a versatile and protective organ, serving to keep body fluids in and foreign agents out, to shield against harmful rays, to help regulate body temperature.

Although it appears to be a simple covering, a single square inch of skin may contain some 70 feet of nerves, 650 sweat glands, 15 to 20 feet of blood vessels, 65 to 75 hairs, and associated muscles, 100 oil glands, and hundreds of nerve endings for detecting pressure, pain, heat and cold.

Three layers form the skin. The outer layer is the epidermis and, because living cells cannot survive exposure to air, the outermost part of the epidermis, the visible surface, is made up of dead rather than living cells. These dead cells are constantly being lost through bathing and rubbing against clothing. They are replaced from underneath by new cells formed in the deeper malpighian layer of the epidermis.

Under the epidermis is the dermis, sometimes called the "true skin." The dermis carries the skin's blood supply and a supply of nerve endings.

The third, subcutaneous, layer is attached loosely to inner body structures such as bones and muscles. The subcutaneous layer contains, along with blood vessels and nerves, fat globules which serve to insulate the body against heat and cold and to cushion inner organs against bumps and jolts. With aging, the fatty tissue in the subcutaneous layer may be absorbed, causing outer skin layers to form uneven folds or wrinkles.

The skin, of course, is subject to many disorders, a few of which sometimes may require surgery.

Warts

Warts, produced by virus invasion, are common, contagious, benign growths of epidermal skin cells. A wart may appear and the infection may persist as a single lesion, or other warts may develop. Complete disappearance may occur after months or years with or without treatment.

Warts are of varied types. Common warts may be round or irregular, firm, rough, light gray or grayish black, and appear most frequently on such areas as fingers, elbows, knees, face, and scalp, but they may spread elsewhere. "Thread" warts are thin elevations that most often occur on eyelids, face, neck, or lips. Flat warts are more common in children and young adults than in older people and are smooth, flat, yellow brown, most often occurring on the face. Plantar warts are common warts on the sole of the foot, where they have been flattened by pressure and may be extremely tender.

Treatment

Many treatments are available; none is completely satisfactory. Warts can be removed, but sometimes the virus remains and the growths reappear at the same or different sites. Many doctors believe that it is better to leave single inconspicuous warts alone.

Various caustic agents—trichloroacetic acid, phenol, or nitric acid among them—may be applied to the tops of warts.

Plantar warts may be treated by first peeling away some of the tissue and then applying a concentrated phenol solution, followed by nitric acid, after which the growth is covered with a 40 percent salicylic acid plaster and adhesive bandage. Often the wart may disappear after three to six or more such treatments given at intervals of about five days.

A 30-second application of liquid nitrogen to freeze a plantar or flat wart may be effective. If warts are not too numerous, they may be removed electrosurgically. After injection of a local anesthetic, a needle carrying electric current is introduced for a short distance into the top of the wart, after which the wart can be removed and soft tissue underneath gently scraped off. A wart also may be incised along the sides and then scraped off.

Moles

Moles, also known as nevi, are fleshy growths on the skin. They vary in color from yellow brown to black, may be small or large, flat or raised, smooth, hairy, or wartlike.

Moles can be removed readily by surgical excision and many are, for purely cosmetic reasons. Excision is recommended when a pigmented mole shows increasing pigmentation, speckling, or a halo of pigment around the base, or when any mole increases in size, bleeds, ulcerates or crusts.

Occasionally a pigmented mole may turn into malignant melonoma, a rapidly spreading type of cancer. Malignant melanoma tends to develop more readily from moles on the lower legs and mucous membranes than from those located elsewhere. When pigmented moles are removed, a wider excision may be used, taking an area of normal skin around the wart and subcutaneous tissue below.

A common hairy mole that does not change in size or color need not be removed. It may not be advisable to remove flat pigmented moles on the soles of the feet since they are common, rarely become malignant, and the scar that may follow removal of a mole from a weight-bearing surface may be painful.

Local anesthesia may be used for mole removal.

Sebaceous Cyst

Thousands of minute sebaceous glands in the skin secrete an oily, colorless, odorless fluid (sebum) through the hair follicles. A sebaceous cyst, also known as a wen, results when the duct of a sebaceous gland becomes plugged, forming a benign tumor of the skin that contains the gland secretions. Sebaceous cysts may occur anywhere on the body except the palms of the hands and the soles of the feet, and are most common on the scalp, back, and scrotum.

The cystic mass is firm, movable and itself seldom causes discomfort. But because bacterial infection with abscess formation is common, surgical removal of the intact cyst sac is the preferred treatment. After injection of a local anesthetic, the skin over the cyst is cut, the cyst is removed, and the skin sutured. Usually this can be done in the doctor's office. In small superficial cysts, called milia, just a tiny slab incision and removal of the contents is often curative.

Boils and Carbuncles

A boil, or furuncle, is a focal inflammation of the skin and subcutaneous tissues, enclosing a central core, caused by bacteria which enter through the hair follicles or sweat glands. Furuncles most often occur on the neck, under the arms, on the breasts, face, and buttocks, but may appear elsewhere. They are especially painful when they occur on skin closely attached to underlying structures, as on nose, ears, and fingers.

Carbuncles, also caused by bacteria, are similar to boils but are larger and more deeply rooted and have several openings. They develop more slowly, are sometimes more painful than boils, may be accompanied by fever. They occur most often in men and most commonly on the nape of the neck.

A single boil may be treated with moist heat to bring it to a head. The boil can then be cut superficially and the central core removed. Anti-infective treatment is used in addition.

When many boils are present, oral penicillin or another antibiotic may be used to start treatment while sensitivity studies are done to determine the most suitable antibiotic, after which that may be used. Seventy percent alcohol rubbed on for a minute or two each day may be used to sterilize surrounding skin.

Carbuncles may be treated with antibiotics and incision and drainage. Surgery, sometimes extensive, may be needed.

Lipomas

Lipomas are fatty tumors under the skin, of unknown cause but quite common. Most produce no pain or other symptoms, and when they do not change in size may be left alone. They may be no bigger than a pea, feel soft, move freely under the skin, rarely become malignant, and give warning before doing so by rapid growth. Lipomas may sometimes grow to large size without becoming malignant.

A lipoma may be removed under local anesthesia. Through an incision in the skin, the tumor is cut out and the skin is then sutured.

Pinched Fat

Pinched fat tissue sometimes may be a cause of back pain. Fat is laid down in the body in patterns, usually separated by layers of connective tissue called fascia. Fat is just below the skin as well as deeper. If a small hole or perforation should develop in a fascial layer because of injury, a small globule of fat may push its way through the hole when the hole is stretched during some movement of the body. When the patient then relaxes so that the hole is no longer stretched, the fat globule may be caught in the hole, pinched, and may then become painful.

Injection of a cortisonelike drug may reduce inflammation and be sufficient to end the pain. In rare cases the hole in the fascial layer may have to be enlarged surgically to end the pinching of the fat. There is usually no need to remove the globule itself unless the pinching has so interfered with blood supply that the fat has become a hard lump of dead tissue.

Excessive Perspiration (Hyperhidrosis)

Generalized excessive sweating frequently accompanies fever. It may also be caused by obesity or excessive thyroid functioning. Occasionally a central nervous system disorder may be responsible. Treatment is for the underlying cause.

Excessive perspiration may be localized, confined to areas such as the palms, soles, groin, or underarms. The perspiration may be malodorous (bromhidrosis), carrying a fetid odor caused by decomposition of sweat and cellular debris through the action of bacteria and yeasts.

For localized hyperhidrosis, the physician may prescribe aluminum chloride solutions and potassium permanganate compresses. A 5 percent solution of formaldehyde may be prescribed for treating the palms and soles.

Treatment for bromhidrosis is basically the same as for hyperhidrosis, and the response is often satisfactory. Scrupulous cleanliness is emphasized. It is usually important to shave the underarm hair, and a topical antibiotic such as neomycin solution may be prescribed.

In excessive underarm perspiration, especially if accompanied by bromhidrosis, surgery to remove a group of the glands in the underarm area may provide relief.

Skin Cancer

Cancer of the skin is common and, fortunately, unless long neglected, is almost 100 percent curable. Skin cancers occur most commonly on exposed areas such as nose, face, or hands. Overexposure to sun is favorable to skin cancer. The incidence in farmers, sailors, fishermen, outdoor sportsmen and sunbathers is related to the amount of exposure. Light-skinned people tend to be most sensitive.

Any sore or ulcer that does not heal; any sudden change in color, size, and texture in moles, warts, scars and birthmarks should be looked upon as a possible warning sign of skin cancer until proven otherwise. Biopsy—examination of a sample of the area under a microscope—may be done in the case of a small tumor by total removal of the tumor and by removal of a sample when a larger tumor is involved.

Some skin cancers may be treated by X-ray or cobalt irradiation. Some small growths may be destroyed by electro-coagulation. Often a skin cancer can be removed completely by knife. If the cancer is large and its removal leaves a sizable opening, a skin graft can be used to close it.

Each year in the United States there are more than 100,000 new cases of skin cancer. Virtually all are curable when diagnosed and treated without undue delay. But yearly 5,000 people have lost their lives to skin cancer which has spread widely and wildly beyond control by surgery. A hopeful development is the finding that a chemical, 5-FU, when applied to advanced skin cancer, is 95 percent effective in completely eradicating the cancer, producing permanent remission, and leaving no visible scars.

SEE ALSO PART II for pertinent information about choice of surgeon, preoperative and postoperative care, anesthesia, costs, and other aspects of your operation.

Plastic Surgery

Plastic surgery is surgery performed to improve the appearance or function of exposed parts of the body that are defective, deformed, or damaged. It is not new. Artificial noses and ears have been found on Egyptian mummies, and the ancient Hindus are known to have reconstructed noses by using skin flaps lifted from forehead or cheek, a technique often practiced because it was a custom to mutilate the noses of persons who broke the laws.

Modern plastic surgery—one of the most rapidly growing branches of medical practice, with almost 200,000 procedures now being done annually in the United States alone —began as a specialty in World War I when surgeons worked to repair scarred and disfigured servicemen. The specialty grew thereafter with the increase in industrial accidents and automobile injuries and with the injuries of the Second World War.

Plastic surgery today covers four major areas: catastrophic surgery for burns and facial and other injuries suffered in catastrophic industrial, automobile, and other accidents; congenital anomaly surgery for babies born with defects such as cleft lip and palate; cancer surgery to reconstruct damaged areas of mouth, throat, skin, and face; and cosmetic surgery to improve appearance.

Only within the last ten years or so has cosmetic surgery —plastic surgery undertaken for reasons of appearance rather than health—become acceptable outside the ranks of aging actors and actresses and wealthy dowagers. Once considered to be a near-sinful frill, today it is sought by the housewife, the businessman, the middle-class youngster, and the ghetto resident.

All of the country's 1,200 board-certified plastic surgeons do some cosmetic operations. There are now about 200 plastic surgeons who do little else. In addition to the American Society of Plastic and Reconstructive Surgeons, a new American Society for Aesthetic Plastic Surgery, started in 1968, includes board-certified plastic surgeons who are members of the older society and who must devote a significant portion of their practice to cosmetic procedures.

Not all cosmetic operations are performed by plastic surgeons. Many facial procedures are done by otolaryngologists and maxillofacial surgeons, and their organization, the American Association of Cosmetic Surgeons, is also open to dermatologists, oral surgeons, and others.

Cosmetic surgery is not inexpensive. The range of fees is great. Generally, fees are highest in New York, on the West Coast, and in Chicago, and lowest elsewhere in the Midwest. The fee, exclusive of the cost of any hospitalization that may be required, ranges from $750 to $2,500 for a face lift; $200 to $1,000 for a face peel; $50 to $600 for dermabrasion; $500 to $1,000 for eyelid surgery; $500 to $1,500 for nose surgery; $500 to $1,000 for breast augmentation; $250 to $1,500 for double chin correction.

Usually cosmetic surgery is not covered by medical insurance although sometimes there may be reimbursement of the patient for part of an operation which also corrects a medical problem, as when a nose operation, for example, involves correction of a deviated septum. The insurance may cover the surgery on the septum but not on the reshaping of the nose.

The choice of a qualified plastic surgeon is important. Not all who practice plastic surgery are necessarily fully qualified. It is wise to get help in making a choice—from the recommendations of your family physician, the local hospital which can provide the names of plastic surgeons who are accepted staff members, and from a check of the Directory of Medical Specialists (see page 352).

Plastic surgery procedures today are notably safe but not 100 percent without risk. There are occasional complications: abnormal scar formation, infection, injury to a nerve.

For the properly chosen patient, the result is almost always satisfactory. Good surgeons take care in choosing patients, fully aware that unrealistic expectations cannot be met. Instant makeovers are not possible. Appearance can be improved, often dramatically, but it is never possible, for example, to make a fifty-five-year-old woman look like a twenty-five-year-old again.

Before undertaking plastic surgery, discuss with the surgeon the probable results of the operation, the risks, the possible complications. Particularly if the procedure is serious and costly, you may wish to see a second plastic surgeon for a second opinion.

Skin Grafting

A common procedure of plastic surgery is skin grafting— the replacement of severely damaged skin in one area with healthy skin from another area of the patient's body or from the body of a donor.

Grafting may be used to prevent the formation of disfiguring scars such as those that may form on the face or elsewhere from severe burns. If burns or other injuries are extensive, grafting can prevent extensive scarring with unsightly tissue and can avoid skin contractures.

Skin can be transferred from another person or from a skin bank as a temporary measure to cover a raw surface for a few weeks. It cannot be expected to last. For permanent coverage, the patient's own skin must be used.

A skin graft may be made by cutting a piece of healthy skin from the back or thigh or other part of the body and stitching it to the injured area. Small arteries from the tissues surrounding the injured area then grow into the graft, nourishing it and promoting normal growth.

A full-thickness graft may be used—or a split-thickness one. For the latter, the outer layers of skin at the donor site are shaved from the deep layers with a special instrument. Three-inch-wide sheets as long as eight inches can be removed. A sheet may be laid as a single piece in the injured area. It is also possible to cut a sheet into patches about the size of postage stamps and to space them at about half-inch intervals in an injured area. The edges will grow to meet each other.

When a split-thickness graft is taken, the deep layers of skin at the site grow a new cover. But when a full-thickness graft is taken from a donor site, new skin will not grow there. It may be possible to suture the site or to fill it with a split-thickness graft taken from elsewhere.

Pedicle grafts are sometimes needed to fill out defects. The surgeon cuts a flap of skin full thickness with the fat layer beneath it, but he only partly frees it from the donor site, letting it remain joined by a nourishing stem or pedicle. He attaches the loose end to the damaged area. Still fed by its natural blood supply, the flap remains healthy while its cut edge grows into and begins to cover the injured site. Meanwhile, the area from which the flap was cut and folded away heals and grows new skin. The flap then can be cut free, and both the graft and the area from which the flap was taken can heal completely.

When the damaged area and the flap are awkwardly located, pedicle grafting can involve inconvenience for the patient. His arm, for example, may have to be strapped against his head to provide a skin flap for his face.

Burns

In the United States alone, more than 70,000 persons are hospitalized each year for the treatment of severe burns. Shock, which accompanies every major burn, once was a major cause of death. In 1940, 34 percent of all extremely severe burn patients died in burn shock during the first forty-eight hours. So great were the strides in caring for shock that by 1955 no burn patients died of shock.

The second great crisis that confronts a burned patient is the possibility of bacterial invasion and massive infection because of the destruction of the normal skin barrier. Skin grafting is of major importance in minimizing this possibility.

Temporary skin grafts may be used on burned areas to provide time for the patient's general condition to improve. As soon as possible, often in about three weeks, devitalized burned tissue is removed and replaced with split-thickness grafts from the patient's unburned areas.

In severe burns, it is often necessary to undertake a long program of scar removal and substitution, which may require additional split-thickness grafts and some full-thickness grafts in certain areas such as eyelids, ears, neck. In some cases, pedicle flaps may be needed to release contractures over joints and allow normal movement. Sometimes, too, ears, noses and fingers must be rebuilt. Reconstructive surgery in very severe cases may require years. Because early burn scars are in a fluctuating state, many plastic surgeons recommend that several months elapse between initial healing and the beginning of reconstructive surgery.

Facial Injuries

After an accident producing serious facial injuries, immediate emergency surgery will remove foreign particles, suture skin edges, and save as much tissue as possible. Almost always, thereafter, plastic surgery is needed to restore function and obtain a satisfactory esthetic result.

Common injuries include those to teeth and jaws, nose, entire mid-face. There may be injuries to bone and soft tissue areas with or without loss of either bone or soft tissue.

Plastic reconstructive surgery is often able to accomplish near-miracles, although the procedures, carried out in stages, sometimes must extend over many months. Broken bones may be threaded together. Useless bone fragments may be removed and new bone grafted, for example, to join the two sides of the lower jaw at the point of the chin, making chewing possible again and allowing normal use of the tongue and, therefore, normal speech and breathing. Voids may be filled with pedicle grafting, a battered nose reshaped, eyelids made to move again, scars stretched.

Cleft Lip and Cleft Palate

Clefts are the most common type of facial malformations, occurring in approximately one of every 600 live births in the United States. They result from failure of the two sides of the face to unite properly at an early stage of prenatal development.

There is a great deal of variation in clefts. A defect may be limited to the outer flesh of the upper lip extending to the nostril—a "harelip," so-called because it suggests the lip of a rabbit—or the defect may extend back through the midline of the upper jaw and through the roof of the mouth. Sometimes only the soft palate, located at the rear of the mouth, is involved.

An infant with a cleft palate is unable to suckle properly because the opening between mouth and nose prevents suction. Feeding must be done by other means, with dropper, cup, or spoon—or an obdurator may be used. This is an appliance which takes the place of the palate and closes the cleft while the baby is suckling. Clefts later can hinder speech because consonants such as g, b, d, and f are normally formed by pressure against the roof of the mouth.

Treatment

Treatment of cleft palate and cleft lip is by surgery and may be followed by measures to improve speech. Repair procedures can vary in detail, depending upon the individual case. Often the plastic surgeon works in consultation with a dentist, orthodontist, speech specialist, and other experts.

Surgery to close a cleft lip can usually be carried out within the first few months of life and if a child is otherwise healthy may even be done in some instances shortly after birth. In the procedure, the floor of the nose may be sutured closed and the edges of the unfused lip brought neatly together. Successful surgery often leaves only a thin scar and a greatly improved ability to form the p, b, and m sounds.

Generally, a good time to reconstruct a cleft palate is when the child is about eighteen months old and before he learns to talk. In the procedure, the separated portions of the roof of the mouth are sutured to the base of the wall that divides the nasal cavities.

Postoperative care

Surgery for clefts may be performed under general anesthesia. Postoperative care is aimed at preventing injury to or infection of the operative site and maintaining adequate nutrition. The child may not be allowed to lie on his stomach until the incision is healed and elbow restraints may be used to keep fingers and hands away from the mouth. The child may be fed with a special syringe with a rubber tip while on a liquid diet for from seven to ten days postoperatively.

The child born with a moderate case of cleft lip or cleft palate can expect a normal life in appearance, speech, and manner if proper action is taken early. This may call for the advice of specialists in medicine, surgery, dentistry, and speech.

Ears

When it is necessary to reconstruct an ear because of tissue loss present at birth or caused by injury, multiple-stage procedures may be required. Cartilage to form a framework may be taken from the chest near the breastbone and pedicle grafting using skin and fat from the neck and scalp may be needed.

Otoplasty, a common form of plastic surgery, is the name for operations to correct ear deformities and is somewhat simpler. Otoplasty may be used to improve appearance by changing the shape and contour of the external ear and by correcting protrusion of the ear. It can be performed at any age. The ears reach mature size before age five and it is therefore possible and advantageous to correct a deformity before a child becomes sensitive about his appearance. While otoplasty is more common with children, an increasing number of adults seek surgical help. Otoplasty is performed by general plastic surgeons and also by otolaryngologists specializing in facial plastic surgery.

For reduction of unusually large ears, some of the cartilage is removed, usually as pie-shaped wedges, and the edges are sutured together. For correction of ear protrusion, enough cartilage is removed to allow the ears to be placed in proper relationship to the face and head. For lop ears, bent over on themselves, some cartilage is removed at the bend and the upper halves of the ears are brought into proper vertical alignment. The operation is done from behind and the scar is hidden.

Otoplasty may require from one to three hours, depending upon the complexity of the case, and general or other anesthesia may be used, depending upon the patient's age, general health, emotional stability, and other factors.

A wraparound bandage is applied after surgery and worn for seven to ten days. After the bandage is removed, until healing is complete, a protective wrap is used during sleep and periods of physical exertion. When the dressings are first removed, the ears may be swollen and discolored but swelling and discoloration usually disappear within a few days. Most patients return to school or work within one to two weeks. In most cases the incision is made behind the ear, where the resulting thin scars are inconspicuous.

The results of otoplasty are usually satisfactory. The goal is improved appearance, not perfection, and perfection is rarely achieved.

Nose

Plastic surgery of the nose, known as rhinoplasty, may be used to improve appearance or to replace a part lost or damaged by disease or injury.

When only the skin of the nose is injured, the defect may be remedied by grafting new pink skin taken from a suitable area such as the ear or back of the ear. Usually arm skin is too pale, abdominal skin too brown.

Much or all of a nose may be missing, usually as the result of gunshot wound, traffic accident, or cancer. When the entire nose is missing, the reconstruction problem is difficult but nevertheless is often solved successfully. Extensive procedures are needed and involve reconstructing a framework for support, a lining, and a cover. A bone graft, taken from a rib, may be used to supply support, and skin flaps taken from the forehead may be used to produce both lining and cover. Thereafter, several shaping procedures are usually needed to produce finally a natural-looking and functional nose.

Cosmetic rhinoplasty

Most rhinoplasties, in which excess bone or cartilage may be removed and the nose reshaped, are performed to improve appearance. Sometimes rhinoplasty may be indicated in cases of increasing disfigurement of the nose as the patient grows older and breathing becomes more difficult. Other patients may have deformities inside the nasal passages which impair breathing and cause headaches, sinus trouble, or other problems, and correction of the deformities may require simultaneous realignment of the external nose.

Procedures

Rhinoplasty often may be carried out under local anesthesia. When considered advisable, other anesthesia may be used.

Ski nose. Working from inside the nose, the surgeon may correct the ski nose by filling in the "scoop" with a piece of a material called Silastic or by using cartilage taken from a rib or from behind the ear or bone taken from the hip. If recontouring of the nose is needed for a natural overall effect, this also may be done from inside the nose. There are no scars.

Saddle nose. The saddle or depressed nose, usually the result of fights or accidents, also can be corrected by using Silastic implant or bone and cartilage to fill in the depression as in the ski nose, and the operation is done in the same manner. The filling-in can be tailored to provide a straight or turned-up profile line.

Thick nose. This type of nose can be improved only moderately. Procedures may include removal of wedges at the sides of the nose and removal of cartilage in the tip. Insertion of a cartilage strut at the tip may provide additional tip projection and definition which can be advantageous. Sometimes a Silastic implant on the bridge may be of value, particularly in the Negro. Basically, the procedures are performed from inside the nose and leave no visible scars.

Button nose. Lengthening a button, or too-short, nose is generally among the least successful of nose operations. How successful the operation is depends upon how small the nose is. There is a shortage of skin which can be overcome, but only to a degree, by separating skin out along the cheeks from underlying tissue and drawing it toward the nose. A slim implant along the length of the nose may be added to provide a more bony shape.

Crooked nose. Straightening a crooked or twisted nose requires straightening twisted cartilage, which stubbornly tends to spring back to its previous shape. By scoring the cartilage with a series of tiny cuts, some of this tendency can be overcome. But while the nose may look straight for weeks or even months, some of the curvature may return, and a perfectly straight nose is not to be expected. The operation is performed from inside the nose and may also entail clearing an air passage, since a crooked nose may have caused blocking. No scars are visible.

Oversized, humped nose. A nasal hump is removed by saw or chisel from the inside. If the nose is too long, it can be shortened by removal of a rectangular piece from the septum. To turn the nose up, a triangle may be removed. These and any other retailoring procedures needed to bring the nose to normal size and desired shape are carried out from inside, and there are no visible scars.

Rhinophyma. The "W. C. Fields" nose, as it is popularly known, or rhinophyma in medical terms, is a nose which, as the result of nodular congestion and enlargement, has become misshapen. In mild cases, dermabrasion, or skin planing, under local anesthesia, may be enough to restore shape. For more severe cases, outer layers of skin may have to be shaved off and after healing a better shape may be achieved. If it is necessary to expose cartilage by cutting, a skin graft is required.

Postoperative care

Rhinoplasty may involve a three- to five-day hospital stay. After surgery, depending upon the procedure used, nasal packing may or may not be required. A splint is applied to the nose and, in some cases, a pressure dressing may be placed over the eyes.

By the end of the first week, much of the swelling and discoloration about the eyes subsides. Some slight swelling of the nose is present in diminishing amounts for several weeks, and the patient is particularly aware of this in the morning on arising but notices a decrease during the day.

If work has been done on the nasal septum, the partition in the middle of the nose, there may be some nasal blockage for several days after the packing is removed.

When dressings are first removed, the nose may appear stiff and turned up too much because of the effects of the bandage and tissue swelling. As much of the swelling disappears within three or four days, the nose begins to approximate its eventual shape. It generally takes upwards of one year for the last 1 or 2 percent of swelling to disappear, but this does not usually bother the patient nor detract from appearance. The thicker the skin, the longer it takes for the nose to assume its final shape. While plastic surgery can alter the shape and size of supporting structures such as cartilage and bone, it cannot change skin that is inherently thick and oily. Such skin limits the amount of correction that can be obtained.

Nasal plastic surgery may be performed by general plastic surgeons and by otolargyngologists specializing in facial plastic surgery.

Face Lift

Probably the most frequently performed plastic surgery procedure today is the face lift, which in recent years has apparently overtaken rhinoplasty. Its purpose is to eliminate sagging skin, including the slack in cheeks and jowls.

While there may be some variations depending on specific problems and an individual surgeon's methods, after the patient is under local or general anesthesia, the procedure begins with an incision in the region of the temple, within the hairline. The incision extends downward and backward to a point immediately in front of the juncture of the upper edge of the ear and the scalp. From this point it is continued downward immediately in front of the ear, around the lower attachment of the ear, then upward and backward to a point within the hairline about midway up the ear, then sharply downward, still within the hairline, to a point on the nape of the neck.

In the second stage of the operation, the facial skin and part of the neck skin is undermined, or separated, from the underlying muscle and tissue. The purpose is to mobilize the skin so it can be pulled upward and backward to remove the wrinkles.

In the third stage, the undermined skin is pulled over its new bed, the excess skin, sometimes as much as two inches, is cut off, and the incision is stitched up. If an unusually fat double chin is present, the surgeon may make a small incision under the chin and remove fat and an ellipse of skin. A pressure dressing is applied. The patient usually stays in the hospital from three to seven days, although some surgeons discharge their patients as early as twenty-four to forty-eight hours after operation.

Some patients are dismayed at how battered and bruised they look immediately after a face lift. But after about three weeks of swelling and discoloration, positive results become apparent. Stitches in front of the ear fade and are readily camouflaged with makeup. Other stitches are usually concealed by the hair.

Not all people scar the same way. Some have tissue with a tendency to form bad scars, and beforehand a responsible surgeon will warn a patient with such skin and may even refuse to take him or her as a patient.

In most face lift cases the results are satisfactory. Improvement is usually most marked in the neck, the jowls, and the lines of the face, in that order. For fine wrinkles around the mouth, which in some cases are prominent, sanding or planing (see dermabrasion) is the only help, although nothing can completely eradicate these lines. Some surgeons use a chemical peel instead.

Beneficial changes in skin tightness from face lifting may last about ten to twelve years before the previous degree of looseness returns. While face lifting can, in effect, set back the hands of the clock, the clock keeps running. Face lifts can be repeated.

Although better operating methods, more specialized training, and other advances have made the face lift safer and more effective, it is a major operation and, as in any major operation, there occasionally are complications. The possible complications include hematoma (a swelling containing blood), damage to skin, damage to a facial nerve, infection.

Face Peel

While a face lift may relieve major creases and sagging jowls, small, spider-web wrinkles often remain. To remove these, the chemical face peel may be used by some plastic surgeons and dermatologists.

With the patient under local anesthesia, the entire face and neck are painted with a powerful chemical such as phenol (carbolic acid) and then covered with adhesive tape to intensify the reaction. The chemical burns away the upper layer of skin and penetrates deeply enough into the subcutaneous layer to harden the connective tissue that has lost its elasticity. In the subsequent process, the face swells, develops a crusty layer, peels, and heals, and in about two months the old skin is replaced by smooth new skin. Blemishes and fine wrinkles disappear or are reduced. The new skin, however, will be somewhat lighter than the rest of the body because the chemical removes some skin pigment. For this reason, blondes and people with reddish hair are the best candidates; those with olive complexions or dark skins may risk a blotchy or uneven result.

Face peeling is to be avoided by anyone allergic to phenol or similar chemicals. Tests and examinations should be made to determine if there is any sensitivity. People with diabetes, high blood pressure, kidney disease, or any other disease which could slow healing or be aggravated by the chemical are unsuitable candidates for face peeling.

Four to six days of hospitalization may be needed for face peeling. In some cases the procedure may be carried out in the plastic surgeon's or dermatologist's office. In such cases, two or more treatments may be given, two weeks apart.

Face peeling is not painless. Individual reactions vary; some patients are not overly distressed while others feel the need for medication to relieve pain.

Although face peeling is obviously a procedure that should be carried out only by experts, it is being used by nonmedical practitioners in some parts of the country who promote the technique as "a miraculous discovery" that produces "baby-fresh skin." Lay practitioners, who may call themselves "facial rejuvenators," often are beauticians with only a high school diploma and a hairdressing course for education. There have been reports of many cases of severe scarring.

Dermabrasion

Used primarily to remove scars from acne or smallpox, this method of scraping the face with a wire wheel or brush has other applications. It is sometimes useful for removing superficial facial wrinkles that are not too deeply furrowed, freckles, moles, and dark spots and may smooth out rough facial skin. To be suitable for dermabrasion, blemishes must be in skin layers near the surface.

In the procedure, which may be carried out in the doctor's office or in the hospital, a freezing spray is applied to harden the skin surface temporarily. In a manner akin to sandpapering, the surgeon moves a rapidly rotating wire brush over the affected area to remove outer skin layers. Dressings are worn over the face until crusting is completed and new skin has formed beneath the crusting, usually within a week to ten days. Rarely are perfect results achieved in eliminating all blemishes; many pits and scars cannot be planed deeply enough to eliminate them; but improvement may be sufficient to justify the procedure.

Chin

Mentoplasty is the term for plastic operation on the chin. In augmentation mentoplasty, the size of an underdeveloped chin is increased. Either of two procedures may be used. In one, the surgeon makes an incision inside the lower lip, lifts tissue off the bones to create an internal pocket, then fills it with a cartilage, bone, or silicone implant. In the other procedure, the incision is made in the crease of the chin and the implant is inserted. The second procedure may leave a visible scar but reduces the risk of infection.

In reduction mentoplasty for a protruding chin, the surgeon can make an incision in the lower lip and use a burr to grind the bone down to desired size. If, however, the bite is abnormal, the plastic surgeon may need the help of an oral surgeon to remove pieces of jawbone, reset the jaw, and wire the teeth, a complicated procedure.

Eyelids

The term used for plastic surgery of the eyelids is blepharoplasty. The operation removes fat and excess skin from either upper or lower eyelids or both, to correct bagginess and wrinkling. Blepharoplasty, which may be performed independently or at the same time as a face lift, is regarded by some plastic surgeons as the most gratifying of all cosmetic operations, for patient and surgeon alike.

In the procedure, which may be carried out under local or general anesthesia, an incision is made in the fold of the upper eyelid and excess skin and fat are removed. With a comparable incision below the lash line on the lower lid, the surgeon can elevate the skin, reach in and remove the fat, and then trim excess skin.

The operation involves a day's stay in the hospital. After surgery, the patient wears a dressing that is kept on when he goes home. He can see through a slit in the dressing. Four days after surgery, the dressing is removed and the stitches are taken out. The scars usually are inconspicuous. An expertly done operation may avoid puffiness and bagginess around the eyes for as long as ten years.

Hair Transplants

Although developed only during the 1960s, hair transplantations are now successfully performed as routine office surgery and are being sought by increasing numbers of men.

Baldness in men, except as a result of a few rare disorders, is inherited. Various patterns of baldness may develop, varying from slight thinning at the temples to virtually complete loss with only a fringe remaining on the sides of the head.

Hair transplantation is based on the fact that hair-bearing scalp, when transplanted from one area to another, retains the characteristics for hair growth of the area from which it was obtained. For example, if a graft is taken from behind the ear to the top of the forehead in a young man who later becomes bald, the transplanted section of scalp will continue to grow hair as long as the site from which it was obtained shows hair growth.

The procedure

Basically a simple procedure, hair transplantation is performed in the doctor's office. The patient is in face-down position, and a local anesthetic is injected to numb the area. With a small instrument connected to a motor-driven drill, small punch grafts are taken. With each punch of tissue, six to as many as eighteen hairs are obtained. The plug of scalp containing the hair follicles is cut off and if necessary the wound is sutured to control bleeding.

In the balding area, holes are made using the same punch or a slightly smaller one, also under local anesthesia. Bald-area plugs are discarded and the holes filled with the hair-bearing grafts.

Usually, in an hour-long session about forty to fifty grafts are placed. A dressing is applied for twenty-four to forty-eight hours. Generally there is only a slight aching during the first twelve to twenty-four hours, which can be relieved by aspirin or other mild drugs. In two or three days, the patient can shower. In most cases no sutures are needed in the front portion of the reconstructed bald region. Sutures in the back of the scalp are removed five to seven days after the operation. Further sessions of grafting are needed until the patient is satisfied with the thickness.

Many of the grafts retain the hairs, but most of the hairs

fall out and for a period of up to three months there is no growth. Then new hair will grow out.

Sometimes, in an extremely bald person, a hairline may be initiated with strips of hair-bearing scalp rather than with individual plugs. The strips, about one-quarter inch wide and up to three or four inches long, are taken from the back of the head and placed one on each side of the forehead. The area behind the strip grafts may be filled in with punch grafts.

Three to six or seven or more procedures may be needed, depending upon how thick the patient wishes the hair to be. The cost of transplants varies from about $5 to as much as $25 a plug, according to the area of the country. Transplanted hair will not usually provide a completely normal look but considerable improvement can be expected.

It is important for the patient to decide with the surgeon at the beginning where he wishes to have the new hairline and the results he wishes to achieve.

"Body Sculpture"

The most controversial of all cosmetic operations are those to reduce excessive abdomen, thighs, hips, and buttocks. Because these procedures can leave large scars and carry some risk of infection or serious and even potentially fatal blood clot, they are usually done in the United States only in cases of lipodystrophia, in which grotesque amounts of fat are deposited between waist and knees.

In an operation to reduce excessive abdomen, performed under general anesthesia, a crescent-shaped incision is made just above the pubic hair, running from hip bone to hip bone. The apron of tissue is pulled up and tissue, including fat, is removed, as much as ten pounds' worth. The apron is then trimmed, smoothed out, and the incision is closed with suturing.

In what is sometimes called the "riding breeches" operation—to correct a heavy, swelling pad of fat on the outer side of each thigh where it joins the buttocks—the patient, under general anesthesia, is placed on the stomach. A wedge-shaped section of skin and fatty tissue is cut out, with the incision running as much as two or three inches deep. Two flaps of skin at the edges of the excised area are created by partially severing these margins of skin from underlying connective tissue, and the flaps are sutured together. The operation may require three to five hours. Recovery is slow and often uncomfortable. For the first few days, the patient is swathed in elastic bandages from waist to knees and can sleep only on the stomach. The patient may go home from the hospital within a week but will not be able to sit down comfortably or return to normal activity for at least two more weeks. The scars will be wide and will look red for about six months.

Angiomas (Birthmarks)

Angiomas, localized skin lesions made up of overgrown blood or lymph vessels, occur in about one-third of new-born infants at birth or shortly thereafter. They vary in size. Many disappear spontaneously, but some persist and may create cosmetic problems.

Capillary hemangiomas, also known as port-wine stains, are flat pink to purplish discolorations. They usually do not fade, though splotchy small discolorations above the nose and on the eyelids may disappear. Many treatments such as ultraviolet therapy, electrodesiccation, cauterization, carbon dioxide snow, and liquid air have been tried and abandoned because of scarring and injury to skin. Many people find it helpful to use a makeup called Covermark, a heavy cosmetic base composed largely of zinc oxide, which covers excellently. In some cases, plastic surgeons have found tattooing treatment helpful; a white pigment is injected to block out the abnormal red in the area. Usually above five treatments at monthly intervals are required.

Immature hemangiomas, also known as strawberry marks, are raised, bright red areas which tend to enlarge slowly, but eventually disappear spontaneously. Treatment is unnecessary except when ulceration threatens or when the lesions are on or near the eye or a body orifice such as the urethra or anus. When treatment is needed, ionizing radiation is often recommended. Surgical removal, electrocoagulation, or application of dry ice may be used.

Cavernous hemangiomas are raised red or purplish marks which, in addition to blood vessels, may also contain fat and connective tissue. They usually do not disappear. Their surgical removal followed by grafting may be considered. Because they are rarely of medical importance, their treatment is justified only for good cosmetic reasons and if a satisfactory result is likely.

Lymphangiomas, elevated marks composed of lymphatic vessels, are usually yellowish tan but may be reddish if small blood vessels are also present in them. Some of the marks appear brownish in color and may be mistaken for warts. Treatment consists of electrocoagulation or surgical excision.

Salmon patches, also referred to as stork marks, almost never require removal. They are flat, pink hemangiomas which may appear in the skin over the bridge of the nose, on the forehead, or at the back of the neck, and usually fade within a year or so after birth, often leaving no indication at all that they ever existed.

Sterilization

Sterilization has become an increasingly popular method of contraception in the United States. Where, in the early 1960s, the total number of sterilization operations was estimated at 100,000 a year, more recently the number has multiplied tenfold.

Most sterilization procedures, until quite recently, were performed on women. Currently, it appears that the majority are being performed on men: it has been estimated that in one recent year, 300,000 female sterilizations were done in the United States, compared to about 800,000 male sterilizations.

As a method of birth control, sterilization is considered to be virtually 100 percent effective. The procedures—vasectomy for men and tubal sterilization for women—are considered to be almost 100 percent safe.

The major limitation of sterilization is its finality. The operations as currently performed cannot be successfully reversed, although there have been some reports of surgical correction and some scientists believe reversibility will be possible in the future. For the present, sterilization must be regarded as a means of ending reproduction and not as a means of child spacing.

According to a comprehensive report, "Voluntary Sterilization," prepared by Dr. Harriet B. Presser, assistant professor of sociomedical sciences at the International Institute for the Study of Human Reproduction and assistant professor of sociology at Rutgers University (published by the Population Council, 245 Park Avenue, New York, N. Y. 10017), a large majority of sterilized men and women are, in general, satisfied with the operation. A large majority also reported no change—neither increase nor decrease—in the amount of their sexual activity or desire after the operation.

When sterilization is requested, both the husband and wife are usually interviewed to make sure they are fully prepared to take the step. Many doctors refuse to perform the procedure on single men on the theory that they may regret the move if they marry later.

The cost of sterilization varies. For a woman, the operation may cost between $150 and $300; for a man, between $50 and $150.

Vasectomy

Male sterilization, or vasectomy, in the hands of an expert is a quick and relatively simple operation. Urologists, who specialize in genitourinary tract surgery, are usually especially qualified to perform it. It may be done in the doctor's office or the outpatient department of a hospital or in a vasectomy clinic.

Vasectomy means cutting of the vas deferens, or sperm duct (one on each side) and may be done under local anesthesia. Somewhat resembling a tiny, flexible soda straw, the vas deferens carries sperm from the testicles, where they are manufactured, to the area of the prostate gland, where they are mixed with other fluids before being ejaculated during sexual intercourse.

To reach the vas deferens, a small incision is made on each side of the scrotum. Through the incisions, each vas deferens is cut. Many urologists remove a small section to make the separation more certain. Each cut end is blocked off. This can be done by tying with nonabsorbable surgical thread, knotting the vas deferens itself, or cauterization. Thus the sperm cannot move through the duct to be ejaculated. With no place to go, the sperm, as with many other cells of the body, including blood cells for example, simply dissolve, and their components are absorbed back into the bloodstream.

Vasectomy takes from fifteen to thirty minutes. A scrotal suspensory is applied and the patient goes home. He may be advised to remain inactive for the rest of the day. After that, he may resume his usual activities, including intercourse.

Right after the operation, many sperm still remain in the duct system. So a supplementary contraceptive method must be used until the doctor is certain that all sperm have been ejaculated. It may take four to six weeks to accomplish this. At the end of this time, the doctor may have the patient provide an ejaculate sample, sometimes two samples, for testing to make certain that sterility has been achieved and other contraceptive methods no longer need be used. The urologist may also suggest examination of ejaculate at six-month intervals for a year or two to make certain that recanalization, the spontaneous growing together of the cut tubes, has not taken place. The incidence of such re-canalization is small, less than one in 200 cases.

Effects of vasectomy

Vasectomy should have no effects on sexual potency unless there are psychological complications which may stem from misunderstanding of the nature of the operation.

The male hormone responsible for virility, libido, sexual potency, and orgasm is produced by the testes. It is absorbed directly into the bloodstream at a site distant from where the operation is performed. The hormone and its functions are not affected by the operation.

The testes produce sperm which are transported through the two tubes to the penis from which they are discharged during orgasm. Vasectomy results only in interruption of the transport of sperm. The testes continue to form sperm which, as already noted, will be absorbed without harmful effects. The constituents of semen come from the seminal vessicles and prostate, and secretions from these organs will continue unchanged after vasectomy. The gross appearance of the semen will be essentially unchanged; the only change will be absence of sperm.

Some men may be emotionally upset by vasectomy. It appears that because virility is mistakenly equated with ability to father a child, sterility is confused with impotence. Most urologists agree that after adequate preoperative counseling, the psychological effects are nil or at most minimal.

Sterlization for Women

In women as in men, sterilization has the same objective: to block the path of reproductive cells so they cannot reach the uterus, where implantation occurs.

In a woman, the usual way to achieve this is through tubal ligation—tying the fallopian tubes, through which ova travel from the ovaries to the uterus.

The most convenient time to perform tubal ligation is immediately following childbirth. At that time, the fallopian tubes are higher in the abdominal cavity, very close to the navel, and thus more accessible. An incision several inches long can be made in the abdomen, the tubes can be reached and tied with sutures, and usually a small segment of each tube can be removed. If a baby has been delivered by Caesarean section, the operation is simpler since the abdomen is already open. In any case, tubal ligation after delivery does not usually prolong the period of confinement.

For a woman who has not just given birth, the standard type of tubal ligation has usually meant a three- to five-day stay in the hospital.

"Band-Aid" sterilization

A new technique now simplifies sterilization for women. It may be done during an overnight hospital admission or even on an outpatient basis. It makes use of a technique called laparoscopy, which previously has been employed for problems of female fertility and for diagnosis in other conditions.

The laparoscope is a fine optical telescope with "cold light" that can be inserted easily through a minute incision to explore the abdominal organs.

For sterilization employing the laparoscope, a general anesthetic may be used. A tiny incision is made below the navel, and the laparoscope is inserted. A second incision, which may be only 1/8th-inch long, is made. A second instrument, combining a tiny forceps and a cauterizing device, is inserted into the second incision.

Carbon dioxide gas is introduced into the abdominal cavity and later is removed through a valve in the laparoscope. The gas helps to push away the intestines so the surgeon has better access to the fallopian tubes.

While looking through the eyepiece of the laparoscope, the surgeon cauterizes each tube and cuts out a tiny piece of each tube. The entire procedure takes fifteen to twenty minutes. Both incisions are small enough to be covered with Band-Aids.

After the procedure, some surgeons report that about one-third of women act "as if nothing has happened," another third experience the equivalent of bad menstrual cramps but are able to resume normal activity, and the remaining third take a few days off to recover.

No sterilization technique is 100 percent successful. A rare failure may be caused by an undetected pregnancy. To avoid this, many doctors recommend that laparoscopy be done in the days immediately following menstruation.

Complications are rare. An occasional hemorrhage usually can be handled through the laparoscope. Laparoscopic sterilization is not usually recommended for extremely obese women or for those with severe heart or lung disorders, hernia, previous abdominal surgery with abdominal scarring or adhesions, or pelvic inflammation.

The operation also is being done with increasing frequency after abortions. It may add only five minutes to the abortion procedure.

The effects

After sterilization by tubal ligation a woman will continue to have normal menstrual periods until her menopause, which will occur just as it would if she had not had the operation. Each month her ovaries will produce an egg but the eggs will be blocked where the tubes have been cut. There, as with male sperm, the egg will disintegrate and be absorbed back into the body. There is no change in a woman's sex hormone production or in her sexual characteristics or satisfaction.

For a woman, no postoperative test is needed, since there is nothing corresponding to the reservoir of sperm in a man.

While there have been reports of occasional successful reversal of sterilization, as of now, for all practical purposes, the operation should be considered irreversible.

Most Blue Cross/Blue Shield, major medical and other medical plans now include voluntary sterilization in their covered services. Many hospitals now will provide the names of physicians who do sterilization procedures and the names of such physicians in individual communities throughout the country may also be obtained from the Association for Voluntary Sterilization, 14 West 40th Street, New York, N. Y. 10018. Information is also obtainable from the nearest Planned Parenthood affiliate, which can be found in your telephone directory.

Transplantation Surgery

Man has long dreamed of a time when diseased or damaged body organs could be replaced with healthy ones. At least part of that dream has become reality in recent years. Corneas of the eye, skin, and bone are transplanted successfully. Kidney transplants are used for patients otherwise doomed to die of irreversible kidney damage.

In efforts to save lives, attempts have been made, too, to transplant livers, lungs, hearts, and other organs, but thus far success has been limited; only a small percentage of recipients have survived for more than a few months. The operations have demonstrated that the transplantation of many vital organs is technically feasible and that transplanted organs are capable of functioning in their new sites.

A major problem to be overcome is the rejection phenomenon.

Rejection

Rejection is part and parcel of a body protective mechanism. When infectious organisms gain entry into the body. the defense system is alerted by antigens, chemicals produced by the organisms. White blood cells are rushed to the site. The white cells produce antibodies, chemicals able to lock onto and destroy the invading organisms.

The same system operates when a heart, kidney, or

321

other organ is transplanted. Organ cells, like bacterial or viral cells, produce antigens, inviting destruction by antibody-producing white blood cells.

At first, for a brief period, a transplanted organ may function well. It has a pink and healthy look. But, as white cells begin to attack, there may be inflammation and the functions of cells within the organ are disturbed, and organ cells may be destroyed. The organ begins to swell and, as an army of white cells infiltrate and overwhelm the transplanted tissue, the organ stops functioning, shrivels, and dies. It has been rejected.

Organs such as the cornea, skin, and bone can be transplanted successfully. In the case of the cornea, blood supply is not involved. In the case of skin and bone, the transplants serve as structual foundations into which new tissues grow.

In the case of intact organs such as kidney, heart, lung, liver, and pancreas, however, generous blood supply is required for their survival. As blood is drained from these transplanted organs, their antigens are circulated, and the rejection process gets under way.

Combating Rejection

Although transplantation efforts date back many years, it was not until 1954 that a successful internal organ transplant was achieved. A kidney donated by one identical twin was implanted in the other. Since they were identical twins, the brothers were identical in genetic makeup, and an organ from one was not looked upon by the body of the other as "foreign." The first successful transplant of a kidney between nonidentical twins came in 1958, and two more years were to elapse before there was a successful transplant between less closely related donor and recipient.

In efforts to prevent rejection, surgeons tried massive doses of radiation. But as the radiation destroyed the tissues that produce white blood cells, the patient was left without defense against disease germs and became prone to death from pneumonia or other infections.

Then, cortisonelike agents such as prednisone and some anticancer chemicals such as azathioprine (Imuran^R) were found to help suppress rejection. Combining these agents with low-dosage radiation, surgeons sought to find a happy medium, some combination capable of keeping an organ from being rejected without so impairing defenses that the patient died of infection. The goal was elusive.

Matching donors and recipients for better compatibility could help. A familiar form of matching is blood typing. Before blood transfusions, red cells of the recipient are classified so donor blood with the same type of cells can be used to avoid transfusion reaction, a kind of rejection process. And blood typing was of some limited usefulness for transplantations.

The matching of white cells proved to be more helpful. The idea behind matching is that the closer the compatibility between organ donor and recipient, the weaker the rejection process is likely to be, the less rejection-suppressing treatment will be needed, and the less likelihood there is of death from infection.

Matching techniques are being improved. More effective methods of combating rejection are also being sought. These include special serums that introduce antibodies directed against the white cells which turn out the antibodies directed against transplanted organs.

Kidney Transplantation

Since the first success in 1954, thousands of kidneys have been transplanted. Kidney transplantation is now the most frequent transplantation procedure.

Each year, thousands of people, many of them young, face uremia and death as the result of severe kidney disease. In uremia, toxic substances accumulate in the blood because of failure of the kidneys to excrete them normally.

Some patients who otherwise would die can be maintained in reasonable health for periods of years by chronic dialysis. Dialysis employs a mechanical apparatus to take blood from one blood vessel, pass it through a system of coils to remove components that would be removed by normally functioning kidneys, then return the blood to another vessel. This must be done one or more times a week.

Dialysis is costly, although costs can be considerably reduced by training patients to dialyze themselves at home. Some patients adjust to the psychological and physical stress and live virtually normal lives. About 80 percent of patients survive at least two years on chronic dialysis.

When transplantation is successful and the transplanted kidney functions properly, the recipient is returned to a near-normal life. At present, many patients receiving kidneys from nonidentical donors can expect to survive for prolonged periods (some possibly, for normal lifetimes, although data as yet are too scanty to determine this).

Chronic dialysis now is often used to maintain life until an optimal kidney becomes available for transplantation or when rejection destroys a transplanted kidney.

The events in kidney transplantation

Since the kidneys are paired organs and one healthy kidney can suffice, a kidney for transplantation may sometimes be obtained from a close relative. But with the increase in transplantation activity, there are not enough living donors. Kidneys from deceased persons must be used more often. Prime sources can be persons dying of brain disease or as the result of automobile and other accidents.

Cadavers can also be the source—and, in fact, must be— for other organs for transplantation, particularly unpaired organs such as heart and liver, which obviously cannot be removed from living people.

In such transplantations, a series of crucial events is involved—organ procurement, organ preservation, recipient finding, and transplant surgery itself. From the moment a donor organ becomes available, the precision timing of these events is essential.

Kidneys—and this is basically true of other organs—must be removed from the donor within sixty to ninety minutes after death. Without the circulation of fresh blood, the organs quickly deteriorate and the chance of their being transplanted successfully rapidly diminishes.

Obtaining viable organs is one of the most difficult aspects of transplantation. Unless a healthy person has specifically agreed to donate at death, the decision must be made by the next of kin when death is imminent.

If the decision is made in time, organs can be removed immediately after death. The surgical removal of the kidneys may take from ten or fifteen minutes to ninety minutes. Immediately upon removal, the organs are perfused with a fluid much like the fluid in cells of the body and are then placed in an ice-packed transporting container, where they can be safely preserved for up to five or six hours until placed in an organ preservation machine, where they may be kept for up to seventy-two hours before actual transplantation.

While the kidneys are being rushed to the preservation machine, lymph glands from the donor go to a laboratory for tissue typing to permit accurate matching of the organs with potential recipients who have the same or similar tissue types. Within four hours after removal of the organs from the donor, the search for "ideal" recipients can begin.

An example of the events involved in kidney transplantation is provided by the Transplantation Section at Rush-Presbyterian-St. Luke's Medical Center, Chicago.

Late on a Wednesday night, a fifty-one-year-old man died of a severe cerebral hemorrhage. When it became apparent earlier in the day that death was inevitable, his family offered to donate his kidneys, knowing that he would have wanted to do so. Twenty-three hours after his death, his kidneys were to become the legacy of life for two people with critical kidney failure.

After the kidneys were removed and preserved and the tissue typing was done, a check for compatibility was made against the records of more than 450 people in the Illinois area waiting for kidney transplants.

A perfect, or "A" match was found for one, but the potential recipient could not be reached; he was with his family somewhere in the South trying out their new camper-trailer. If he had been found, he would have had to make an immediate critical decision about leaving his family and flying at once to Chicago for surgery. On Thursday afternoon, another man with a close but not perfect match received the kidney.

At approximately the same time, the other kidney went to a thirty-two-year-old woman. When she was contacted by phone early Thursday morning in her home in Barrington, her blood was being filtered through a dialysis machine. Her physician told her to leave the machine and get to Presbyterian-St. Luke's Hospital within two hours.

While she was on her way, the operating room was prepared on an emergency basis for 4 P.M. A room was reserved on a floor with nurses specially trained to care for transplant patients. Six units of "washed" frozen blood were ordered from a blood bank. Because blood is in short supply and must be prepared for transplantation through a special "washing" procedure, it is prepared only just before surgery so that if surgery should be canceled no blood is wasted.

As surgery began, the blood was delivered to the operating room. Midway through the six-hour operation, the donor kidney arrived and was transplanted in time. Six to eight weeks later the woman was able to return to her family, and in about a month after that she was able to resume a fairly normal life, since all went well. The chances were four out of five that the kidney would function and could be kept functioning without rejection.

When a kidney transplant is rejected, dialysis may be used again until a second suitable kidney becomes available. Repeated kidney transplant operations are not common.

Heart, Liver, and Lung Transplantation

At this time, the kidney is the only vital internal organ that can be routinely transplanted with expectation of success. Transplantation of heart, liver, lung, and pancreas has been attempted with varying success.

Transplantation of these organs presents more difficult problems than those for kidneys. Being unpaired, except for the lungs, they cannot be taken from living donors. While lungs are paired, the risk and disability involved in lung donation for a living donor make it impractical. Cadaver organs are mandatory.

Replacement of such organs as the heart, lungs, and liver is also made much more difficult by the fact that there are no machines, as there are for kidney problems, to sustain a patient for many months until a suitable substitute organ can be found.

The first heart transplantation, which took place in Cape Town, South Africa, in 1967, used the heart of a girl automobile accident victim and added eighteen days to the life of a man dying of an irreversible heart condition. Since then, there have been more than 220 heart transplants. Only 41 recipients have survived beyond one year.

The disappointing record is a matter of medicine's inability so far to deal as effectively as necessary with rejection; it is not a matter of insufficient surgical technique.

Many years of laboratory research preceded the first human heart transplant. Repeatedly, animal hearts were transplanted with successful immediate results. A dog with a damaged heart, for example, could be placed on a heart-lung machine (see page 408), the heart could be removed, a healthy heart from a donor dog could be stitched in place, and with one quick electric shock the donor heart could be made to start beating effectively.

As a technical procedure, human heart transplantation was expected to be even simpler than dog heart transplantation because the human aorta, the great artery coming out of the heart, is sturdier than the dog aorta. If a dog aorta could be connected to a transplanted heart, it seemed likely that the human aorta could be. Additionally, there had been successful experiments in which hearts removed from people who had just died of massive brain injuries had been perfused with blood and stored for an hour, then made to beat again. As expected, when the Cape Town operation was performed, there was less trouble than with dogs but, as expected, the big problem was rejection.

There have been a few notable successes with heart transplants. Several patients have lived as long as five years. The exact reason for such occasional long-term successes is not known. There is some likelihood that by chance these patients were sufficiently similar genetically to the heart donors, in ways that may not yet be fully understood, so that the rejection process was unusually weak and could be combatted without unduly disarming the defense system.

Because of past inability to cope adequately with rejection, heart transplant procedures, 101 in 1968, were reduced to 47 in 1969, and to as few as 17 and 18 in subsequent years. More recently, however, there has been some increase in the number of procedures.

One reason for the revival is a system of selection that seems to assure that half or more of recipients can live at least a year. Preferred candidates for transplant are patients under fifty-five years of age, with effectively functioning kidney, liver, and other major systems, able to stand up to the shock of major surgery.

Another reason is what appears to be a significant technical advance—an instrument called a biotome. Essentially a length of wire with a clipper at the end, the biotome can be threaded into and through the jugular vein in the neck to the heart, where it takes a small sample of heart tissue. By allowing direct judgment of the rejection reaction through study of the heart tissue, the biotome helps avoid excessive use of drugs to combat rejection. In so doing it helps avoid crippling of the defense system against infection.

Another potentially promising development is antithymocytic globulin, which appears to be a more precise antirejection drug than another, antilymphocytic globulin, used earlier.

Surgeons working in the field of transplantation dream of the day when biochemists can produce an exquisitely precise antirejection drug that will protect transplanted hearts, kidneys, lungs, livers, and other vital organs, yet leave unweakened the body's ability to combat infection. Because many people are working on the problem, there is a growing conviction that the day may not be far away.

If liver transplantation should become routinely feasible, thousands of people yearly could benefit—people with diseased livers made useless by infections, cirrhosis, tumors, bile duct diseases, and other disorders. Similarly, effective lung transplantation could benefit thousands with crippling or fatal lung diseases.

Other Transplants

Children born with bone marrow disorders may be helped by bone marrow transplants from closely matched relatives. The marrow, the soft spongelike material in the cavities of bones, produces red and white blood cells. If the body's demand for white cells is increased because of infection, the marrow responds immediately by increasing production. It does the same if more red cells are needed, as in hemorrhage and some types of anemia. Bone marrow may be transplanted by mincing it and injecting it into a recipient's vein. Most of the marrow moves from vein to bones and settles in the marrow cavities where it is needed.

Successful thymus transplants have been achieved. The thymus, a gland in the neck, is involved in the body's system of defense against infection. When the thymus is defective, there may be inability to fight off pneumonia or other infection. To overcome this, donor thymus tissue has been inserted into an abdominal incision. More recently, a much simpler technique has been used with success. It involves injecting into the patient's thigh muscle thymus tissue from a twelve- to twenty-week-old fetus. Only a local anesthetic is required. The relative ease with which the transplant can be performed makes it possible to repeat it until it is successful and the patient can fight off infection. If the procedure is a success, the thymus will be rejected at some later time but the injected thymus fragments are expected to survive long enough to do their job, which is to "teach" the patient's own bone marrow cells how to fight common infections. Since the marrow cells have a long life span, they may protect for ten or more years, after which another thymus transplant may be done.

The Future

With the intense research now being carried out, it is almost certain that organ transplantation will become increasingly useful.

Under study are new techniques that may make possible longer preservation of donor organs, and new and more certain methods of matching, as well as more refined techniques for combating rejection. Also under study are computerized information storage-and-retrieval systems to facilitate transplants. As the results of transplantation procedures improve, there is likelihood of more people willing their bodies for transplantation use after death. In time, it is likely that the transplantation of many organs will become as feasible and routine when needed as other essential surgical procedures.

PART TWO

Some Important Basic Facts About Surgery

Surgery has become a modern giant of the therapeutic art. Perhaps no other single form of treatment deals definitively with so large a volume of painful, crippling and life-threatening diseases.

Between 40,000 and 50,000 operations are performed every day in more than 5,700 U. S. hospitals with surgical facilities. Surgery is the reason for more than half of all hospital admissions. Each year one in thirteen Americans has an operation.

At its best, American surgery is very good—quite possibly the best in the world.

There are virtually no age barriers any longer to surgical intervention if it is needed. In a single recent year for which figures are available, 1,998,000 children under age fifteen were discharged from hospitals after at least one operation. Many were young children, infants, even newborns, for whom surgery to correct congenital defects meant the difference between life and death.

In that same year, 4,718,000 people aged fifteen to forty-four years underwent surgery, as did 2,641,000 aged forty-five to sixty-four. Also in that year, 1,583,000 men and women aged sixty-five years and over benefited from operative procedures.

333

Surgery for the Aged

The ability of many elderly people to tolerate extensive modern surgical procedures is becoming established.

A recent study in a Louisiana community showed that of 131 elderly patients undergoing surgery for gallbladder disease, for example, 98 percent experienced marked improvement. Among the patients was a seventy-two-year-old woman who, in addition to gallbladder removal, required surgery for an abdominal aortic aneurysm, a dangerous weakening and ballooning out of the body's main trunkline artery; the diseased section had to be removed and replaced with a graft. She also required another procedure to remove a clot in a leg artery. She came through both quite well.

So did a sixty-five-year-old man who required gallbladder operation, removal of a duodenal ulcer, broadening of the passageway from stomach into duodenum, a nerve resection to reduce stomach acid secretion, closure of a perforation of the small intestine, and closure of a duodenal fistula.

The first open-heart operation on a patient over sixty was performed in 1957. Since then, at one institution alone, Texas Heart Institute in Houston, 292 such operations have been performed in patients from sixty to eighty-four years of age, with the results indicating that a patient of advanced age who needs open-heart surgery has a better than 85 percent chance of benefiting from it.

Older people, in addition to being susceptible to illnesses younger people may develop, are particularly susceptible to cancer and to degenerative diseases of the kidneys, heart, blood vessel, and pulmonary systems. Many of the disabling and life-threatening problems that affect the elderly can be corrected only by surgery. While age no longer, in and of itself, is a contraindication to a needed operative procedure, other disease conditions may be present and, if untreated, may increase the risk of surgery. Therefore, emergency operations tend to be riskier for the elderly in general than operations that can be done electively, with some preoperative preparation. The great majority of emergency operations do end successfully. But when time is available to bring under better control other conditions that may be present and to build up strength and recuperative power, the likelihood of success can be enhanced.

The Many Functions of Surgery

One function of surgery, of course, is to remove diseased tissues or organs. In any one year, among the millions of operations performed, there are 300,000 to remove diseased gallbladders, 350,000 to remove diseased uteri, about the same number of breast removals, and 225,000 intestinal operations.

Surgery has other functions as well. There are skin graft procedures to add needed tissue; a wide variety of birth or developmental deformities—harelip, cleft palate, clubfoot and many others—to be corrected; cosmetic procedures to remove moles or warts and more complex plastic surgery procedures for altering facial or other features. There are also vital-parts replacement procedures: diseased sections of blood vessels to be removed and replaced or bypassed with synthetic vessels; malfunctioning or nonfunctioning heart valves to be repaired or replaced; useless eye corneas to be replaced.

Safety

Surgery carries risk. There has been notable progress in reducing them.

A study at Columbia-Presbyterian Medical Center in New York City, shows a more than 80 percent decrease in surgical mortality for gastric ulcer in a ten-year period. At Baylor Affiliated Hospitals in Waco, Texas, the ten-year drop in mortality in peptic ulcer operations was greater than 80 percent. In children undergoing surgery for intestinal disorders, the mortality rate declined by two-thirds in three decades.

A study of more than 9,000 major operations performed in one medical center showed a steady decrease in surgical mortality spanning a period of three decades. The mortality rates for digestive and genital tract surgery fell 60 percent; and during the most recent five-year period covered by the study, the rate was consistently below 1 percent.

It is all the more impressive that the hazards of surgery have decreased—and continue to decrease—despite the greatly broadened scope of surgery that now includes conditions once considered inoperable, despite the increased complexity of some newer operative procedures, and despite the more frequent use of surgery for both infants and the aged.

There are many reasons for this: better training of surgeons; sophisticated new tools for use in surgery; improved methods of anesthesia that allow more time to be taken to insure precision and thoroughness in any procedure; new understanding of body processes and how best to maintain them even during extensive surgical procedures; improved methods of preparing patients for surgery, of preventing infections, and of helping them to recuperate afterward.

Recently a distinguished American medical journal editor at age eighty-two reviewed his own experience as a recipient of surgery, after having been at various times "scissored from stem to stern."

He recalled his tonsillectomy in 1912, a primitive knife-and-scissor operation. Only one tonsil was removed because of his loss of blood, which required an extended hospitalization. As he noted, a physician who had observed the tonsillectomy remarked that, "Here is a hell of a lot of blood but damned little surgery." Twelve years later, his other tonsil was removed in an efficient, quick, and relatively bloodless procedure with a snare.

In 1928 he had hemorrhoids removed. Because of the subsequent pain and swelling he required such immense doses of medication that he developed a serious, even potentially life-threatening, blood abnormality.

In 1956, in what he considers to be his "biggest performance as a surgical patient," he occupied the operating room for eight hours while his spleen was removed, six polyps were severed from his bowel, and a hernia was repaired. No problems.

Nor were there any when at eighty-two he required an operation for another hernia. Within ten days, even at that age, he was resuming the ordinary activities of a busy life.

The Natural Margin for Safety

Engineers designing machines like to build in overload capacity, a considerable extra margin for safety. Nature does too. It is the continuing discovery of how much safety margin Nature has built into the human body which has encouraged surgical approaches to problems not long ago regarded as hopeless—and it has allowed increasingly successful solutions to such problems.

The great reserve provided by the presence of doubled organs in the body—as in the case of kidneys, lungs, ovaries, testes—is obvious. But there have been insights into less obvious reserves. A fifth of a normal liver, for example, is enough to preserve life—and even less may do. It is now known that we can manage, if necessary, without a stomach, without a large bowel, and with less than a yard of small intestine!

It has been known that life can be maintained despite severe restrictions disease imposes on heart function. But no one ever dreamed that anyone could get along without the presence of two heart valves—the mitral and pulmonary —supposedly vital to keep blood flowing through and out of the heart and to prevent blood backup. Yet patients who have recently had one or both removed without prosthetic replacement are doing well.

Elective and Emergency

We touched briefly on elective versus emergency procedures in discussing surgery for the aged.

There are instances in which there is no alternative to immediate surgery. Victims of severe trauma—people hurt seriously in accidents, for example—often require surgery without delay to stop life-draining internal bleeding or damage to organs that can be fatal if not immediately countered. The least amount of delay offers greatest hope for many who have ruptured appendices, perforated ulcers, serious internal hemorrhaging from any cause.

But most surgical procedures—90 percent or possibly more —need not be rushed even when vital to save life. When, for example, a malignancy is amenable to surgical treatment, a delay of many weeks or months may add greatly to the danger or even prevent cure that might otherwise be possible. However, this is not true of a delay of days when such delay is needed to better prepare the patient for operation.

The elective category of surgery includes many types of operations for which there may be delay without undue risk—delay to a time when surgery is more convenient for the patient in terms of work or family situation, delay to provide time for medical correction of any other nonsurgical conditions that may be draining the patient's vitality, delay to provide time, even when such conditions do not exist, to nourish and otherwise prepare the patient optimally for the operation.

The elective category also includes surgery for conditions for which there may be medical alternatives. Medical advances have opened, and undoubtedly will continue to open, new opportunities for therapy that may, at least in some cases, avoid need for surgical intervention. Not long ago there was little other than surgery to control severe, rapidly advancing high blood pressure; now, even the most severe pressure elevation can often be controlled medically. Surgery is no longer the only practical means for attacking some serious thyroid gland problems. It is now possible in many cases to reduce the elevated fluid pressure of glaucoma within the eye with medical measures, avoiding operative intervention. There are now useful medical alternatives for other problems for which surgery once was essential—such as acute mastoid disease, or diabetic complications that once almost inexorably produced gangrene in and required amputation of one or both feet or legs.

Is Your Operation Really Necessary?

Recently a New York City labor union which administers its own health and welfare benefits found that it could reduce the amount of surgery performed on its members by having a second doctor review each recommended operation before it was performed. The second opinion resulted in 19 percent fewer operations than had been originally recommended. Of 289 members who had been told that they required surgery, 51 were later told that they need not undergo an operation.

The extent to which operations that aren't really essential are being performed has been the subject in recent years of many articles and books for the public and also of numerous articles in professional medical journals. A 1972 American College of Surgeons survey found that the great majority of surgeons who responded considered that unnecessary operations in their hospitals are either "very rare" or "uncommon" (occurring less than once a month). But 11 percent indicated that "operations of questionable value" take place in their hospitals once a week or oftener!

No one has any real doubt that the great majority of the approximately 15 million operations performed annually in this country are honestly recommended and skillfully performed. And there is little reason for most patients to worry when faced with need for emergency surgery or for obviously desirable nonemergency surgery.

But there is also little doubt that some operations not

340

really necessary are performed—and for many possible reasons.

The Decision For or Against Surgery

There are emergency situations, as noted in the preceding chapter, in which there is no choice but immediate surgery.

In other situations, however, the decision for or against surgery should be made logically, with full consideration of reasons pro and con.

How effective is medical treatment likely to be? How safe? How effective is surgery likely to be? How safe? Everything considered—including possibly age and general health and other factors pertinent for the individual patient—where does the best hope lie, the greatest possible gain?

Factors in Unnecessary Surgery

In surgery, as in other areas of medicine and in all professions and occupations, there are practitioners, relatively few, who can be considered outright charlatans, performing needless operations simply for the fees and, perhaps in some cases, because of an egotistical need to maintain full operating schedules.

There are also practitioners, relatively few again, deficient in what one critic, a surgeon himself, has called "surgical conscience." By that he means that, although judgment should be made exclusively on the basis of the needs of the patient, some surgeons may take other considerations into account and may, for example, be more likely to operate on insured than on uninsured patients.

Additionally, some surgeons perform unnecessary operations because they may know no better; they have not kept up-to-date on possible alternatives, on newer, nonsurgical methods of treatment.

There is another aspect to the problem.

A Kind of Parkinson's Law

One operation a year for every thirteen people—the overall rate in the U. S.—may seem like a considerable amount of surgery. And, in fact, it is twice the rate in England and Wales, for example. Not surprisingly, there are proportionately twice as many surgeons in this country as in England and Wales.

Why such a remarkable difference in surgical manpower and operative frequency? Do American surgeons operate too often or do British surgeons not operate often enough? It may well be that both are true to some extent. "It seems reasonable to assume that the United States, as a wealthier country, can afford the luxury of operations that are desirable but not essential," suggests Dr. John Bunker, Professor of Anesthesia at Stanford University.

That wealth is a significant factor in the distribution of surgeons within the U. S. is apparent. For example, the states of Alabama, Arkansas, Mississippi, and South Carolina have proportionately half the per capita income and half as many surgeons as the states of California, Connecticut, Massachusetts, and New York.

Prof. Charles Lewis of the University of California at Los Angeles, studied surgeons and operative rates in eleven population regions in the state of Kansas and discovered three- and fourfold variations in rates for such common procedures as appendectomy, gallbladder removal, hernia repair, and tonsillectomy. Lewis established that the numbers of operations varied directly with the numbers of surgeons and hospital beds. He suggests that this may indicate a kind of Parkinson's Law: as more health services are offered, more are used.

If that seems inconsistent with the public image of medicine as a precise and scientific discipline considering each illness as calling for a specific remedy, the image is not entirely accurate. Medicine is increasingly scientific. Its efforts are increasingly toward preciseness. But specific guidelines are not invariably available.

"In the absence of specific guidelines," observes Dr. Bunker, "doctors tend to favor active intervention. When in doubt, it is always preferable to do something rather than nothing —whether the something is operating or prescribing a drug."

Actually, guided by the strictest medical ethics, doctors can have differing opinions and approaches. Some tend to be more conservative than others about recommending surgery; some are more inclined to operate than to use nonsurgical methods. Both groups base their opinions and approaches on honest professional judgments.

The Patient Factor

It is unfortunately a fact that many patients do not know how to judge their needs or the quality of medical care they get. One study, carried out several years ago in a large number of hospitals in the New York City area by Columbia University researchers, found considerable differences in the quality of treatment. The study also discovered that three-fourths of the patients whose care was less than optimal felt they had received the best care possible.

When they are unable to judge needs or quality of care, patients often may consider that more care is better care, and their demands often tend to increase as their affluence does. "Again," says Dr. Bunker, "where there is doubt, doctors are apt to accede to their patients' demands."

Moreover, the blind faith of many patients, their failure to investigate the competence and background of surgeons, and their failure to exercise their right to question and explore a recommendation for surgery, may permit practitioners so inclined to get away with surgical exploitation.

Efforts to Reduce Unnecessary Surgery

There are controls over flagrantly unnecessary operations.

All hospitals accredited by the Joint Commission on Accreditation of Hospitals have tissue committees to review specimens of tissue taken from surgical patients as a check on whether operations that are performed are necessary. In such hospitals, there are often other procedures for regularly reviewing operations and for guarding against unnecessary surgery. A surgeon who performs unnecessary surgery may get by with a few flagrant violations, usually not many, before he is called on the carpet and warned that if he should continue to do such operations, he may lose his operating privilege in the hospital.

Of the more than 7,000 hospitals in the country, almost 5,000 are accredited. In the remaining hospitals, there may or may not be procedures for trying to control needless surgery.

The American College of Surgeons makes contributions to the control of unnecessary surgery through its representation on the Joint Commission on Accreditation of Hospitals and in other ways. It has stringent professional requirements for its membership, who are certified and privileged to use the letters F.A.C.S. (Fellow of the American College of Surgeons) after their names. The college may institute disciplinary proceedings against any Fellow charged with persistent unnecessary surgery. Through its sponsorship of continuous training for surgeons, the college also tries to assure that its membership keep abreast of latest developments in surgery and of medical advances that may help to determine need for surgery.

It is only realistic to recognize, however, that while much is being done to minimize needless surgery, the patient can and should do his part to insure that he is not rushed into an operating room without real need.

What You Can Do to Help Make
Certain Your Operation Is Necessary

Except possibly in dire emergency, don't be stampeded—or stampede yourself—into surgery.

Don't take for granted that surgery is essential; it may or may not be.

When possible, consult your family physician first rather than deciding on your own that you may need surgery and going directly to a surgeon. The family physician can exercise professional judgment, and if he finds that surgery may be advisable, can send you to a surgeon.

When you see the surgeon, ask him, without hesitation, to outline both the alternatives to the operation and the possible benefits and complications. If a surgeon seems to want to rush you into surgery in a situation that is clearly not an emergency, without discussing nonsurgical approaches or possible complications, be wary. You may do well to avoid a surgeon who is too busy to give you enough time and attention to answer your questions.

It is helpful to remember that a good ethical surgeon is usually not interested in increasing an already adequate work load and that he spends much of his time both in carefully selecting patients who really need and can benefit from surgery and in recommending nonsurgical treatment when in doubt about the effectiveness of surgery.

You may have read of tendencies to perform too routinely certain classes of operations—among them, hysterectomies, hemorrhoidectomies, and tonsillectomies. Others sometimes mentioned include removal of symptomless varicose veins, thyroid surgery, and spinal disk surgery. If yours is to be one of these operations, you may want to be especially convinced that it is really necessary and the gain to be expected outweighs whatever risk may be involved.

The risk factor should not be brushed aside. As we have seen earlier, with advances in surgical and anesthetic techniques, the hazards of surgery have been drastically reduced, in some cases almost to the vanishing point.

But even minimal risk should be considered, especially when there is any doubt about real need for an operation. Even a tonsillectomy carries some risk. There were more than 1 million tonsillectomies performed in the U. S. in 1972; only 300 patients died as a result of these operations. But that is small consolation if your child is one of the fatalities, especially if the operation was not really essential.

If you have any doubts remaining about the need for a recommended nonemergency operation, don't hesitate to get a second opinion. A second independent surgeon whom the first surgeon or your family physician may suggest may see some aspects of your problem in a different light and may see it as solvable by nonsurgical measures. It could be all to the good, too, if, like the first surgeon, he considers that an operation is advisable, thus helping to resolve your doubt so you can prepare for and enter into surgery more confidently.

Do you have a right to consultation or second opinion? You certainly have. Competent, ethical surgeons will be among the first to tell you so. In no uncertain terms, Dr. William R. Barclay, assistant executive vice-president of the American Medical Association, advises: "Patients should realize that they're the boss, since they are purchasing a service. If the patient wants to get another doctor's opinion, he should feel no embarrassment about it."

Some authorities suggest that you can be guided by a surgeon's reaction to your request for a second opinion: if he indicates you have insulted him by such a request, that the request indicates lack of confidence in him, such a reaction may be all the more reason for seeking a second opinion and, if operation is still indicated, another surgeon to perform it.

On the other hand, do not let such a reaction steer you from a surgeon who, you have established, is technically best equipped to perform the operation. Some topflight surgeons feel that unquestioning patient confidence is essential in their relationship.

When you're convinced that surgery is necessary, check out your surgeon's qualifications. You will find information about how to do this—and about considerations that may enter into choice of the hospital—in the following chapters.

Choosing the Surgeon

The most important single factor in the success of any operation is the choice of a surgeon. Yet most people are uncertain about how to make the choice. Often the recommendation of a friend or neighbor is accepted and an appointment made without further investigation. Sometimes a name is chosen at random out of the classified telephone directory.

Under ordinary circumstances, it is best to have a family doctor and to call upon him first in every illness. If surgery may be needed, he will suggest a surgical consultant to confirm the diagnosis and perform the operation. If you have a well-established relationship with a family physician and confidence in him, you will have a considerable degree of confidence in the competence of a surgeon he suggests. Even then, you may wish—and it is entirely proper—to reassure yourself by checking on the surgeon's qualifications and evaluating him in other ways.

But you may not have a family physician. This is the case for many families who move from one community or neighborhood to another where there may be a shortage of family doctors.

Thus, it is important to know what qualifications to seek in a surgeon and how to go about making a wise choice.

Erroneous Image and True

Movies and television often convey an oversimplified image of surgery. It is an image of doctors and nurses, masked and gowned, huddled over a patient in a floodlit operating room.

Even dictionaries may underscore this image, defining surgery as "the art, practice, or work of treating diseases, injuries, or deformities by manual operation of instrumental appliances."

Yet surgery, while often portrayed only in an operating-room setting, is much broader and deeper in scope. It is really total medical care. In addition to problems and challenges unique to the operating room, the surgeon must master those which confront all physicians. He must accurately diagnose the patient's condition, determine whether an operation is needed, and if it is needed, which type of operation is most suitable. Only when he and the patient are in the operating room does the surgeon primarily use deft fingers and manual skills.

Once the operation is over, the surgeon's responsibility does not stop. He is charged with managing the patient's postoperative care and with following the patient to full recovery.

In short, the surgeon should be a physician, trained and experienced in total patient care, and who is also an expert in surgery.

Who Are Surgeons?

After earning his M. D. degree, any doctor can legally operate. He is licensed as a "physician and surgeon." Only about 60,000 of the country's 300,000 physicians have had special training in surgery.

Once surgeons were shamans or priests; then, barbers; during most of the last century in this country, they were self-taught. The change from do-it-yourself training and qualification to special licensing and certification took many years.

Every physician does, in fact, receive some training in certain aspects of surgery during medical school and internship. In the past, such general training plus experience gained in practice was considered enough to allow physicians to carry out at least simpler procedures such as tonsil or appendix removal.

But as surgery has broadened its domain to include every body area, as surgical techniques have become increasingly complex, more and more training has become essential.

Today, to qualify for specialized practice in general surgery or in one of the surgical specialities, a young medical school graduate goes on to four or more years of special training and in many instances may take still more training.

After completing specialized training, the surgeon is eligible for examination by one or another of the boards in the various surgical specialties or for Fellowship in the American College of Surgeons.

The Boards

Beginning in 1937, American Specialty Boards were set up by prominent surgeons, mostly medical school professors of surgery, to examine and certify surgeons for the one purpose of providing for the public, hospitals, medical schools, medical societies, and the medical profession lists of specialists meeting high standards of education, training, and competence.

Each specialty board carries out rigorous examinations. oral, written, and clinical, for candidates, who must have completed required surgical residencies before they are permitted to take the examinations. Some boards send out representatives to observe the operative skills of candidates. It is not unusual for a specialty board to fail as many as one-third of applicants on their first attempt at qualifying.

A doctor who has completed his prescribed hospital residency and is in the process of examination is "taking his boards." If he passes and is certified, he "has his boards," and is referred to as a diplomate of the particular board.

To assure the proper functioning of the individual boards, there is an overall Advisory Board for Medical Specialties, made up of representatives from the Association of American Medical Colleges, American Hospital Association, American Medical Association, Federation of State Medical Licensing Boards, and the National Board of Medical Examiners.

The principal surgical specialties include:

General Surgery: operations for the most part within the abdominal and chest cavities and occasionally other specialized procedures.

Neurological Surgery: operations involving the skull, brain, spinal cord, and nerves.

Obstetrics and Gynecology: childbirth and operations on the female reproductive organs. Since some problems of the reproductive organs may produce symptoms indistinguishable from those produced by diseases of other abdominal organs, the work of gynecologist and general surgeon may sometimes overlap.

Ophthalmology: operations on the eye and optical structures, including removal of cataracts, relief of glaucoma, correction of crossed eyes, and other eye and eye muscle disorders in children and the young, and repair of eye injuries.

Orthopedic Surgery: surgical treatment of injury and diseases of the musculo-skeletal system, including reconstructive operations for disabling conditions of spine or extremities and treatment of fractures, dislocations, and other injuries to bone.

Otolaryngology: surgery of the ear, nose, and throat, including removal of diseased or enlarged tonsils and adenoids, operations to relieve hearing impairment and other disorders and to remove tumors of larynx, mouth, and nearby areas, and reparative and reconstructive operations.

Pediatric Surgery: Operative treatment of diseases of children.

Plastic Surgery: Operative treatment to repair, restore, correct, or improve defects of the body.

Proctology: Treatment of colon and rectal conditions.

Thoracic Surgery: Operations within the chest, such as those on heart, lungs, and great blood vessels.

Urological Surgery: Operations of the kidneys, ureter, and bladder, and male genital tract.

F.A.C.S.

The American College of Surgeons, established in 1913, admits as Fellows only well-trained surgeons whose backgrounds, ethical standards, and professional abilities have passed review. Through local and national meetings and many postgraduate courses given under its auspices, the college encourages continuing education of its Fellows.

Checking a Surgeon's Qualifications

The qualifications and backgrounds of surgeons are matters of record. There are various directories, one or more of them to be found in most public libraries, which you can consult to determine a surgeon's age, educational background, board certification, and whether he is a Fellow of the American College of Surgeons. The directories include the American Medical Association Directory, the Directory of Medical Specialists, the Directory of the American College of Surgeons, and directories of special surgical societies and associations.

Board certification and Fellowship help to assure competence. But a surgeon who lacks certification or Fellowship is not necessarily a poor one. He may be a brilliant young surgeon, already highly experienced, even though he has not passsed through all the steps on the way to certification and Fellowship. In some cases, he may be an older man who, because of special circumstances, has not taken his boards but has earned the respect of the local medical community, including your own personal physician, for his excellence.

Other Factors in Choice of a Surgeon

Sometimes the choice of a surgeon may be influenced by desire to have an operation performed in a particular hospital. Surgeons, like other physicians, have staff privileges in certain hospitals, not necessarily in all. And if the desire to go to a particular hospital weighs heavily with you, you will need to choose a surgeon who has staff privileges at that hospital. Your family doctor may be able to recommend such a surgeon or the hospital in question can do so.

Some surgeons have acquired great fame for their accomplishments. Sometimes, while they have achieved excellent results, their skills may in reality be no greater and their results actually no better than those of many other surgeons. Their fame may have stemmed from the fact that they operated successfully on celebrated patients.

You may wish to employ a famed surgeon and travel a distance to do so. Should you? There is no simple answer. Many things have to be taken into consideration. Your family physician may believe strongly that one or another of several competent local surgeons can do well what needs to be done. Finances may be a consideration. Your insurance coverage may or may not extend to costs of travel. There is considerable likelihood that a nationally renowned surgeon has a very busy schedule and there may be a delay before he can get to you. Is your condition such that the delay is of no consequence?

Certainly the skill of a surgeon is a most important consideration but other factors enter into the wise choice of a surgeon.

As in medicine, so in surgery, rapport between doctor and patient plays no small part in a successful outcome. If the rapport is good, if you have a feeling of confidence in the surgeon, your mental and emotional outlook in advance of and after surgery is likely to be good and helpful in making things go more smoothly.

It may not always be possible to warm in an instant to a surgeon, nor is that a prime requisite. But if he rubs you the wrong way, if anything about him, about his attitude toward you, about the way he examines you on your first visit with him, bothers you, you may do well to consider another choice. You are not obligated to use him as your surgeon. You may pay his bill for the consultation, indicate that you wish to think over the operation, and go on to see another surgeon.

Just as do other medical men and in fact all people, highly competent surgeons differ in the way they relate to people. Some take refuge in surgical mystique, preferring to keep their work a mystery. If their patients cannot understand what they are talking about, they won't ask questions, and there is that much less bother.

Ideally, a good surgeon should try to spell out things simply for his patients. Many patients make better recoveries when they understand what a surgeon tells them.

Some doctors, surgeons among them, are guilty of a kind of unmeant male chauvinism, which some women may find annoying, even to a considerable degree. As one surgeon has observed quite honestly, when confronted with a man with a stomach ulcer requiring surgery, he will spend fifteen minutes, half an hour, all day if necessary, explaining the problem to him and the proposed treatment. "He's a man and I feel he wants to know and has a right to know all the facts. On the other hand, if I see a woman who needs her gallbladder removed, I'm inclined to take a paternal attitude. I'll tell her, 'Just leave everything to me.' Then, when she has left, I'll call her husband and explain everything."

"This," the surgeon acknowledges, "is medical protectionism: the doctor taking a paternal, protective attitude toward his women patients while treating his men patients as equals." As he sees it, this seems to many male doctors the natural thing to do: to shield female patients from worries. "But," he adds, "it's unfair and it has to change. Women have as much right as men to know what's going on in their bodies, what the doctor proposes to do about it, and why."

If you're a woman and a surgeon treats you in what you consider a male chauvinistic way, the chances are that he doesn't realize he is doing so and may well accede graciously to your request to treat you as a first-class citizen. If not, and you are considerably disturbed by his attitude, you can find another surgeon.

It is worth noting here that adverse comments of friends or relatives about a surgeon may have to be weighed carefully. People sometimes are influenced, mistakenly but understandably, in their view of a surgeon by their own hospital experience. Even a minor unpleasantness unrelated to the surgeon—a brush with a nurse or nurse's aide or an orderly or anyone in the hospital hierarchy, for example—may so color the whole experience that it is reflected in a dim view of the caliber of the surgeon.

Even for what you may consider a minor operation, you have every right, and will do well, to choose your surgeon thoughtfully rather than on impulse—giving heed to the informed recommendation of your family physician and perhaps to the recommendation of knowledgeable friends or relatives, checking for yourself on the surgeon's background and qualifications, and considering, too, your own feelings of confidence and liking.

Should your operation be performed by a general practitioner? Some general practitioners may be competent at some types of surgery even though they have not had the extended formal training and experience of the specialist.

If your personal doctor advises an operation and suggests that he can perform it himself, you might ask several questions: How many times has he performed that operation? Does he feel that he can do as skillful a job as a specialist in surgery? What are the risks? You may find that you have doubts after getting the answers, including possibly some doubts about the necessity for the operation.

You can always insist upon seeing a specialist for his opinion or upon going to the nearest medical center for examination and recommendations even if you have to travel some distance to the specialist or center. You may be told that the operation is, indeed, needed, and that your doctor and the local hospital facilities are equal to the task, and if so, fine.

The fact is that in some areas general practitioners remove tonsils, gallbladders, appendices, and uteri and may perform other operations as well. But training does count. I recall the comment of a distinguished physician, the head of a major medical center, not a surgeon and with no particular ax to grind: "In the hands of a gynecologist, a woman with a cancer of the cervix has an 80 percent chance of a cure; in the hands of someone who is not specially trained, the chances are only 50 percent."

The Hospital

A surgeon can operate only in a hospital where he has staff privileges. So if yours has privileges in just one hospital, you must accept that hospital or look for a different surgeon. Often, however, a surgeon has multiple appointments, and he may state a preference—perhaps for a hospital convenient to his office, perhaps for one with special facilities that may be helpful in your case. Patients usually follow a surgeon's recommendations, but the ultimate decision is yours.

Famed Hospitals

In any discussion of outstanding hospitals—and such discussions are often found in newspapers and magazines—one invariably hears such names as these:

Massachusetts General, Boston; Johns Hopkins, Baltimore; St. Mary's, Rochester, Minn. (used by surgeons of the Mayo Clinic); University of Chicago, Chicago; Columbia-Presbyterian, New York City; New York Medical College, Flower and Fifth Avenue Hospital, New York City; New York Hospital, New York City; Mount Sinai, New York City; Barnes, St. Louis; Henry Ford, Detroit; Palo Alto-Stanford, Palo Alto, Calif.; Yale-New Haven, New Haven, Conn.; University Hospital, Ann Arbor, Mich.; University of Minnesota Hospital, Minneapolis; Duke Hospital, Durham, N. C.; Montefiore Hospital, New York City; University Hospitals, Cleveland; Michael Reese, Chicago; Cedars-Sinai, Los Angeles; Methodist Hospital, Houston; Peter Bent Brigham, Boston; Strong Memorial Hospital of the University of Rochester, Rochester, N. Y.; Hospital of the University of Pennsylvania, Philadelphia; University Hospital, Seattle; University of California Medical Center, San Francisco; Presbyterian-St. Luke's, Chicago; University Hospital, Birmingham, Ala.; Cleveland Clinic Hospital, Cleveland; New York University Medical Center, New York City; Vanderbilt University Hospital, Nashville; Baylor University Medical Center, Dallas; Beth Israel Hospital, Boston.

This is by no means a complete list of celebrated hospitals, most of which have certain things in common. They tend to be large; with few exceptions, they have between 500 and 1,000 beds. They have a full scope of services. They are nonprofit hospitals. They are also teaching hospitals, connected with medical schools. With bright, alert, always questioning young residents and interns looking over specialists' shoulders, in teaching hospitals there is a kind of fishbowl atmosphere, with everything under scrutiny.

Not so many years ago, only the largest cities could provide facilities where major surgery could be carried out with adequate skill and safety. If a small city did have a well-trained surgeon, it might lack a hospital with sufficient laboratory and other equipment to enable the surgeon to provide the best of care.

Today, however, in many smaller cities there are excellent hospitals. They may not have all the facilities of large hospitals in major metropolitan centers, and for certain types of operations—for example, brain surgery, special orthopedic operations, or surgery of the heart—they may refer patients to the large centers. But, with such exceptions, many smaller hospitals can provide facilities with which skilled surgeons can work well.

Community Hospitals

Of the more than 7,000 registered hospitals in the U.S., more than 5,000 are community hospitals supported by contributions and charges for services. Almost 90 percent of these have 300 or fewer beds. Most are located in small cities and towns.

Although the achievements of the major medical centers are renowned, the average citizen still gets his health care and often his surgery in his hometown hospital. How good that care is depends upon a number of factors: the caliber of the hospital staff; the capabilities of the administrators; the work of volunteer boards of managers and trustees; public support for equipment. How good the care is may well depend, too, upon whether or not the hospital is accredited (see below).

Ownership

There are three basic types of ownership—government, voluntary, and proprietary.

Government-owned hospitals include federal hospitals, which usually limit admission to certain categories of people such as veterans and servicemen; state institutions, which are largely mental hospitals; and municipal hospitals, which admit anyone in need of their care, with payment expected from those who can afford to pay.

Voluntary hospitals are private but nonprofit. Their primary reason for existence is to provide care and, in some cases, to teach physicians and other health professionals.

Proprietary hospitals are operated for profit. They may be owned by a large corporation or by an individual or group of people, often doctors.

Authorities often argue that because voluntary hospitals do not need to make a profit, they are unlikely to cut corners, whereas perhaps some proprietary hospitals may do so. They suggest too that there is some possibility for conflict of interest in physician-owned proprietary hospitals if a doctor, in addition to a fee for treatment, makes a profit from hospitalization. Yet physicians sometimes have no choice but to build their own proprietary hospitals when funds for a voluntary hospital cannot be raised by fund drives, taxes, or bond issues.

Teaching Hospitals

A hospital may be closely affiliated with a medical school. Its services are run or supervised by the medical school faculty, and its staff must meet standards of the school. Generally, standards in a school-affiliated hospital are high.

A school-affiliated hospital is often a teaching institution. Medical students may be assigned to it for instruction. The medical school faculty may regularly provide continuing education for the hospital's doctors. It may have internship and residency programs.

There are teaching hospitals which are not affiliated with medical schools. They have internship and residency programs, which must be approved by the American Medical Association and a specialty board. Teaching hospitals, affiliated or not, must have a staff of attending physicians of high enough quality to teach interns and residents who provide care for hospital patients when senior doctors are not present. Standards in such hospitals are likely to be high.

Accreditation

Both voluntary and proprietary hospitals can be accredited.

An accredited hospital is one which has been approved by the Joint Commission on Accreditation of Hospitals, and the accreditation means that the hospital has met and continues to meet a series of standards that promote the delivery of quality care and help safeguard the patient.

The commission is sponsored by four organizations in the hospital and medical fields: the American College of Physicians, American College of Surgeons, American Hospital Association, and American Medical Association, each of which has representatives on a twenty-two-member Board of Commissioners.

Standards set by the commission cover areas of hospital operation ranging from a hospital's board of directors to its meal service.

To help insure safety and cleanliness, the commission requires fire-resistant construction and use of equipment as close to fireproof as possible; it also sets cleanliness standards that apply to personnel and to bathrooms, kitchens, laundries, hallways, and other physical facilities.

Since a hospital houses patients with a wide variety of problems, infection is an ever-present possibility and its prevention and control are considered continuing responsibilities. Each accredited hospital is required to provide a mechanism for investigating any infections and finding ways to control and prevent them.

Joint Commission standards require that every patient entering a hospital have a medical record established for him which must include a health history and report of physical examination, diagnosis of cause for admission, results of tests and examinations, documentation of all surgical procedures and medical treatments, reports on all tissues removed during surgery, notes by physicians and nurses on the patient's progress during the hospital stay.

One reason for the medical record is to make certain that if a physician cannot continue care, either because of illness, death, or other circumstance, another physician can quickly familiarize himself with the patient's problems and continue necessary treatment.

The record also permits committees of the medical staff to review the care given and to make recommendations about how individual physicians as well as the entire staff can improve quality of practice.

One of the committees which an accredited hospital must maintain is a tissue review committee. In most hospitals, the committee is made up of at least three doctors from the staff, one being the hospital pathologist, whose specialty is the recognition of abnormalities in tissue caused by various diseases. All tissue taken from a patient during surgery is checked by the pathologist to determine whether the preoperative diagnosis is confirmed by the tissue findings, a check which indicates to the tissue review committee whether the surgery was justified.

If an error was made and healthy tissue was removed without cause, the surgeon is asked to explain his actions to the committee. A surgeon who performs several questionable operations may be called before the executive committee of the hospital medical staff. If violations are flagrant, the surgeon may be barred from further practice at the hospital. While a tissue committee is not infallible, the presence of one helps over a period of time to make unnecessary operations less likely.

Under accreditation requirements, a hospital must have an organized medical staff which develops by-laws, rules, and regulations. A physician who wishes to admit patients to the hospital must first apply for membership on the staff. His application is considered on the basis of his professional experience, ability, judgment, and competence. The hospital decides not only whether to admit him but also as to which treatments and procedures he is competent to perform. In some cases, he may be permitted to perform certain procedures only under direct supervision of a more qualified physician who can take over completion of the procedure if complications should develop.

Where a surgical operation may represent an unusual hazard to life, the Joint Commission requires that at least two physicians be present, one who performs the operation and a second designated as qualified to assist by the appropriate committee of the medical staff. The operating surgeon determines whether an unusual hazard to life may be present; his decision is subject to review by a Surgical Evaluation Committee; a surgeon who repeatedly abuses the requirement faces disciplinary action.

Generally, you can consider that accreditation is more important to you than the fact that a nonaccredited hospital may have an imposing building or be reputed to serve excellent meals. Your doctor or the county or local medical society can tell you whether a hospital is accredited. You can also obtain this information from the Joint Commission on Accreditation of Hospitals, 200 East Ohio Street, Chicago, Illinois 60611.

New Developments in Hospital Care

Faced with the problems of rising costs and also recognizing the continuing need to find better mechanisms for providing good care, many hospitals try new approaches. Sometimes the experiments do not work out and are abandoned. Sometimes an experiment's results are so quickly and clearly seen to be desirable that other hospitals very rapidly adopt the procedure. At other times the spread of use is slower, so what we discuss here may not always be generally available.

A Seven-day Work Week

A seven- rather than a five-day work week for hospitals has been suggested as a way to greater effectiveness of service and control of costs.

Among the possible advantages of a full work week are: reduction of delay in waiting for services, more efficient use of beds and equipment, shorter average patient stay, fewer beds needed to care for the same number of patients, more even distribution of nurses' work loads.

There are obstacles. Trying to change local customs of working Monday through Friday is often not easy. In some cases there is also a problem of shortage of personnel.

Pre-admission Testing

Commonly, whatever the reason for hospital admission, a patient has first been admitted and then put through a necessary series of tests. But increasingly it is now possible for patients to have these tests made on an outpatient basis before admission, and insurance plans that once did not cover such testing now do so.

Pre-admission testing can save the cost of room and board for one or more days of testing after admission. It also reduces the length of separation from home and family. Sometimes, too, the tests may indicate that no inpatient care is needed and thus may avoid unnecessary hospitalization.

Early Discharge

Some hospitals have been finding that after certain operations a considerable proportion of patients can be discharged without ill effect much earlier than long thought possible.

In the experience of many hospitals now, the postoperative stay of many patients undergoing appendectomy, gallbladder removal, hernia repair, or hemorrhoidectomy can be shortened by one-third to one-half of the customary hospital convalescence, when the patients live in favorable socio-medical environments.

In many hospitals, some patients who need certain types of surgical procedures, including women who need dilation and curettage (D & C) and patients requiring minor plastic surgery, can enter the hospital in the morning, leave the same evening, and in between get all the services, including anesthesia, laboratory testing, and recovery room care, available to inpatients. Some hospitals have also found that one-day surgery, in in the morning and out in the evening, is feasible and even desirable for some children requiring ear, hernia repair, or minor plastic surgery procedures.

Minimal Care Units

More than 400 hospitals now have minimal or self-care units for patients hospitalized for diagnostic tests, surgery preparation, minor surgery, convalescence and long-term care. Since they do not need the same type of care as acutely ill patients, they should not have to pay the same costs.

In a self-care unit, an alternative for the walking patient, costs may be cut almost in half. In most such units, patients are encouraged to bathe and dress themselves, get their own meals in a central dining room, in some cases administer their own medications, and in some cases attend classes related to their illness.

In addition, some hospitals with such units provide accommodations, at minimal cost, to a patient's family members, who may want to stay overnight or longer to learn any home-care procedures that may be needed after hospitalization. And at least one hospital has a self-care unit with a kitchen where patients can prepare their own meals if they choose not to use the hospital cafeteria!

Special Provisions for Children

Recently, an increasing number of hospitals have been taking steps to make hospitalization an experience less likely to arouse undue fears and anxiety in children. Many measures are used and they may differ from one hospital to another, but all are helpful.

An outstanding example of the trend is the program at Johns Hopkins in Baltimore, which has a staff of nineteen psychiatrists, pediatricians, nurses, and others devoted solely to children's psychic needs before and during hospitalization. The effort is to make a child see his hospital stay as an adventure.

To help allay fears before admission, each child receives an attractive coloring book at home, explaining in simple terms how the hospital is set up, what his room will look like, and how various instruments and procedures are used to help children get well. The book's tone is positive and cheerful but also forthright. For example, in one picture a little boy about to get an injection is shown in tears and the accompanying text advises: "Yell 'ouch' if you want to but try to be very still. It helps to grit your teeth or hold tightly to something."

Upon admission, a child is introduced to doctors and nurses who will care for him and, if scheduled for surgery, is taken on a tour of operating and recovery rooms. He is told, sometimes with the aid of puppets, what will be done and how he will feel. He is allowed to touch and even play with a stethoscope and other objects that may be used in his treatment. If, sometimes an older child facing a heart operation or other serious operation has questions about the risk, they are answered; he is told that the objective is to operate so he can lead a normal life, and the child usually agrees that the risk is worth taking.

In the Hopkins program, a parent is allowed to "room in" with the child. The arrangement, available in many hospitals now, permits the parent to sleep in the child's room in a chair that converts to a cot. Rooming in, in many cases, has proved helpful for a child undergoing surgery. But much depends upon the parent and his or her ability to be cheerful, optimistic, reassuring. If you are such a parent and feel strongly about the desirability of rooming in, availability of the arrangement may be a factor in your choice of a hospital.

Arranging for Hospital Admission

Except in an emergency, your surgeon will arrange for your admission to the hospital. Usually, you will receive in the mail a pre-admission form from the hospital for you to complete and return in order to save time when you are admitted. When you go to the hospital on the pre-arranged day and hour (sometimes the hospital may call you on the day of admission to tell you exactly when to come), you sign in at the admissions office, check any valuables you may have forgotten to leave at home, receive your identification bracelet, and are taken to your room.

Upon arriving in your room, familiarize yourself with your surroundings. Many hospitals provide printed information about hospital services, meal times, mail delivery schedule, telephone use and cost, smoking restrictions, and other matters; if such printed information is not available, ask questions of the person who takes you to your room.

What to Take Along

For one thing, bring your hospital insurance card or policy. You will probably want some cash for newspapers, magazines, stationery, stamps, other incidentals—but not a large sum. Bring your checkbook to settle your bill.

Hospitals provide gowns but you can, if you like, bring your own nightgowns, or pajamas and it is a good idea to bring your slippers and a bathrobe, toiletries, writing materials, reading matter, and a small clock. Leave valuables at home. Usually, a radio or TV set is provided, sometimes for a small rental fee, which is usually indicated in literature that comes with your pre-admission form.

What Kind of Room

In many hospitals, you may have a choice ranging from a private room with bath to a multibed ward. If you have a distinct preference for a private room, you may be able to arrange for that.

It is a good idea to discuss the matter of room choice with your surgeon not only on the basis of what you would like and can afford but also what you may need. For example, if after surgery your care will require frequent visits by nurses and technicians around the clock, a private room may be indicated.

If finances permit and you are a person who prefers complete privacy, you will, of course, do best to choose a private room. Many people, however, prefer not to be alone and if you are one of them, you may wish to choose a semiprivate room or ward.

Most hospital insurance coverage provides for semi-private room accommodations, and you will usually be required to pay the difference between the cost of a semi-private and a private room if you prefer the latter.

Who's Who: The Hospital Hierarchy

Your own doctor has prime authority for your case, and all other hospital personnel assist in whatever is necessary according to his instructions.

There will be many people in the hospital whom you will never see: dietitians, bookkeepers, laboratory workers. But you will come into daily contact with a certain number of people.

You will get to know staff doctors—residents and interns—in a teaching hospital. Their functions include caring for you as necessary according to the directions of your doctor when he is not in the hospital.

Next in the chain of command under the staff doctors are nurses and aides. The registered nurse, or RN, is the senior professional among them. After at least three years of formal training in nursing, she has been required to pass a state examination. She usually wears white, with a cap and insignia indicating her nursing school. (Increasingly now, men are entering the nursing profession and are proving highly effective.)

The licensed practical nurse, or LPN, next in order, has had at least one year of formal training and in most hospitals, he or she too, wears white. Nurses' aides, who help both RNs and LPNs, are nonprofessionals with on-the-job training. Usually they wear colored uniforms and no caps.

There are likely to be volunteer workers—older volunteers trained by the Red Cross and known as "Gray Ladies" because of the uniforms they wear, and younger teenage volunteers often called "Candy-Stripers" because of their uniforms. In some cases, volunteers trained by the hospital may wear pink, blue, yellow, or green uniforms and are given such names as "Ladies in Yellow," etc.

If the hospital is associated with a nursing school, you will also see student nurses, wearing white aprons, colored blouses, and caps decorated to indicate how far along they are in training. You may also see housekeeping personnel in colored smocks, identifiable by their name tags which also indicate job classifications.

Sometimes, men or women in white may be confusing. While making hospital rounds practicing physicians usually wear white coats over street clothes. In teaching hospitals, they are often followed by an entourage of doctors-in-training. The residents in postgraduate training may wear knee-length white coats, which distinguish them from interns, who may wear short jackets. But a white jacket alone may not be reliable identification because pharmacists and male volunteers may also be garbed the same way.

You won't, of course, insult anyone by referring to them as doctor or nurse. Any hospital worker is likely to be flattered.

No member of any of the groups is allowed to try to do something beyond his tested competence. Only an RN, or a physician, and in some states only a physician, may administer narcotics, for example, and most states prohibit a nurse's aide from administering even an aspirin tablet.

The Patient's Friend: The Hospital Ombudsman

A common criticism about many hospitals, particularly large ones, is that they seem to be indifferent to the patients' individual personal problems as distinguished from their medical needs. Now patients with complaints can get someone to listen to them in the increasing numbers of hospitals which have appointed ombudsmen, or patients' representatives, to hear complaints and to adjust them whenever possible.

To be sure, some of these appointments may be little more

than token responses to rising demands, and the appointees may have little authority to act. But many hospitals are actively seeking to improve relations with patients.

For example, at one large hospital the patient representative is a twenty-six-year-old former nurse with a broad understanding of hospital procedures. She is a member of the hospital's administrative structure and has broad authority to investigate and, when necessary, do something about patient complaints.

Some complains arise out of misunderstandings. Unfamiliar with hospital activities, some patients may not realize that a nurse who seems brusque and has no time for a chat actually must take a dozen more temperatures and perhaps as many blood pressures within a specified period. On the other hand, some complaints, in the experience of patient representatives, are well justified, and they include complaints about doctors and nurses. Hospital personnel sometimes tend to forget that a patient is upset by his illness, worried about his work, his children, his bills; he needs someone to listen to him and explain things to him. Often patient complaints can be resolved by the representative's chat with nurses or doctors.

Whether or not there is a patient representative, you have a right, even an obligation, to report any incompetence to the nursing supervisor, hospital administrator, or your physician.

It is important to understand a basic fact: that hospital personnel who may not seem obliging may in many cases be restricted by instructions given to them by your physician; they have no leeway.

A nurse, for example, never can accommodate a patient who requests an unauthorized sleeping pill or who doesn't want to take one that is ordered. She can never allow visitors in a sickroom which the doctor has placed off limits to them. She can never augment a restricted diet or let a patient out of bed if the doctor specified he must remain there. Your only recourse is to argue these matters with your physician, and usually it is possible to work out problems with him.

A *"Patient's Bill of Rights"*

In 1973 the American Hospital Association issued a twelve point Bill of Rights for patients and urged hospitals to distribute copies to incoming patients. Actually, these rights are reaffirmations of long-established principles known to health professionals but not to many patients.

Knowing about those rights may be of great value to you.

As a patient, you have the right:

1. To considerate and respectful care.

2. To obtain from the physician complete current information concerning diagnosis, treatment, and prognosis, in terms you can understand.

3. To obtain from the physician information necessary for informed consent before any procedure or treatment is begun; to information on significant alternatives; and to know the name of the person responsible for the treatment.

4. To refuse treatment to the extent permitted by law and to be informed of the medical consequences of refusal.

5. To every consideration of your privacy concerning your own medical care; persons not directly involved in your care must have your permission to be present at case discussion, consultation, examination, and treatment.

6. To confidentiality of all communications and records pertaining to you.

7. To expect that within its capacity a hospital make reasonable response to your request for service and not transfer you to another institution except after you have been given reasons why.

8. To obtain information concerning any relationship of your hospital to other health services so far as your care is concerned, and to the existence of any professional relationships among individuals who are treating you.

9. To be advised if the hospital proposes to engage in

human experimentation affecting your care and to refuse to participate in such research.

10. To reasonable continuity of care, including postdischarge follow-up.

11. To examine and receive an explanation of your bill no matter who pays it.

12. To know what hospital rules and regulations apply to your conduct as a patient.

Fees, Costs, and Insurance

Even when covered by insurance that may pay a large share of the cost, patients want to know what the expense of an operation will be. Surgery is reputed to be expensive and when every charge that may enter into an operation is considered, it can be. Usually, the bulk of the expense is for hospital care rather than for professional fees.

Determining the Cost of Your Operation

The way to find out how much your operation is likely to cost is to ask the surgeon, and possibly the simplest way to do so is to say, "I'd like to talk about your fee," or, "I'd like to talk about how much everything will cost."

You have the right to such a discussion in advance of surgery. Medical and surgical organizations advise and urge it. In an emergency, there may be no time for it; in most cases, however, there is time.

Some doctors may bring up the subject of cost routinely, Others hesitate, not because they wish to avoid going into it but because they worry that some patients may be offended. Almost without exception, if they do not themselves bring up the matter, surgeons will welcome your bringing it up and will be glad to go into it with you.

It is not always possible for the surgeon to provide an absolutely firm figure. Occasionally, unexpected complications may arise. Yet, if you request it, he can usually provide a reasonably good approximation of what the operation will cost. He can indicate that if yours is to be an operation for a peptic ulcer or a gallbladder removal and if nothing else is found to require attention or no complications arise, the fee will be about so much.

Fee Variations

In the past, surgical fees often were based to a considerable extent on ability of patients to pay. Essential operations were performed whether or not a patient could pay anything at all. As many as one-third or more of operations performed by most surgeons were without fee at all or at a very nominal charge. To make up for this, wealthier patients were expected to pay more, since they could afford to do so.

Today the situation is different. Most patients have some form of financial coverage for surgery, through insurance or governmental agencies. As a result, except in some cases where patients or their families may be unusually demanding, surgical fees are essentially the same for all. In hardship cases, however, many surgeons will adjust their fees downward.

Surgeons' fees vary. They may vary geographically, tending to be lowest in the South, higher on the East and West Coasts, somewhere in between in the Midwest. Fees also may be as much as 10 percent higher in large metropolitan areas than in rural areas.

There may be variations from one surgeon to another. Each surgeon can set his own fees and what one may establish as his usual fees may be quite different from those of another surgeon in the same community.

For example, the most recent survey* by a professional publication, *Medical Economics*, found the median fee for an appendectomy for all fee-for-service general surgeons was

---

*Copyright © 1973 by Medical Economics Company, Oradell, New Jersey., 07649. Reprinted by permission.

$250, but the range of fees is considerable. Ten percent charged $350 or more; 4 percent, $325; 8 percent, $300; 6 percent, $275; 23 percent, $250; 15 percent, $225; 25 percent, $200; 6 percent, $175; 3 percent, $150 or less.

For a gallbladder removal (cholecystectomy), the median fee for self-employed general surgeons under age sixty-five in 1971, the last survey year, was $350. Twenty-three percent charged $350–$374; 40 percent charged less than $350; and of these, 9 percent charged $250 or less; on the other hand, 37 percent charged more than $350–$374; and of these, 5 percent charged $600 or more.

For partial stomach removal (subtotal gastrectomy), the 1971 median was $500, with 21 percent of general surgeons charging $500–$549. Fifty percent charged less, with 4 percent charging as little as $300–349. Twenty-nine percent charged more than $300–349, with 10 percent charging $750 or more.

For a inguinal hernia (unilateral) operation, the median fee in 1971 was $200, with 31 percent of general surgeons charging from $200 to $224. Twenty-six percent charged less, with 9 percent charging as little as $150 to $174. Forty-three percent charged more than $200–$224, with 4 percent charging $400 or more.

For a total hysterectomy, the 1971 median fee was $350, with 29 percent ·of general surgeons charging from $350 to $374. Twenty-eight percent charged less, with 7 percent charging under $300. Forty-three percent charged more than $350–$374, with 3 percent charging $700 or more.

It is virtually impossible to provide in a book any valid indication of what the fee for a particular operation for a particular patient at a particular time is likely to be. Not only will the fee depend upon the patient's specific problem and the possible difficulties to be expected during and after operations, and the individual surgeon's customary fee structure, fees change as the surgeon's expenses are affected by the economy.

It is possible only to provide rough guidelines, the approximate range of fees for various relatively common operations. For example:

Bone fracture, open reduction, and internal fixation	$300–600
Breast, partial mastectomy	$100–150
Cystocele	$300–500
Dilation and curettage (D & C)	$90–150
Disc surgery	$500–900
Exploratory laparotomy	$200–400
Gastrectomy (partial stomach removal)	$400–800
Hemorrhoidectomy	$200–400
Hydrocele	$175–300
Nasal septum	$175–300
Prostatectomy, transurethral	$475–800
Tonsillectomy/adenoidectomy	$100–150

In some areas, medical organizations have established suggested guidelines for surgical and other fees in the form of relative value scales. A first office visit, which involves the taking of a medical history and physical examination, may be assigned a base value of 1. Fees for various operations may then be assigned relative values which are multiples of the base value and take into account the relative complexity of the operation, time required for surgical care, and skill and experience required to perform the operation.

Thus, an appendectomy, for example, may be assigned a relative value of 30, meaning that the fee for that operation may be 30 times the fee for a first office visit. If the latter fee is $10, the charge for the appendectomy may be $300.

The following are examples of relative values proposed in some areas:

Appendectomy	30
Breast, cyst removal	15
Breast, removal	30
Breast, radical mastectomy	60
Brain tumor removal	100
Cataract	70
Cholecystectomy (gallbladder removal)	60
Closed heart operation	100
Colon and rectum removal	100
Esophagus, diverticulum removal	60
Hernia, inguinal	30
Hemorrhoidectomy	30
Hip fracture	60
Hysterectomy, abdominal	60
Hysterectomy, vaginal	70
Intestine, large, removal of portion	80
Intestine, small, removal of portion	60
Laparotomy, exploratory	40
Lung removal	100
Larynx, removal for cancer	150
Myringoplasty, eardrum repair	60
Nephrectomy, kidney removal	75
Prostate, transurethral resection	70

Rectum, removal for cancer 90

Spleen removal 60

Stapes (ear) surgery 70

Stomach, partial removal 80

Septum surgery, nose 40

Tonsillectomy 15

Thyroidectomy 60

Tympanoplasty (middle ear repair) 100

Relative value scales, which are subject to revision, are usually only suggestions on which surgeons may base their fees.

By all means, discuss in advance with your surgeon what his fee is likely to be—and also fees for others assisting in the operation. Major surgery may require a surgical assistant and in some cases more than one assistant.

An assistant's fee may be a percentage of the fee charged by the surgeon. A rough rule of thumb is that the assistant's fee will be about 20 percent of the surgeon's fee.

Another rough rule of thumb is that charges for anesthesia will run 20 to 25 percent of the surgery charge.

Your family physician may need only visit you in the hospital on a friendly basis to see how you are doing and to reassure you of his continuing interest. On the other hand, if you have a medical problem in addition to the problem for which surgery is to be performed, he may need to attend you while you are in the hospital, and you may need to consider the charges he will make for this.

It is often assumed that part of the surgeon's fee is paid back to the referring physician as a "commission" for referral. But such fee splitting is strictly prohibited among ethical doctors. They feel it is contrary to a patient's best interests since it provides an inducement for a referring physician to send his patients to the surgeons who pay the highest percentage rather than to those he considers best qualified to make the diagnoses and perform the operations.

Ethical doctors are pledged not to pay or receive payment for referrals; accredited hospitals bar access to their facilities to physicians who split fees; some states have laws forbidding fee splitting and the practice is now forbidden by Federal law. Nevertheless, some fee splitting may still go on.

Hospital Costs

Bills for hospital stays have been skyrocketing in recent years. It is not unusual today for the hospital bill for a one-day stay for a tonsillectomy to run as much as $250 or more, for a stay of up to five days for an appendectomy to cost as much as $600 or more, for a week-long stay for a hysterectomy or cholecystectomy to run as much as $800 or more.

Charges include those for room and board, floor nursing care, use of operating room and its equipment, use of hospital laboratory and X-ray departments, drugs and medications, and blood transfusions if needed.

Costs may vary to some extent from one hospital to another in a community, and from community to community. Cost in a teaching hospital is usually higher than in a community hospital because of the added expense of training nurses, physicians, and other health workers, and because of the generally higher cost of caring for patients with the more complex illnesses usually referred to such institutions.

Increased costs reflect many things, including increasingly complex but more and more effective care. It is worth noting that a man suffering a heart attack, for example, in 1920 would have stayed for as long as eight weeks at one major teaching hospital for a total cost of $180; in 1930 he would have stayed six weeks for $210; and in 1970 he would have stayed four weeks for $3,500 (which would have included $1,500 for ten days in the intensive-care unit and $2,000 for twenty days in a regular bed). Of 100 patients treated for heart attacks in 1920, however, 40 died; of 100 treated in 1930, 30 died; but of 100 treated in 1970, only 18 died.

But there has been marked inflation of medical care costs. In a recent three-year period, while the Consumer Price Index rose 13 percent, hospital daily service charges increased 54.6 percent.

Increasing efforts are being made to bring hospital costs under control, to reduce personnel turnover which is costly, to make use of more effective management techniques, systems analysts, computers and automatic machines. There is also an increasing tendency to shorten hospital stays, to get patients home earlier when this can be done without jeopardy. The evidence is that it can be done often, not only with safety and financial savings but also with benefits to patients. These include earlier reunion with families and possibly even quicker recuperation.

If your surgeon indicates that your hospital stay can be shortened, that it can be less than a minimum indicated in the description of your operation earlier in this book, it will be because trials have established that what once was considered to be an invariable minimum stay is not so in many cases, and you are likely to benefit financially and otherwise from a quicker return home. Similarly, if he suggests that the procedure you need may be done on an outpatient basis—in and out of the hospital the same day—it will be because evidence will have indicated that this is feasible and even of benefit for someone undergoing your operation.

Insurance Coverage

The chances are that, like the vast majority of American families today, you have some type of health insurance protection. As of 1971, the most recent year for which complete records are available, 179,900,000 persons had hospital expense protection; 165,449,000 had surgical expense coverage; 144,442,000 had regular medical expense protection; 80,067,000 had major medical expense protection; 58,850,000 had short-term and 12,011,000 long-term disability income policies. In 1971, Americans spent 3.1 percent of their disposable income for health insurance premiums.

Types of Policies, Medicare

Hospital expense plans provide benefits toward the expense of hospital room and board and other charges. Surgical expense insurance provides benefit payments usually made according to a schedule listing surgical procedures and maximum benefits for each procedure covered. Regular medical expense insurance provides benefits toward physicians' fees for nonsurgical care given in the hospital, home, or physician's office, and some plans also provide benefits for diagnostic X-rays and laboratory expense. Major medical expense insurance, which is growing rapidly, from just 108,000 persons covered in 1951 to almost 81 million, provides benefits toward virtually all kinds of health care prescribed by a physician, helping to cover the cost of treatment given in and out of hospital, special nursing care, X-rays, prescriptions, medical appliances, nursing home care, ambulatory psychiatric care, and other health care needs. Loss of income—or disability income—protection provides regular weekly or monthly cash payments in the event wages are cut off as the result of illness or accident. The coverage may be short-term, with the maximum benefit period running up to two years, or long-term, with benefit periods greater than two years.

Benefits paid by insurance companies are primarily provided through indemnity payments. The insured is paid a specified sum of money toward his covered expenses; such payments also can be made directly to the provider of the care through an assignment-of-benefits arrangement. Blue Cross, Blue Shield, and other hospital-medical plans usually make direct payments for covered services to the participating hospital or physician.

Although most people now have some form of coverage, few are familiar with the details. If possible, you should review your contract before talking with your surgeon about it.

Some policies include a list of common operations and amounts to be paid toward them. But in some group insurance plans, such lists and payment schedules appear only in a master contract, in which case you can obtain information from your employer about the amount to be paid in your case. If yours is an operation not included in the list, the surgeon or his secretary usually can tell the approximate amount that will be paid and also the amount, if any, the surgeon will charge in addition to the insurance payment.

Patients over sixty-five are covered by Medicare, the government health insurance plan, which has two parts—hospital insurance and medical insurance. Every person over sixty-five registered for Medicare has the hospital insurance coverage, but only those who have requested and paid for the medical insurance are covered for doctors' services as well. The Medicare card indicates whether one or both kinds of insurance are in force.

With the Medicare medical insurance, you pay the first $60 charged for medical services in any calendar year. Beyond that, the insurance covers eighty percent of accepted fees as set by Medicare (which may be lower than the average doctor's fees) and you pay the remainder of the charges. Many older people covered by Medicare also have "Medicare supplement" insurance coverage to help pay amounts not included in Medicare.

Although, overall, insurance pays a substantial fraction of medical bills and an even greater share of hospital expenses, individual coverage varies widely. Your coverage needs to be considered when you discuss costs with your surgeon. If you have doubts about the extent of your coverage, he may be able to resolve them for you.

If the surgeon's fee, beyond what insurance will cover, is large enough so you will have difficulty in paying it in full when the bill is presented, you can discuss this, too, in advance of the operation and usually a reasonable schedule of payments can be agreed on. If you have no insurance and are unable to pay for hospital costs and the surgeon's fee, he can usually arrange for you to see a social agency that may provide financial help.

Preoperative Care

Upon your admission to the hospital, you will receive preoperative care as ordered by your surgeon. Under some circumstances, the surgeon may make suggestions for steps you can take at home that will contribute to successful surgery.

Home Preparation Measures

Weight

If you are markedly underweight, perhaps as a consequence of the problem for which surgery is indicated, and if there is time enough, diet suggestions may be made. The objective may be not so much to add pounds as to improve nourishment and build strength.

Obesity is not a bar to successful surgery. To some extent, however, surgery may be simplified if there is less fat to be cut through at the start of an operation and less to be sutured afterward. Healing may proceed a little more smoothly in the nonobese. If there is time and weight reduction can be achieved without undue psychological trauma, your surgeon may suggest a diet for you to use in the period before the operation.

Exercise

If you have led a nonsedentary life and have kept in good physical condition, that is all to the good. Healthy muscle condition may help to speed healing after operation. Some degree of muscle deconditioning is to be expected during even a short stay in bed, and if you start with good muscle condition, you are a bit ahead of the game and may recover muscle strength and tone more rapidly.

So if there is time and he deems that it may be helpful, your surgeon may advise preoperative exercises. He may also suggest deep breathing exercises.

Smoking

As any heavy smoker knows, one consequence of excessive smoking may be large amounts of mucus in the breathing passages accompanied by wheezing, particularly in the morning.

A few weeks, sometimes even just a few days, without smoking or with smoking cut to the lowest possible amount, may do much to minimize mucus buildup and also to increase vital capacity, or the amount of air and oxygen you can get to your lungs with each breath you take.

Medications

No matter what prescribed drugs or over-the-counter remedies you may be taking, let your surgeon know about them. He can decide whether there are likely to be any possible undesirable interactions between them and any medication that may be required during the course of your hospital stay. He can also decide whether such medicine-taking should be curtailed prior to the operation or whether certain measures should be taken during or after surgery to accommodate those medications.

Preoperative Hospital Care

Before surgery, regardless of the type of operation, certain routine tests are carried out.

While there are some procedural variations among hospitals, generally a blood sample will be taken and tested for hemoglobin, the oxygen-carrying pigment of the blood; a hemoglobin determination aids in discovering anemia if present. There is likely to be a count of red and white blood cells and, in some hospitals, a routine test for syphilis. If there is the slightest possibility that a blood transfusion may be needed, the surgeon will order that your blood be typed so it can be cross-matched with donor blood to increase the safety of transfusion.

A urine analysis will also be done. The urine will be tested for the presence of sugar, blood, pus cells, crystals, and other materials.

Beyond routine tests done for all patients, your surgeon may order special tests—X-rays or pathology laboratory tests as described elsewhere in this book—as an aid to the operation or to help confirm the diagnosis or to determine whether there might be other possible conditions present beyond the one for which surgery is scheduled.

Both routine and special tests may be carried out very soon after your admission to the hospital or, as we have noted earlier, they may be done prior to admission in the PAT, or preadmission testing, programs more and more hospitals are adopting as a means of shortening hospital stays.

You can expect that soon after admission, a nurse will record your temperature, blood pressure, pulse and breathing rates on your chart, and this will be repeated many times during your stay. Every time you are given medication or treatment of any kind, it will be recorded on the chart.

Other Measures

Because there may be temporary interference with normal intestinal functioning after some forms of surgery and the bowels may not move for several days, an enema may be given in advance of operation to clear out the bowel.

Usually there will be a ban on eating and drinking for about twelve hours before operation so that surgery can be performed on an empty stomach. You may have a light evening meal and then nothing by mouth after midnight the night before surgery.

The skin and hair are harborers of organisms that may cause infection, and so they require special attention before surgery. The particular area to be shaved and cleansed will depend upon the wishes of the surgeon and accepted hospital procedure. Usually it is desirable to shave and cleanse with an antiseptic an area larger than the proposed incision. In some types of orthopedic surgery, skin preparation may start as much as twenty-four hours before operation. The operative site may be wrapped in sterile towels or dressings and in some cases the dressings may be removed at regular intervals and an antiseptic applied.

Because of attention to such detail in preparing patients —and to the scrupulous and lengthy scrubbing of surgeons and nurses prior to operation—what once was a fairly common hazard no longer is. In the 1920s as many as 5 percent of surgical wounds became infected. Now such infections are rare and in many hospitals where thousands of operations are performed annually, not a single death may occur from wound infection.

Sometimes, when tests indicate that a patient does not have quite normal blood chemistry, when there is a deficiency in one or more components of the blood such as protein, sugar, vitamins, and minerals such as sodium, potassium, or calcium, the deficiency may be overcome by administration by vein prior to surgery.

If the condition for which you are to undergo surgery is

one that has produced anemia or loss of blood—or if there has been blood loss or anemia for any other reason—you may receive preoperatively a transfusion of blood to restore the level toward normal.

Generally, there are three types of drugs that may be used prior to surgery. Sedatives, such as one of the barbiturates, may be given to promote relaxation and rest. A good night's sleep before operation is helpful and a sedative may help you sleep well despite normal anxieties about the operation.

Another type of drug that may be used is a drying agent such as atropine or scopolamine to decrease secretion of mucus in the mouth and throat.

Not long before you go up to surgery, you may receive a narcotic such as morphine or Demerol® or a tranquilizer to promote relaxation and enhance the effects of the anesthetic.

Usually you will know the day before the operation the exact time for which it is scheduled and will have time to let your family know. Depending upon the rules of a particular hospital, it may or may not be possible for your family to see you off to the operating room. In most hospitals, there is a waiting room not far from the operating room and as soon as the operation is completed, they may meet and talk with the surgeon there.

Anesthesia

The Crude Origins

Late in 1841 in the small rural town of Jefferson, Georgia, an itinerant showman aroused much interest when he gave a gas, nitrous oxide, to volunteers in his audiences and produced curious antics. Looking for excitement, the young men of Jefferson asked the town's physician, Crawford W. Long, then twenty-six, to make some of the gas for their use. Long didn't have the equipment to do that but he remembered that while a medical student in Philadelphia he had experienced "ethereal" effects from sulphuric ether and had seen traveling showmen use ether much as the itinerant showman in Jefferson had used nitrous oxide. And so, Long produced some ether and its inhalation for "kicks" soon became fashionable, not only in Jefferson but in the surrounding countryside as well.

Then, on March 30, 1842, Long ventured to try ether as a surgical anesthetic while removing a tumor from the back of the neck of James Venable, a student at a local academy. In 1843, he employed it to remove a tumor from a woman's head and in 1845 to amputate a finger of a slave boy.

Anesthesia has come far since. For many years after Long's trials, the production of surgical anesthesia was makeshift and for the sole purpose of avoiding pain. Little consideration was given to a patient's condition, and the patient's life often depended not only on his ability to recover

389

from the operation but also from the effects of well-meant but crude administration of such compounds as ether, chloroform, and nitrous oxide. The anesthetist's attention was focused on getting and keeping the patient unconscious during operation, and there was little knowledgeable concern about oxygen needs, heart action, or blood pressure. Often, in fact, the anesthetist was an orderly or someone without medical background.

Anesthesiology remained relatively crude until well into this century. A major step forward took place during World War II, when armed forces experience demonstrated the vital importance of trained anesthetists, and they were given equal rank with other specialists.

Anesthesiology Today

Anesthesiology now has as only one of its goals the alleviation of pain. It is concerned with relieving anxieties beforehand, increasing safety in the operating room, providing optimum conditions for the surgeon during the actual surgical procedure, and then helping to assure complete and comfortable recovery afterward even for patients who not long ago would have been considered poor surgical risks because they were too young, too old, or too feeble.

The modern anesthetist has available a wide array of agents from which to choose: sedatives, muscle relaxants, analgesics, narcotics, gases, and more. On some occasions he may need to use only one or two. On other occasions, he may use half a dozen or more, some administered in pill form, some injected, others given through a face mask or a tube down the windpipe. By employing combinations, he makes use of a phenomenon known as *synergism,* through which one drug reinforces another and lesser total amounts are needed, which means that undesirable reactions are minimized.

Through his choice of combinations, the anesthetist can also produce selective effects. For example, he can paralyze, temporarily, skeletal muscles without dangerously interfering with the heart muscle's activities; such muscle paralysis can be vital in many delicate chest and abdominal operations.

What You Can Expect

If you remember a personal experience many years ago or have heard stories of operations long ago in which a mask was suddenly placed over the face and the patient was held down while ether was poured into the mask, or in which a long needle was thrust into the back for spinal anesthesia, you can forget that now. However unpleasant and even terrifying the prospect of anesthesia and anesthesia induction may once have been, anesthesia today is entirely different.

The anesthesiologist may come to your room the evening before surgery and his visit will have several purposes. Aware of the anxieties of many patients and of old tales they may have heard, he will want to ease any anxiety you feel, explain what will happen, and answer questions.

He will have purposeful questions of his own. Do you have any allergies that you know about? Any sensitivity to any drug? What medications, if any, are you taking? Do you have any illnesses beyond what the operation is for?

He may volunteer information—and if not, you can ask— about the next day's procedure, including the drugs to be used, what, if any, discomfort to expect, when you will go to sleep and have no awareness of what is going on, and when you will regain consciousness.

In addition to visiting your room, the anesthesiologist will study your medical history and all available medical records and will consult with the surgeon about the operative procedure and the material and method of anesthesia most suitable for the operation and for you.

On the Day of Operation

An hour or so before the operation, while you are still in your room, you may receive a barbiturate to make you drowsy. You may also be given other medication, an agent such as atropine or scopolamine, to dry up mucus and salivary gland secretions as an aid to facilitating anesthesia.

An orderly will roll a bed-high surgical cart into your room, transfer you to it gently, and take you to the surgery floor. By now, you will be drowsy and relatively calm and relaxed.

The anesthesiologist may insert an intravenous (IV) needle to provide a quick and easy route for administering any drugs that may be required during operation. The anesthesiologist may then inject Pentothal® and within seconds you will be asleep. By testing a reflex, he can make certain you are well enough asleep so you will have no awareness of a mask being placed over your nose and mouth or, if an endotracheal tube is to be used, that you will be unaware of its being passed down your throat. The passing of the tube can be achieved readily after injection of a short-acting muscle relaxant. Through either mask or tube, an inhalation anesthetic, a gas or vapor, and oxygen can be administered. For most major operations now, the tube is preferred, and it is often attached to a mechanical device that assists breathing.

In addition to the anesthetic, other drugs may be needed during the operation and these can be introduced readily through the intravenous needle that was inserted before surgery. The needle is joined to a length of flexible tubing attached to a bottle hanging over the operating table and drops of whatever drug may be needed, when released into the tube, will flow immediately into the bloodstream.

Through the tube can be administered, as needed, an analgesic to raise the pain threshold, the level of pain that must be reached if it is to be felt; a sedative that does not affect pain threshold but can extend unconsciousness; a muscle relaxant; and much more.

All through the operation, the anesthesiologist will be closely scrutinizing your condition. He will monitor your blood pressure, pulse rate, temperature, and the electrocardiographic recording of the action of your heart. As needed, he can administer through the tube glucose, plasma, whole blood, various other drugs.

The Forms of Anesthesia

General. General anesthesia, which produces complete unconsciousness, is used in most surgical procedures. It can be controlled to achieve only the desired depth—light when surgery involves only superficial areas of the body or deep enough to permit operations within the abdomen and even within the heart.

The anesthetic is combined with oxygen so that the same ratio of oxygen as is found in the air we breathe and needed by body tissues, normally about 21 percent, is maintained.

Many gases are available for general anesthesia. One of the oldest and most commonly used is nitrous oxide, also known as "laughing gas." Also in use are cyclopropane and ether, a liquid which becomes a gas upon exposure to air. Chloroform, once in wide use, is employed less often now with the availability of other agents. A number of newer agents, including Penthrane®, have the advantage of being nonexplosive.

Intraveous. Agents which can be dripped into a vein in the arm or leg at a controlled rate to induce sleep very quickly, often within seconds, are in increasing use. They include pentothal which is often used, too, in dental surgery.

For some short operations that are relatively minor in nature, an intravenous anesthetic may be the only one used. Intravenous anesthetics are often employed as an aid in regional or local anesthesia, allowing a light sleep while pain is prevented by the regional or local agent. Sometimes, in what is called balanced anesthesia, an intravenous agent may be combined with a spinal or local as well as a gas.

Spinal. Spinal anesthesia can be used to anesthetize completely a specific part of the body. A needle is inserted between the vertebrae in the back and controlled doses of an anesthetic agent such as Novocain® are injected into the spinal fluid. If organs in the upper or mid-abdomen are to be operated upon, the injection can be administered high up in the back. A low spinal injection can be used when lower abdominal organs are to be operated upon.

With spinal anesthesia, a desirable level of anesthesia can be produced and the patient, although no longer sensitive to pain at the surgical site, can remain fully conscious. Increasing expertise in this form of anesthesia makes it both effective and safe. There is a side effect in about one of every twenty patients: a headache, which may persist for several days to a week or more.

When a patient does not wish to remain conscious, he can be put to sleep during spinal anesthesia or any of the other regional or local methods of anesthesia, by injection of a barbiturate into a vein after the anesthetic has been injected.

Epidural and caudal. Somewhat similar to spinal anesthesia, these variations place the anesthetic agent outside the spinal canal. A greater amount of drug is required and it takes somewhat longer for the full effect to be obtained, but epidural and caudal methods avoid the possibility of post-anesthesia headache.

Regional. Just as a dentist can inject Novocain® to deaden pain in a specific area when it is necessary to extract a tooth or do extensive drilling, so the anesthesiologist can inject an anesthetic at a specific site, temporarily blocking or deadening specific nerves through which pain impulses are transmitted from the site.

A hand, an arm, the neck, or the side of the face, for example, can be anesthetized when surgery is to be confined to that area. With localized anesthesia, there is no effect on heart, lungs, blood pressure, and general condition, and this is often advantageous, particularly for high-risk patients.

Topical. Spraying or painting an anesthetic on mucous membranes is useful for some procedures, particularly those involving eye, nose, and throat. In some cases it may be used to produce superficial pain deadening and may be followed by injection of a local anesthetic. Topical anesthesia is often used to help pass tubes into the windpipe or esophagus.

Thus, today, there is often a choice of suitable methods of anesthesia. For tonsil removal, for example, either a general or local may be used, although a general is usually preferred for children. For major breast surgery, a general is commonly employed, but for a minor breast procedure either a local or general may be used. For abdominal surgery, a general or spinal may be employed.

For prostate, bladder, and kidney surgery, spinal, epidural or general may be used. For surgery on the spine, spinal or general may be used; for bone surgery on an extremity, either spinal, regional nerve block or general may be chosen; for leg surgery, low spinal, local, regional, or general; usually for heart and lung operations, general is used.

The Anesthesiologist

As already noted, the anesthesiologist can play many vital roles not only in selecting and administering suitable anesthesia for a patient but also in monitoring and supporting the patient. Particularly in the last twenty years, anesthesiology has become a major medical specialty.

In 1955, only 34 percent of those administering anesthesia were members of the American Association of Nurse Anesthetists (registered nurse anesthetists) and 18 percent were members of the American Society of Anesthesiologists (physician anesthesiologists) for a total of 52 percent. By 1965, AANA members giving anesthesia in operations in U. S. hospitals had increased to 46 percent and doctor anesthesiologists to 39 percent for a total of 85 percent. In a ten-year period, the number of nonspecialty doctors, nurses, and others administering anesthetics had declined from 48 percent to 15 percent. Since 1945, the American Association of Anesthesiologists has increased in membership by 377 percent but there is still a shortage in this specialty.

As a patient scheduled for surgery, you can participate in

selecting your anesthesiologist. Customarily, the choice is left to the surgeon or the personal physician. But no good doctor resents a patient who investigates a colleague's credentials. If your local medical society's records or a medical directory show that a doctor is a Diplomate of the American Board of Anesthesiology, he has completed at least two years of specialized graduate training beyond medical school and internship and, after two to four years of clinical practice, has passed qualifying tests. If he is listed as a Fellow of the American College of Anesthesiologists, his proficiency has been certified by the college's Board of Governors after qualifying tests.

Any lack of formal endorsement does not necessarily mean that a man is incompetent; he may be an expert in anesthesia as the result of long experience. A trained nurse-anesthetist, too, can be most competent.

It may be possible for you to participate in deciding on the form of anesthesia to be used. You can discuss any feelings and desires you have. If you think you will not like some particular kind of anesthesia, you can indicate so. If you don't wish to be conscious during surgery even though you will feel no pain, you can indicate that.

The anesthesiologist's major concerns in the choice of anesthesia will focus around the nature of the operation, the needs of the surgeon during the procedure, your particular physical needs. But whenever possible—and it is often possible because there are now sufficient alternatives—he will take your desires into consideration.

Some Common Questions About Anesthesia

Often patients wonder how long anesthesia can be maintained safely. Expertly administered, anesthesia can be maintained for eight hours or even more when necessary, but this is rarely the case. However, a major reason for the ability of surgeons to achieve superior results in many operations and to carry out some procedures once considered virtually impossible is that they now can take their time, proceed carefully. No longer is there the time pressure that once prevailed when much depended upon getting an operation over with as quickly as possible in order to minimize the trauma of anesthesia. More time can be taken now not only because of advances in methods of anesthesia but also in the monitoring of patients during surgery and the ability to use drugs and other measures to maintain body balance and normal or close-to-normal functioning all through anesthesia and surgery.

Some patients are concerned that they may babble away under anesthesia, perhaps telling things about themselves that they don't wish others to hear. This need be no cause for concern. With a mask over mouth and nose or a mechanical airway tube in the throat, talking is difficult, if not impossible. Later, in the recovery room, even with mask or airway removed, it will take time before you are able to make any but the most indistinguishable sounds.

You can dismiss another fear: that the operation may begin before you have become completely insensitive to pain. Before any surgical procedure starts, tests are made to make certain that you can feel no pain.

Once the operation is completed, it may be minutes to hours before you awaken, if general anesthesia is used. The anesthesiologist can so control administration in the last stages of surgery that anesthesia will be maintained at a level to keep you insensitive to pain until the final steps are completed and will thereafter wear off at a desirable rate. With local, regional, or spinal anesthesia, the effects usually wear off within one to three hours after the operation. To maintain pain relief, drugs may then be given.

Like anything else in medicine or surgery, or in fact in life, anesthesia is not 100 percent free of risk. Deaths do occur as the result of anesthesia, but they are remarkably few, especially considering that many operations have to be performed on an emergency basis with no time for what might be ideal preparation of the patient, if there is to be any chance of saving life.

It would be too much to say that no anesthesia deaths ever occur as the result of mistakes or improper management.

Some do. But the likelihood is constantly being reduced through increased training for those allowed to administer anesthesia and through the increasing use of physician and nurse anesthesiologists.

In the Operating Room

On Your Way

You may be surprised to find yourself moving toward the operating room not with feelings of apprehension but relaxed, perhaps even carrying on a joking conversation with the attendant wheeling you there. That will be because of the relaxing medication given you in your room beforehand.

Because you may be drowsy, you make take in few details of the operating room itself and you may get the impression, common to the unfamiliar eye, that it is an awesome, bewildering room, full of lights and shiny surfaces and much equipment. Everything, of course, is there for a purpose and while there are some differences in detail between operating rooms in various hospitals, they have much in common.

Equipment

There will be the operating table, centrally located in the room, and above it the operating light. The table, a complex piece of equipment, can be tilted in virtually any direction and adjusted to elevate or lower head, body, or extremities to any necessary position. The overhead light, too, is a complex and costly piece of equipment, designed to produce

399

a strong, shadowless beam over the operating field and be readily adjustable.

If a gas anesthetic is to be used, there will be a portable stand with tanks of anesthetic gases and oxygen near the head of the table.

There will also be one or more instrument tables containing every possible instrument that might be needed. Almost always there is a surplus of instruments, and if an operation commonly requires, say, a dozen clamps, there may be several times that number just on the off chance that something unforeseen may arise requiring their use.

In addition to the main instrument table or tables, there will also be a special stand which can hold many of the instruments needed during the operation and which can be moved into place over the operating table, close at hand.

Among other equipment will be a suction machine to be used if necessary to remove fluids from the operative site or from the throat; a small table holding soap, alcohol, other antiseptics, gauze pads; a sponge stand; a stand or rack for containers of blood, plasma, or other fluids that may be administered during the operation; and supplies of sutures, dressings, and other needs, all sterilized and ready for use.

Also present in the operating room will be electronic equipment for continuous monitoring of blood pressure, pulse, blood, and the heart, designed to provide surgeon and anesthesiologist with a continuing picture of the patient's condition throughout surgery. In more and more hospitals now, a computer is used in conjunction with the electronic equipment to produce instant analyses and even forecast of what is likely to be a patient's status several minutes later.

As a safeguard, modern operating rooms have floors covered with electrically conductive material or conductors built into the floors, and everybody in the operating room except the patient who never touches the floor wears shoes with conductive soles. As a result, any static electricity that may develop is safely removed.

Antisepsis

If you were to examine human skin under a very high-powered microscope, you would find it a strange terrain—full of clefts, pits, occasional forests or swamps, and areas where scales of skin can be found drying, curling, and ready to float away.

It's a well-populated terrain. Within the womb, our skins may be sterile or relatively so. But, with birth, the human skin quickly becomes a site always occupied by bacteria, viruses, yeasts, and fungi, usually living together peaceably. Studies have shown that on the surface of your forearm, for example, there may be as many as 4,500 living organisms per square centimeter and, in the armpit, as many as two million.

As a rough rule of thumb, you can figure that the number of bacteria populating your skin is equivalent to the number of people on earth. Ordinary washing makes little dent in their numbers. They come and go because we constantly shed skin scales. In the course of a month, you shed your entire skin surface, much of it ending up in the vacuum cleaner! Shed skin is the chief component of the dust that collects atop bedroom furniture and under beds. Thousands of scales are loosed from the skin every time you undress, and each scale carries with it a cargo of clinging organisms.

We have some idea today about the ecology in our macroscopic world, the balance in nature between flora and fauna. Ecological influences affect our skins as well: many harmless organisms live there, with some potentially harmful ones always mixed in, but there are usually enough of the harmless to keep the harmful from multiplying out of hand and causing trouble.

While ordinary washing of the skin does relatively little to reduce the skin populations, hard, prolonged scrubbing can reduce the numbers of organisms temporarily, as may some antiseptics, And so, before operation, the skin over the surgical site is scrubbed and prepared, the operating team is well scrubbed, and every instrument and anything else that touches the patient is antiseptic.

And yet, while relative antisepsis is attained, complete antisepsis is a goal still to be reached. Trying to come closer to it, many hospitals now have operating rooms designed so that air changes quickly (as often as every ten seconds) to eliminate any particles and organisms that somehow manage to be present on and escape through surgical gowns and masks. If infection should develop, modern antibiotics can control it in the vast majority of cases but still the objective is to make them unnecessary.

The Operating Team

The surgeon in the operating room is supported by a staff of trained assistants. Depending upon the type of operation, there may be, in addition to the anesthesiologist, one or more surgical assistants who take part in the surgical procedure; an operating room supervisor or chief operating nurse who is in charge of other nurses on the operating team and supervises preparations for the operation; a scrub nurse (sometimes two) who keeps instruments and other materials in order on the supply tray over the operating table and hands them as needed to the surgeon; a supply nurse who sees to it that all instruments and materials are properly prepared and ready for use; a circulating nurse who is available to help the others, to get additional supplies if needed, and to handle any other requirements that may come up.

During the operation, the surgeon's assistants carry out many tasks to facilitate the surgeon's work. While he is occupied with using tweezerlike forceps, scalpel, scissors, needles, and clamps, the assistants use other instruments to spread tissues and retract overlying muscles so the surgeon has a clear field in which to work. They also sponge away blood, tie the ends of blood vessels to control bleeding.

In complicated procedures such as those in which the chest is opened for operations on the heart or lungs, the surgical team also includes engineers, biomedical technicians, and others who may be needed to set up and operate the heart-lung machine and other devices to safeguard the patient. During heart or major blood-vessel surgery, a cardiologist, or heart specialist, may also be part of the team, concerned with monitoring heart action and breathing.

Sponges play an important part in many operations. They are layered gauze pads used to blot up blood from the operative site to enable the surgeon to see clearly what he is doing. Sponges may be used to cover and to separate tissues and, when placed deep in the surgical site, they may be lost to view. But there is a safeguarding ritualistic sponge-counting procedure. Usually, the circulating nurse hands sponges as needed, in packages of five, to the scrub nurse, who then opens a package, counts the sponges while the circulating nurse watches. As sponges are used and then removed, the circulating nurse picks them up, groups them in fives, and fastens them together. Before the surgical wound is sutured, both nurses check the sponge count and give the tally, sponges used and sponges retrieved, to the surgeon. And there is much the same kind of counting procedure for instruments and other supplies used in the operation.

The Operation

Even as you are being prepared in your room on the day of operation and are being wheeled to the operating room, everything in the way of instruments and supplies is being set out in the operating room, which has been thoroughly cleaned since the last operation. The operating team is going through a ritualistic, prolonged scrubbing, then donning sterile caps, gowns, and masks.

After you have received the anesthetic and have been covered completely with sterile drapes except for the operating site, which has been cleaned and to which an antiseptic solution has been applied, and when surgeon and anesthesiologist are satisfied that you are well asleep or, if conscious, unable to feel pain, the operation begins with an incision. During the procedure, the scrub nurse at her tray slaps smartly into the surgeon's hand, as he needs them, as many as two dozen or more instruments; she is usually so expert that she can anticipate his needs and have the right instruments selected and ready before he can speak.

The climax of the operation comes, of course, when a necessary repair is made or a diseased area is tied off, cut free, and lifted out with forceps. At this point, as well as before and after, the anesthesiologist will be carefully regulating the depth of anesthesia, watching vital signs, making any adjustments needed, keeping the patient supported in every possible way. Finally, there is the careful suturing or sewing back together of the various layers of skin and other tissue that were cut to reach the site of trouble.

We have touched on it before but it deserves repeated emphasis: there is still a common idea that a successful operation is a short one and if it lasts three, four, five hours, or longer, is must be because there were unexpected difficulties and the outlook is dire. Once, years ago, this might have been true; surgeons had to work under time pressure, completing an operation as fast as possible in order to spare patients the shock of prolonged anesthesia, then relatively crude, and the shock, too, of much loss of blood. Now, however, hurry, rather than anesthesia shock and blood loss, is considered to be a hazard. Modern anesthetic methods minimize shock even when anesthesia is prolonged; bleeding control is more effective; and, when necessary, blood can be transfused to make up loss.

Working calmly, carefully, without hurry, examining anything he may find that looks the least bit suspicious, calling in the hospital pathologist to check suspicious tissues, the surgeon can usually remove an appendix in about half an hour, may take an hour or so for a hernia, one to two hours for a gallbladder operation, two to four hours for a stomach or intestinal operation, six hours or more for operations on the heart or lungs.

Blood Transfusions

Each year a small river of blood—six million or more pints—is run into the veins of the sick in the U. S. Because of blood transfusions, tens of thousands of lives are saved. Not all transfusions are connected with surgical procedures. Blood may be transfused in many other situations. In severe anemias, for example, transfusions may be urgently needed; they may be urgent, too, after severe accidents.

Today's surgical procedures do often require transfusion; indeed, many of them have been made possible only because of it. When much blood is lost during an operation, it must be replaced. For blood serves many purposes in the body. If you're an average adult, you have twelve or thirteen pints of it circulating through some 60,000 miles of blood vessels, carrying essentials of life—oxygen from the lungs, food from the intestinal tract—to all tissues of the body and carrying away their wastes for disposal. Blood also distributes the heat produced by working muscles, acting as a body temperature regulator. It also serves as a guard against disease: in addition to its red cells which transport oxygen (of which the average man has 30 trillion and the average woman about 27.5 trillion), it has white cells (about one of them for every 600 red cells) which are part of the body defense system. They engulf invading bacteria, each white cell being capable of swallowing as many as twenty.

The more extensive an operation, the more blood is likely to be lost. Lifesaving cancer surgery, for example, in which whole organs and sometimes even large areas of adjacent tissue must be removed, depend heavily upon transfusions. So do other complex and lengthy procedures. Many of the remarkable feats of heart surgery today—operations to correct defects within the heart and operations to route more blood to the heart muscle when original arteries have become narrowed by disease—are possible only because the heart is temporarily bypassed and the blood is pumped through a heart-lung machine. For this technique, extra blood is essential; twelve to fifteen pints of fresh blood sometimes may be needed.

Blood transfusions have become increasingly safe as refined methods of typing and matching have been developed so that there is little if any risk that the body will reject the transfused blood as alien.

The way for blood matching was opened by the discovery just before the turn of the century that there are four basic types of blood: O, A, B, and AB. Each of these divides into two factors, Rh positive and Rh negative. Generally, of every hundred people, forty-five have group O blood, (thirty-nine Rh positive, six Rh negative); ten have group B (eight positive, two negative); forty have group A (thirty-five positive, five negative); and five have group AB (four positive, one negative).

For successful transfusion, patient blood and donor blood must match as to major group and Rh factor.

Nature makes the donation of blood easy enough. The usual amount withdrawn at one time, about a pint, is restored by the body within a few weeks. The drawing, by needle and tube from a vein in an arm, requires from four to ten minutes.

One problem has been the occasional transmission via transfused blood of viral hepatitis, a disease that may damage the liver. Because of concern over hepatitis transmission—which has affected about 30,000 patients of the two million yearly receiving transfusions—a number of efforts have been undertaken.

For one thing, tests have been developed which detect hepatitis-tainted blood in at least some cases. The tests look for an antigen, or agent, which appears in the blood of people who have serum hepatitis. They detect about 25 percent of tainted blood; they cannot detect blood from donors who may be carrying the disease without realizing it and whose blood does not contain antigens. The tests represent a major advance because, even though they fail to detect all tainted blood, it is antigen-associated hepatitis which is the more serious form of the disease.

Research is continuing to find additional tests and other

methods of preventing hepatitis transmission through blood. Research has been indicating, for example, that freezing and "washing" of blood are useful in removing disease-causing agents. There have been promising early results, too, in immunizing against infectious hepatitis.

On another front, efforts are increasing to recruit volunteer donors, reducing the need for blood from donors who sell it to commercial blood banks. Studies indicate that blood sold to commercial banks is two to ten times more likely to transmit hepatitis than blood from unpaid volunteers. Authorities believe this may be due to the fact that many drug addicts, alcoholics and derelicts give blood for money. As the result of the unsanitary conditions in which many of them live and, in the case of addicts, because of use of unsterilized needles, their blood is more likely to be contaminated.

On still another front, there have been promising preliminary results with an autotransfuser designed to eliminate need for banked blood during surgery. The device, a disposable plastic unit attached to a pump, sucks up blood as it is lost during surgery, cleans and stores it, and then pumps it back to the patient.

Still another development holds promise. Patients who are to undergo elective surgery can donate their own blood in advance for use during their operations. As much as four pints of blood may be taken within ten days before surgery and by the time of surgery, the blood supply has been well built up again. Then, during surgery, the patient's own blood may be returned to him. The method has been used successfully in open heart surgery.

If yours is to be an open heart operation, you will want to know something about the heart-lung machine that will make it possible.

The Heart-lung Machine

One day in January, 1931, Dr. John H. Gibbon, Jr., then a young surgical fellow in a Boston hospital, was called to the bedside of a fifty-three-year-old woman who had undergone a serious operation fifteen days before. Now she had sharp pain in her chest; her breathing rate was greatly accelerated; her blood pressure was far down. She had a clot in a lung blood vessel. For the next seventeen hours Gibbons stayed at her side, taking blood pressure and pulse readings every fifteen minutes. Next morning, a senior surgeon in a desperate attempt opened her chest and removed a massive blood clot from a pulmonary artery, but the patient died on the operating table.

In his notebook, young Dr. Gibbon wrote: "During those seventeen hours at the patient's side, the thought constantly recurred to me that her condition could be improved if some of the blue blood in the distended veins were withdrawn into an apparatus that would cleanse it of carbon dioxide, reoxygenate it, and pump it back into the patient's arteries. This would also lend support to the circulation during the embolectomy (the removal of the clot).

From this episode came the inspiration for the heart-lung machine, which has saved scores of thousands of lives. Gibbon built his first machine from a collection of second-hand equipment, including an old air pump and rubber corks out of which he fashioned valves. He used a cylinder that revolved and kept a film of blood on its inner surface as it revolved so the blood could be aerated.

With his primitive Queen Mary, as Gibbon called the device, he had proved by 1935 that during complete blocking of a pulmonary artery he could maintain life in cats for periods up to forty minutes. Five years of further study and trials revealed that after heart-lung bypass, animals could recover and resume normal life. It took still more years before Queen Mary could be applied to the first human patient, an eighteen-year-old girl with a defect within her heart. Later Gibbon recalled that during the twenty-six minutes on that day in 1953 when the machine pumped blood and breathed for the girl while her heart was successfully repaired, "I used up all my courage."

Dr. Gibbon was always a quiet, reticent man. But when, in 1935, he was able to achieve the first complete heart-lung bypass in an animal, he broke down and wrote: "My wife and I threw our arms around each other and danced around laughing and shouting. Nothing in my life has ever duplicated the joy of that dance round and round the laboratory of the old Bullfinch Building at the Massachusetts General Hospital."

Until the heart-lung machine became available, the problem of trying to operate on the heart without disrupting circulation to vital organs seemed almost impossible to solve. To be sure, working blind, introducing a finger into a heart chamber, a surgeon could give a patient some degree of relief from a heart valve obstruction. But more complex heart problems could not be solved until it became possible to work on the open heart under direct vision and with time enough for intricate repairs.

Today's heart-lung machine can take over the pumping job of the heart and the oxygenating job of the lungs for several hours. Usually, blood returning from the body via the veins is carried through tubing into the lung part of the machine where carbon dioxide is removed and oxygen added. The blood is then pumped through another tubing connection into the patient's artery system. With the machine at work, the heart does not have to pump and can be stopped and opened, and repairs can be made.

There are limitations to how long the machine can be used without producing some damage to blood. It has been used successfully for as long as four hours, but many surgeons prefer to use it for three hours at most whenever possible. This is commonly possible because the machine need not be used during early stages of surgery when the

chest is being opened and the way paved to reach the heart
nor need it be used once work on the heart itself is completed. During later stages, when closing up is done, the
heart and lungs can be working again.

Postoperative Care

Recovery Room

Immediately after surgery, you will usually be transferred to a recovery room rather than to your own bed. Your postoperative care begins even while you are under the effects of the anesthetic.

Many patients require no special care immediately after surgery, except possibly for an injection of a pain-relieving drug timed to take effect as the anesthetic wears off. Others may need close watch to make certain that breathing is adequate so that if it is not, oxygen may be administered or other measures taken until it returns to normal.

Routinely as a safeguard, whether they need special care or not, patients are checked frequently for blood pressure, pulse rate, breathing, and other vital signs at least for a time in the recovery room, which is staffed with personnel experienced in this type of care.

The recovery room is a special unit within the operating area. In many hospitals, especially larger ones, the term "postanesthesia department" is used in place of recovery room since the patient load requires more than a room-size area.

If your operation is early in the day, you will go to the recovery room or postanesthesia department; if later in the day, you may be taken instead to an intensive care unit, which operates around the clock for medical as well as sur-

411

gical patients. The recovery room or postanesthesia department in some cases may not be kept open through the night.
In any case, the care will be essentially the same. Your
anesthesiologist is likely to accompany you and stay with you
long enough to see that you are settled there.

Your stay there will be for only as long as necessary to
make certain that all is well. Unless the operation has been
a complex one and extended intensive monitoring and care
are required, you may be back in your own bed in an hour
or so.

As you begin to regain consciousness, things may seem
hazy and vague. Until the anesthetic has worn off completely, you may experience some disturbances in hearing and
vision, which should be no cause for alarm. You may also
feel drowsy and have an urge to go back to sleep; and if so,
fine. You can count on being awakened when it is time for
any medication to be administered or something else to be
done if needed.

After some operations, drainage tubes may be left in place
for up to several days. They are important for assuring success of the operation and avoiding complications. Tubes are
usually positioned securely so as to allow you to move about
in bed without great constraint. If you should have any
difficulty with them—if, for example, they tug unduly or
cause some discomfort—you can and should let your nurse
know, and adjustments can be made.

Usually, after recovery from the anesthetic, patients are
encouraged to change position often and move the legs, thus
stimulating circulation, making for deeper breathing, and reducing the likelihood of blood clot formation.

Ambulation

In recent years, it has become clear that early ambulation
—getting the patient to sit up as soon as possible and then to
get out of bed, sometimes even on the first or second day
after surgery—can speed recovery. Early ambulation is not
always possible; because of the nature and extent of opera-

tion, some patients may have to remain in bed for a week or longer, but most can be up and about long before that. Muscles tend to weaken fairly quickly when not used; the earlier up and about, the less opportunity for such weakening, and the quicker the ability to engage in normal activities returns.

Discomfort

You can expect some degree of discomfort for two or three days after the operation. You don't have to be distressed unduly by pain. Pain-relieving agents can be administered and your doctor will order as much of them as he thinks advisable under the particular circumstances. While drugs can be used to wipe out all traces of pain in many cases, large amounts of them may have some tendency to depress breathing and interfere with other vital functions. The objective will be to give you as much comfort as possible without sacrifice of vital functions and recuperative powers. It may therefore be necessary for you to put up with a little discomfort. But you should not hesitate to let your doctor or nurse know if the pain becomes substantial, for there is some leeway and it may be possible to provide additional pain relief without undue penalty.

After an abdominal operation, distention of the stomach with air can be distressing. A tube may be inserted through the nasal passageway into the stomach to provide relief; sometimes the tube may be inserted before the operation.

Food

Often, patients may be allowed fluids as soon as they feel like having them. They may begin to sip water or tea within a few hours if they have not undergone stomach or intestinal surgery. After a stomach or intestinal operation, fluids and food may have to be avoided for forty-eight hours or more, after which frequent small meals may be allowed. If there has been nausea following operation, sometimes a result of the anesthetic, it may be a day or two before the patient can comfortably start taking fluids and food, but this need be no cause for concern since adequate nutrition in the meantime can be supplied by vein.

Other Measures

Sometimes there is some difficulty with urination for the first twenty-four to forty-eight hours after operation, especially when spinal anesthesia has been used or when the operation has involved lower abdomen, female genitals, or rectum. Medication may be used to stimulate urination and, if necessary, the bladder may be emptied by passing a tube or catheter into it. Usually, spontaneous urination is resumed within a week.

Sick or well, many people labor under the misconception that a daily bowel movement is essential for health. Failure to have a regular daily movement often arouses worry among postsurgical patients. The fact is that there is no necessity to move the bowels in the first days after operation. Often, by the third or fourth day, normal bowel function returns. If not, an enema may be administered.

In the first several days after operation, hospital personnel will be making frequent visits to check on temperature, pulse rate, blood pressure, breathing rate, and other functions, in addition to giving medication prescribed by your doctor.

There are variations between hospitals. In some, if you occupy a private room and would like to have a member of your family stay with you the first night or two after operation, you may have him or her do so. If you should need more care than can be supplied by floor nurses, you may be able to have private-duty nurses, although there has been some trend, with the development of intensive care units, for physicians in such cases to prefer the latter.

Deep breathing deserves emphasis. You may be advised repeatedly by doctor and nurses to take deep breaths soon after operation. By doing so, you fill lung air sacs which otherwise would remain collapsed and might stick to each other, making possible unnecessary complications. Sometimes, as an aid to breathing, you may be asked to breathe in oxygen. Sometimes, a humidifying mist may be used to add moisture to the air. For patients who have chronic respiratory problems such as asthma or emphysema, positive pressure breathing treatments may be ordered to assure that the lung sacs are properly filled.

The need for changes of dressings varies greatly. Some wounds without drains can be left alone until it is time to remove the stitches. Draining wounds, or infected wounds, may call for daily dressing changes by surgeon, intern, or nurse. With few exceptions, changes can be accomplished without much pain. When pain is to be expected, medication may be administered beforehand.

Skin sutures, or stitches, may be removed from about the sixth to tenth day after operation, depending upon the location of the wound and the extent of firm healing. In some cases, metal clips may be used instead of sutures, and these are usually removed within four to six days. Suture or clip removal usually entails little discomfort. In some cases, self-dissolving sutures may be used; they require no removal.

Going Home

How soon you will go home after surgery follows no firmly fixed schedule. It is determined by the nature and extent of operation, your progress in the first days afterward, and to some extent by your home situation. Given a family able to provide any special care you may need in the first days at home, you may be able to go home earlier than if you live by yourself.

Your surgeon usually can give you some idea before operation of the likely range of time you can expect to stay in the hospital; when he has had a chance to observe your progress after operation, he can provide a closer approximation of when you will probably be going home. In the absence of infection or other complications, surgeons almost uniformly now encourage early activity and early discharge from the hospital—even discharge in as few as four or five days after operations that just a few years ago were thought to demand at the very least two weeks of complete bed rest.

When you're ready to go home, your surgeon may tell you, in effect, that you can be as active as you wish, provided that you don't overtire yourself. Usually, you can expect that the ban against becoming overtired will put some healthy limits on your activity for a few weeks. Before you get home, you may tend to think you have regained far more strength than you really have. For you may not realize that much is done for you in hospital, and what you do have to do for yourself is often more easily done there than at home, including dressing, washing, eating, going to the bathroom.

Don't be surprised if, when you first get home, you feel a letdown and every movement, even the most routine, seems somewhat formidable for the first several days. Some of the feeling of lethargy and fatigue may be psychologically rooted. If you recognize that it is not necessarily abnormal but rather almost predictable, that will help you get over it. Your mental state will also improve as you gradually regain your physical vitality, which does take time after surgery, especially major surgery. What activity you can accomplish without becoming overtired will be to the good.

Your surgeon will undoubtedly give you instructions about diet, any prescriptions you may need, and suggestions about bathing, exercises, and other matters. He will indicate before you go home or at some point later—and if not you can ask —when you can resume specific activities such as driving, and when you may best return to work full-time.

Physical Therapy

Many patients require no physical therapy at all. Some are helped by passive movement of joints in the early days after surgery. After some operations, in which important muscles may have had to be disturbed or removed, there may be need for extensive muscle reeducation.

After extensive breast surgery, for example, in which muscles at the front of the shoulder may be removed, reeducation of muscles is important. Shown how to begin to do simple exercises in the hospital and to carry on with them at home, many patients are able within a few months to use remaining muscles not only to carry on all normal routine activities but also to engage in tennis, bowling, golfing, swimming, and other sports activities.

Extended physical therapy, provided by a specially trained technician called a therapist or by a physician trained as a physiatrist, may be needed to restore muscle strength and avoid joint stiffness after some orthopedic operations and may be of great value after some other operations as well.

Radiology

Until 1895 when X-rays were discovered by Wilhelm Conrad Roentgen, a German physicist who received the first Nobel prize for physics for his work, nobody had ever "seen" inside the human body without surgery. Today, almost every part of the body can be visualized, and radiology, which uses X-rays, radioactive substances, and other forms of radiant energy, has become a vital branch of medical science, contributing to more certain diagnosis and in some cases to treatment.

Very likely, radiology played an important role in the diagnostic workup that determined your need for surgery. It may be used in the operating room as an aid during the surgical procedure. In some cases it may be used as a supplement to surgery to enhance the effectiveness of treatment.

In its early days, radiology was regarded as good only for visualizing "bones, stones, and bullets." Today, as the result of new radiological procedures, many of them less than twenty years old, more than 800 different disorders can be diagnosed.

Through injection of special contrast materials, including air and gases, virtually every organ in the body can be outlined for X-ray study. The spleen, the bowel, the liver, the kidney, the adrenal glands can be seen. The inside of the heart, the brain's circulatory system, different areas of the brain can be visualized. Brain disturbances—blood clots, blood vessel malformations, tumors—can be detected

418

through use of a special radioactive isotope, technetium 99. Radiologists can see inside joints, visualize the salivary glands with their ducts that have a diameter no greater than that of a hair, and, by injecting a dye into a groin artery, can determine if a liver is cancerous and if the cancer is still localized or has become widespread.

How X-rays Work

Think of firing a shotgun at a wire fence. The fence would stop or deflect some of the buckshot; other shot would get through. Similarly, some X-rays travel right through the body while others are deflected or stopped.

However solid the body may appear, it is partly empty space. Different parts of the body, moreover, vary in density; the air-filled lungs, for example, are much less dense than the bones of the rib cage.

If you could balloon up a body many times normal size, you would be able, with the naked eye, to see through certain empty spaces, see at least a little through areas of low density, and not see at all through other areas of high density. This is what radiation does.

Newer Techniques

One of many significant advances is body section radiography. It can make a single horizontal plane of the body—such as the front part of a lung—be seen without obstruction from organs or bones in front or behind it. For this, a special machine is used to move the X-ray tube and the X-ray film in opposite directions, a maneuver which leaves the single section of the body in focus but blurs other areas.

Many of the most important diagnostic advances of recent years involve the use of contrast media, as we've noted. Such media, substances taken by mouth or injected, can make a specific organ temporarily opaque and therefore make it stand out on X-ray film. These media act much as does milk when it coats the inside of a glass so you cannot see through it.

If brain surgery is under consideration, an opaque solution can be injected into a carotid artery in the neck leading to the brain. The solution moves up through the carotid into brain arteries, allowing them to be visualized on X-ray film, permitting the surgeon to come to a more knowledgeable conclusion about the need for surgery and the exact site of operation. With much the same technique, kidney blood vessels can be visualized as an aid to determining whether a tumor is present.

When an opaque material, barium, is swallowed, the upper portion of the gastrointestinal tract can be visualized; with a barium enema, lower areas of the tract can be studied.

The heart and its blood vessels can be seen with contrast material. Under a local anesthetic, a small incision is made in a blood vessel in an area such as the crease of the elbow. A long, thin flexible tube or catheter is introduced and, as its course is followed on a fluoroscope screen with the aid of a special image-intensifier, the catheter is maneuvered up through the vessel and into the heart itself. The patient feels nothing while this is going on nor when contrast material is injected into the catheter and reaches the heart. X-ray films taken at intervals then can show the heart and blood vessels and in addition can reveal heart activity, the motion of the valves inside the heart, and the flow of blood.

Is a ruptured disk actually present in the spine? Before proceeding to operate, the surgeon wants to see X-rays. By injecting an opaque material into the spinal column and tilting the X-ray table, the surgeon and radiologist, watching a fluoroscope, can see the movement of the material in the spinal canal and how, if a ruptured disk is present, it slows progress of the material.

X-ray equipment is standard in surgical suites. Instant Polaroid X-rays can be developed only a few feet from the operating table so that a surgeon can, for example, quickly double-check bone position before joining broken pieces. During gallbladder surgery, a thin plastic tube can be threaded into the main bile duct and X-ray pictures, called cholangiograms, can be made with the X-ray tube focused straight down into the open abdominal cavity to determine whether a stone may be present in the duct.

The Remarkable New X-ray Scanners

Introduced only as recently as 1973, a new device called an EMI brain scanner is producing a profound change in neuroradiology. And extension of the principle so the whole body can be scanned in the same way promises to mean sweeping changes for the better in the diagnosis of many diseases.

The way the new scanning devices work: Without special preparation, the patient lies down and a water-filled section of equipment goes around head or body and rotates 180 degrees. As it moves, an X-ray beam shoots out to 160 different areas of the head or body and the radiation coming through is picked up by a crystal.

The crystal feeds data on radiation quantity received to a computer which, after instantly solving 28,000 simultaneous equations, turns out a picture. But, unlike conventional X-ray devices which provide only a two-dimensional picture, this is three-dimensional.

The brain scanner shows, among other things, the difference between white and gray matter brain areas (not possible with conventional X-rays); damage to the optic nerve (also never visualized before); brain tumors and blood clots difficult to see with conventional diagnostic techniques.

The brain scanner is costly (more than $300,000) but it provides savings for patients, greater safety, increased likelihood of accurate diagnosis and effective treatment. With it, exposure to X-rays is actually minimal; no dyes, air or gas need to be injected into the brain for visualization; and cost to the patient is less.

The body scanner promises to be even more widely useful. Standard X-rays can picture bones and other hard substances such as gallstones but can show up internal organs only when dyes are used. Without dyes, the body scanner provides even sharper and more detailed pictures of the heart, lungs, kidneys and other organs, exposes the patient to less radiation, is less expensive for the patient (although the cost of the equipment to the hospital runs about half a million dollars), and can be used on an outpatient basis.

The brain scanner has been under successful trials in some eighty major medical centers and hospitals in the United States and it undoubtedly will be purchased and put into use by hundreds of others in coming years. That is also likely to be the case with the even newer whole body scanner.

Radiation Therapy

Radiation is used increasingly for treatment. Sometimes it may be employed in place of surgery, sometimes to supplement surgery.

When X-rays were first discovered, attention was focused on their ability to visualize parts of the body. Then, as investigators experimented, they found that X-rays could be dangerous if not used with care; they could burn an experimenter's hands. Such accidents served to arouse curiosity. If X-rays in large doses could damage tissue, might it not be possible to use them in controlled and carefully directed doses to destroy malignant tissue? It turned out that they did have value for that.

Since World War II, there has been major progress in the therapeutic use of radiology. During the war, scientists interested in splitting atoms built high-powered cyclotrons, betatrons, and linear accelerators—machines that use millions of volts of electricity instead of the mere thousands that X-ray machines use. They also developed radioactive cobalt with the power of millions of volts. The machines and the cobalt speeded up electrons to almost the velocity of light and the high-speed beams could be used to produce megavoltage radiation which differed markedly from previous radiation.

X-rays from previous kilovolt machines concentrated their

most intense power on the skin surface. To try to reach tumors deep within the body, therapists had to be extremely careful and had problems with dosages. To get the rays to the cancer within, they sometimes had to give considerable radiation to the skin, and years ago it was not uncommon for a patient's skin to be severely burned and scarred as the result of efforts to destroy an internal cancer.

But powerful megavoltage beams concentrate below, instead of on the skin, leaving that vital organ unaffected. Therapists can use much more radiation in their efforts to destroy internal cancers and are often much more successful now in doing so. In hospitals where megavoltage therapy is used frequently, severe skin damage rarely if ever occurs.

Nuclear Medicine

Recently nuclear medicine has become a subspecialty of radiology, useful in both diagnosis and treatment.

Nuclear medicine makes use of compounds "tagged" or labeled with radioactive isotopes. An isotope is a chemical element variant. It has the same atomic number, i.e., the same number of nuclear protons, as the standard chemical element, but a different atomic mass, i.e., a different number of nuclear neutrons. Radioactive isotopes may occur naturally or may be produced by bombardment in the nuclear reactor. They are unstable and give off radiation which is similar to X-rays.

Radioactive isotopes in small doses can be administered by mouth, by injection, or by inhalation, and the radiation they give off can be traced with a detector just as radiation in the earth can be located by a Geiger counter. Tracings, called "scans," can show the distribution of the isotope and, in so doing, indicate the condition of an organ, because the concentration of the isotope varies in healthy and diseased tissue.

With radioactive isotopes it has become possible to study organs of the body, such as the liver and thyroid gland, that cannot be seen effectively with X-rays. Their use can also complement standard X-ray examinations of kidneys, bones, brain, and circulatory system.

Radioactive isotopes are also useful in treating thyroid conditions, some forms of leukemia, and other blood diseases.

The Radiologist

There are now more than 7,500 radiologists certified by the American Board of Radiology. After graduation from medical school, the physician who wishes to specialize in the field goes through a three- or four-year residency in radiology, which includes training in diagnostic and therapeutic radiology, radiation physics, radiobiology, and nuclear medicine. A year after completing his residency, he can sit for the board's qualifying examination.

Radiologists practice in hospitals and in private offices. They are assisted by technologists who have completed two-year courses in approved schools of radiologic technology.

When you have a routine X-ray examination, the film in all probability is taken by a technologist but the radiologist "reads" it. For fluoroscopy or more complex procedures, the technologist may assist the radiologist. Radiation therapy may be administered by a technologist under the radiologist's direction and supervision.

Laboratory Tests

Science now has developed more than 300 blood tests alone, and there are scores of other laboratory tests. These tests are relied upon increasingly as aids to diagnosis and also as aids to treatment, including surgical treatment.

Some 53,500 clinical laboratories in the country—7,000 in hospitals, 6,500 operating independently, another 40,000 in in clinics and doctor's offices—perform an estimated 1.4 billion tests annually.

The number of tests is growing at the rate of about 15 percent a year. In one general hospital, the number of tests tripled in a fifteen-year period during which time hospital admissions increased by only 10 percent.

Routine and Special Tests

If you are the usual surgical patient, in general good health for your age despite the specific problem for which you require surgery, you are likely to have only a few preoperative laboratory tests. Some of these may be administered to you because it is the policy in more and more hospitals to require them routinely for all patients on admission. Such tests may include those to uncover previously unsuspected or newly developed high blood pressure or diabetes, for example. They are of great value in uncovering disease early, before much damage has been done and when control may be easiest. In some situations, the results of such tests may influence the way the surgeon goes about the operation and what extra precautions he may take.

If your operation is to be under general anesthesia, your surgeon may think it necessary to have a BUN (blood urea nitrogen) test made. It provides an indication of how well the kidneys are working and can stand up to surgery and anesthesia. If necessary, measures, including use of intravenous fluids, can be used to make you better prepared for operation.

If your problem has caused loss of appetite, vomiting, or diarrhea, your blood can be checked for levels of salt and various minerals such as potassium, calcium, phosphorus, and magnesium, and if these are too low, they can be restored to normal.

During operation, laboratory tests sometimes may be required. If infection, usually in the form of an abscess, is found, a sample of pus from the area can be taken and sent immediately in a test tube to the laboratory, so that the type of causative organism can be determined and the most effective antibiotic can be chosen to combat the infection.

If a tumor is found or sometimes if an abnormal-looking area, perhaps a sore or eroded spot or what appears to be an inflamed and swollen area, is discovered, a laboratory check can determine whether it is benign or malignant. A piece of the suspect tissue is removed and sent to the laboratory where it is quick-frozen, then cut into extremely thin slices for microscopic study by a pathologist. In fifteen minutes or less from the time the tissue is removed—the procedure is called a biopsy—the surgeon will have word about the nature of the tissue, whether benign or malignant.

Explanation of Some Common Tests

Here are a few of the more common of the many hundreds of tests:

Acid phosphatase. This is an enzyme which is normally present in the blood in small quantities. In about two-thirds of patients with cancer of the prostate, the amount in the blood is elevated. Testing of a small sample of blood can be used both to help diagnose prostatic cancer and to determine the effectiveness of treatment (as shown by a fall of acid phosphatase to normal levels).

Alkaline phosphatase. This enzyme occurs in bone, liver, kidney, and other tissues and is present in small amounts in blood. When testing of a sample of blood shows increased levels in the blood, this can be an aid in the diagnosis of a number of disorders such as hepatitis, infectious mononucleosis, cirrhosis of the liver, and some bone diseases.

Albumin, serum. Albumin is one of the principal proteins in the blood. A blood test for it is useful because an abnormally low level of albumin may indicate the possibility of a problem such as chronic infection, kidney disease, or liver damage.

Amylase, serum. When a blood test shows this substance to be elevated in the blood, the patient may have acute pancreatitis, an inflammation of the pancreas.

Bilirubin, serum. Bilirubin is a pigment normally present in the blood in small amounts. When a blood test shows abnormally high levels present, the patient may have liver disease or an anemia.

Bone marrow. The marrow is the soft, spongelike material within bone which serves as a major factory for blood cell production. A sample of bone marrow can be removed with a needle after a local anesthetic is injected. Examination of the marrow is helpful in assessing anemia and other suspected or known blood problems.

BUN (blood urea nitrogen). In this blood test, the amount of urea nitrogen in the blood is determined. Urea nitrogen is a compound of urea and nitrogen, both of which are end products of the body's use of proteins. Normally, the end products are excreted by the kidneys and given off in urine. When the kidneys are affected by disease, they may fail to remove enough of the products from the blood and the BUN test will show an elevated level in the blood. The BUN also may be elevated when there is massive gastrointestinal bleeding or excessive breakdown of proteins in the body such as may occur in infections, untreated diabetes, and some cancers. The BUN level is low in severe liver disease and malnutrition.

CBC (complete blood count). From a sample of blood, a series of laboratory analyses can be made. The numbers of red and white blood cells can be determined. The amount of hemoglobin, the substance which transports oxygen, can be measured. The CBC can be valuable in many ways. An increase in white cells indicates the presence of infection; a decrease may indicate that a drug or chemical is having a damaging effect on the bone marrow where the white cells are produced and its use should be stopped. A decrease in red cells indicates anemia, sometimes the result of chronic bleeding from hemorrhoids, excessive menstruation, or another cause. An increase in red cells may indicate chronic lung or heart disorder. Decreased hemoglobin indicates anemia, which may be due to excessive blood loss, or simply to inadequate dietary intake of iron which is needed to form hemoglobin.

Cholesterol, serum. An excess of cholesterol in the blood is believed to be associated with increased risk of artery disease. When a blood test shows high cholesterol levels, a low cholesterol, low fat diet may be advised. Also, a high cholesterol sometimes may be associated with kidney disease, hypothyroidism or underfunctioning of the thyroid gland, pancreatitis, an inflammation of the pancreas, or diabetes. Thus, it indicates the need for further tests to determine if any are present and require treatment.

Creatinine, serum. Creatinine is a nitrogenous compound formed in small amounts in muscle. It passes into the blood and is carried to the kidneys for excretion in the urine. Small amounts may normally be present in the blood, but large amounts indicate that kidney function may be disturbed.

Cystoscopy. A cystoscope is a hollow metal tube which can be passed into the bladder through the urethra, the canal extending from the bladder to the outside of the body. At the end of the instrument, there is a light to illuminate the bladder interior and by means of special lenses and mirrors the bladder can be examined for inflammation, stones, or tumors. A catheter or tube can be passed through the cystoscope into the bladder or, if necessary, beyond, into ureters and kidneys to obtain samples of urine for diagnostic purposes. Also, contrast materials, or dyelike substances, can be injected into the bladder or ureters for X-ray films of the urinary tract.

Cytology. This is the study under the microscope of body cells in order to detect malignant changes. In *cervical* cytology, also known as the Pap smear, the cells are in fluid obtained from the uterine cervix. In *gastric* cytology, the cells are in juice obtained from the stomach by means of a stomach tube. In *sputum* cytology, the cells in the sputum are examined.

Frozen tissue section. A specimen of tissue removed during surgery can be quick-frozen, cut by a fine knife into a thin section, stained, then viewed immediately under the microscope for rapid diagnosis of possible cancer. It gives the surgeon immediate information which may determine how the operation should proceed.

GI (gastrointestinal) bleeding. Chronic small-scale gastrointestinal bleeding may not be obvious. But by injecting radioactively-labeled red blood cells, such bleeding can be detected when radioactivity appears in the stool.

Glucose, serum. Glucose is a sugar into which carbohydrates in the diet—sugars and starches—are converted after digestion, and it is a normal constituent of the blood. When a blood sample is taken two hours after eating, the glucose level can be measured to see if it is normal. A higher-than-normal level may indicate the possibility of diabetes or, rarely, other diseases such as an overactive thyroid gland or overactive pituitary gland. A lower-than-normal level may indicate the possibility of underactive gland functioning, kidney or liver disorder, or excessive insulin administration in the treatment of diabetes.

Glucose tolerance. When diabetes is suspected or is suggested by the serum glucose test, a special test, the glucose tolerance test, is used. A definite amount of glucose is given in a carbonated drink or other palatable preparation and at hourly intervals for the next several hours blood samples are taken and blood glucose levels are measured. Abnormal levels help to confirm the diagnosis of diabetes.

LDH (lactic dehydrogenase). LDH is an enzyme found in various body tissues. It appears in the blood in increased amounts when these tissues are severely injured. A study of LDH in a blood sample can be helpful in the diagnosis of a heart attack and of disorders of liver, lung, muscle.

Pheochromocytoma screening. A pheochromocytoma is an adrenal gland tumor, which is usually benign, not cancerous. It produces hypertension, or high blood pressure, and may also produce other symptoms such as severe headache, sweating, and visual blurring. A test for the presence in the urine of certain specific substances such as vanillylmandelic acid helps in the detection of pheochromocytoma.

PBI (protein-bound iodine). The thyroid gland secretes a hormone, thyroxine, which contains iodine which is bound to blood proteins. Measurement of the amount of protein-bound iodine in a sample of blood helps to determine whether the thyroid gland is functioning normally or abnormally. In hypothyroidism, or underfunctioning of the gland, the amount of protein-bound iodine in the blood is below normal. In hyperthyroidism, or overfunctioning of the gland, the blood level of protein-bound iodine is above normal.

Proctoscopy. The proctoscope is an instrument designed to be passed through the anus for inspection of the lower part of the intestine. Such an examination is usually done prior to rectal surgery and it may be part of the physical examination of patients with hemorrhoids, rectal bleeding, or other symptoms of rectal disorder.

SGOT (*serum glutamic oxaloacetic transaminase*). SGOT is an enzyme normally present in the blood and in various tissues, especially the heart and liver. Because the level in the blood rises in some heart, liver, and muscle diseases, and also after use of some drugs such as aspirin, codeine, and cortisone, measurement of the amount of the enzyme in a blood sample can be valuable in diagnosis. After a heart attack, for example, the level goes up, usually in about twelve hours, then return to normal in four to seven days. The level also may rise when the heart muscle is inflamed as the result of rheumatic fever or viral or bacterial infection. It is also increased greatly with liver damage from hepatitis or carbon tetrachloride poisoning and is high in some forms of muscular dystrophy, and moderately high in infectious mononucleosis and cirrhosis of the liver.

Scanning procedures. Various materials, called radioactive isotopes, are available. When specific isotopes are injected, they have the ability, to concentrate in specific organs or tissues such as brain, kidney, or thyroid gland. They give off emissions which can be picked up by an instrument and which help show the size and shape of a specific organ and whether it is functioning normally or abnormally.

Stool examinations. Studies of the stool can provide much information of value in diagnosis. Blood streaking may indicate a local disturbance such as hemorrhoids. When blood in stool is tarry black, the indication is that the blood, digested on the way down, has come from the upper gastrointestinal tract, perhaps the stomach or duodenum. A foamy stool may indicate a pancreatic disturbance. Studies under the microscope may sometimes reveal amoebas, bacilli, worms or worm eggs or segments, or other disease organisms as causes of trouble.

Urinalysis. Several valuable tests are performed on a urine sample. Urine is commonly acid. A bladder or other infection may make it alkaline. The specific gravity—the weight of urine compared to the weight of water—provides a clue to kidney function. If the urine is too watery, with low specific gravity, the kidneys may be doing a poor job of concentrating wastes. If the urine is too heavy, diabetes or kidney inflammation may be present. Acetone is a compound produced in abnormal amounts in diabetes and its presence in the urine suggests that disease. If albumin is found in the urine, it may indicate malfunction of the kidney, heart failure, or toxic conditions. The presence of blood in the urine suggests damage to tissues somewhere along the urinary tract. The appearance of pus cells indicates infection in the urinary system, as does the presence of bacteria or other organisms. If the bile pigment, bilirubin, appears in the urine, it may indicate liver disease or obstruction of the bile ducts leading from the liver or gallbladder.

The Progress of Surgery and Recent Advances That May Help You

Some Background on the History of Surgery

Surgery has come very far very fast. There were crude attempts among the ancients to treat superficial wounds and bone fractures. But modern surgery, going far beyond the superficial, may well have begun to emerge only in 1809 in the small town of Danville, Kentucky, when Emphraim Mc-Dowell operated on Jane Todd Crawford for the removal of a huge ovarian cyst.

McDowell had no medical degree. A good medical education at that time ideally consisted of one or more years, if possible, in a medical school and a medical preceptorship under a good practitioner. McDowell studied under a Staunton, Virginia, physician, Alexander Humphreys, and then spent two years at the University of Edinburgh. In 1795 he entered practice in Danville.

In December, 1809, McDowell was called to see a Mrs. Crawford in a small town sixty-three miles from Danville. She was forty-five, had a large and growing abdominal tumor and pain. Her doctors thought she was pregnant and unable to have the baby. After a careful examination, McDowell concluded she was not pregnant but had a large ovarian cyst.

433

In concluding that the cyst was operable and that he should try to remove it, McDowell made a decision which changed the course of surgical history. It was the uniform opinion of authorities then that to open the abdomen meant death due to inevitable infection and peritonitis.

McDowell explained to Mrs. Crawford what he was certain she had and that what he had to offer as the only alternative to a long and painful illness ending in death had never been done before. With remarkable courage under the circumstances, Mrs. Crawford said simply: "Doctor, I am in your hands."

She was to come to McDowell's home in Danville for the operation. She made the three-day-trip on horseback, resting her bulging lower abdomen on the pommel of the saddle. On Christmas Day, McDowell operated, making a 9-inch-long incision in the left lower abdomen. There was no anesthetic. The cyst was too large to get through the incision and the surgeon had to cut into it and withdraw 15 pounds of fluid before he could remove the ovary, which still weighed 7½ pounds.

The operation would almost certainly have been deadly in the hospitals of Europe. Those hospitals were known as "pest houses," where infection was rampant and surgeons kept their operating coats, covered and soaked with blood and pus from previous patients, hung on pegs in the operating room—never cleaning them because the more blood and pus the more obvious the great experience of the surgeon. But there was no infection in McDowell's house. Five days later, the patient was up and making her bed, and she lived for thirty more years.

McDowell's work—before long he had done a dozen other ovary operations with only four deaths—led to the development of intra-abdominal surgery which ultimately covered all organs. Following the advent of anesthesia in 1842 and later the discovery of antisepsis by Lister, surgery could begin to blossom, but it took time.

An interesting record of what surgery consisted of late in the nineteenth century is in a report made by a committee of physicians in 1886 to the Texas State Medical Association. The report covers 4,293 surgical procedures. Almost all were for lesions on the surface of the body: there was not a single appendectomy or gallbladder operation, and only two on the thyroid.

The records of Charity Hospital in New Orleans for 1888 show thirty amputations of the extremities, eight hernia repairs, two hysterectomies, three ovary operations, and five breast operations. Only three abdominal operations other than gynecologic were recorded, all three for penetrating wounds of the abdomen. There were no gallbladder operations, no appendectomies, no colon or gastric operations.

In just the last several decades surgery has had its greatest growth and development, thanks to more effective methods of preoperative preparation and postoperative care, and also thanks to vastly improved techniques of anesthesia and support for the patient during operation, because they have removed the need for desperate hurry.

And within very recent years, there has been a whole series of other major advances, one or more of which may be applicable to your operation.

Microsurgery

The inability of the human eye to pick out fine detail in very small objects has been a limiting factor in many areas of surgery, including the reconstruction of small blood vessels and nerves.

To try to surmount this limitation, surgical investigators began to experiment years ago with a variety of magnifying glasses and ocular loupes. But these were unsatisfactory. The magnification was too low. After much work, a binocular surgical dissecting microscope was developed. With a 6- to 40-power magnification, it proved highly satisfactory in repeated animal experiments. In their early trials with it, Dr. Julius H. Jacobson II and his coworkers at Mount Sinai Hospital in New York were able to ream out clogged sections of neck arteries in dogs. These researchers were working in areas measuring three to four millimeters in diameter.

Otologists, that is, ear specialists, were among the first to use microsurgery in human patients. It is estimated that without the microscope, 80 percent of ear surgery now successfully performed couldn't even be attempted. The operating microscope has permitted reconstruction of the middle ear, with its eardrum and three tiny bones that transmit sound vibrations to the inner ear. It has allowed surgeons to remove acoustic nerve tumors and tumors of the pituitary gland at the base of the brain. It is being used increasingly now for delicate surgery on the brain and nervous system, to repair nerves damaged by birth injuries, and to help babies with congenital cysts at the base of the spine.

For use in microsurgery, special suture materials almost invisible to the eye—one-quarter the thickness of a human hair—have been developed. So delicate are the sutures that a surgeon can put more than thirty stitches along a ¾"-incision in an artery only 1/10" in diameter.

Whereas once, when confronted with an injured nerve, a surgeon could only sew up the outer sheath around the nerve and hope that the tiny fibers inside would line themselves up, now he can see the fibers and can join their ends so that they align properly.

Power Instruments

High-speed surgical power tools now available not only speed surgery and decrease anesthesia time, which is all to the good; they are so precise that they virtually eliminate risk of accidentaly cutting a blood vessel, and so maneuverable that some operations once considered almost impossible now can be performed routinely.

There are power drills to help in reconstructing hips damaged by arthritis or injury; power saws to get through bone and tissue with care; planelike devices for stripping off skin to be grafted; rasplike devices for filing off skin blemishes; and many others. Most are powered by compressed gas, thus keeping them spark-free. They are far lighter and smaller than home workshop tools and have infinitely more sensitive controls. Some of the tools cost as much as $800 each.

As an indication of how precise the tools can be, one of them is capable of cutting off a section of the shell of a raw egg without damaging the membrane immediately beneath.

Pediatric Surgery

Someone once said it well: "The adult may safely be treated as a child but the converse can lead to disaster."

To meet the needs of children, pediatric surgery has developed as a special field.

The primary concern of pediatric surgeons has been and continues to be malformations in the newborn, congenital anomalies that once were uniformly fatal. A surgeon undertaking the treatment of a four-pound premature infant with an imperforate anus or absence of the normal opening of the rectum, for example, needs to know the types of this deformity, other anomalies that may be associated with it, the proper operation and the correct timing. He must be comfortable and expert with miniature instruments and tiny structures.

Where not very long ago physicians trying to treat major congenital anomalies anticipated only failure, today they assume success. Since 1950, pediatric surgery has advanced to such an extent that survivors of some of the most life-endangering defects, including absence of normal intestinal and esophageal openings, have increased from 35 percent to 80 percent, and in most cases functioning is normal. Pediatric surgical advances also include increasingly effective methods of helping older children, some with conditions that only occur in their age groups and are rarely seen by experienced general surgeons, and some with other conditions that occur in adults but manifest themselves differently in children.

In the last twenty-five years or so, there has been a tenfold increase in the number of surgeons primarily interested in children's surgery. Initially, pediatric surgeons were almost entirely to be found in children's hospitals. Now pediatric surgeons who have graduated from children's hospital programs are to be found in most medical centers.

Hypothermia

Hypothermia means low temperature. And *induced* hypothermia—deliberate lowering of body temperature—is now being used for some types of surgery. It is based on the principle that lowered temperature enables living tissue to survive with very little oxygen for a short time. The time can be long enough to allow surgery for which the interruption of blood circulation is essential.

Hypothermia was used, for example, for a three-month-old child with a congenital heart defect which was draining her life away. Doctors gave her, at best, only a few weeks to live. There seemed very little chance that she could tolerate the heart-lung machine.

Because her condition was so grave, a surgical team decided to try open-heart surgery to repair the heart defect without using the machine. Instead, they used a technique of body cooling.

The child was anesthetized, placed on a plastic sheet, lowered into a cooling tank where she floated on ice water. Bags of crushed ice were packed around her. When her rectal temperature reached 78° F, she was removed from the tank and placed on the operating table. Her temperature continued to go down until it reached 68°. At this point an injection was used to stop her heart. And for thirty-two minutes, while surgeons corrected the defect inside the heart, it remained still. Then it was restarted. Now three years old, the girl is healthy, lively, growing normally, and has an IQ of 140!

Deep body cooling, used successfully in other infants requiring corrective surgery for heart defects, promises to have other applications.

Brain surgery may be aided. The brain's large endowment of blood vessels and its exquisite sensitivity to arrest of circulation have limited brain operations in many cases to those that can be performed within four minutes and preferably less.

Profound cooling, or hypothermia, slows brain metabolism and thus provides protection against damaging effects from circulation arrest. To achieve it, additional cooling techniques may be coupled with surface cooling.

In one method, for example, after the body is cooled, a tube is inserted into a neck artery and a salty liquid at freezing temperature is pumped in slowly. Much of the cold liquid flows up through the brain, dropping the temperature to as low as 59° F.; the rest of it flows down to the heart, liver, kidneys and spinal cord, further cooling and protecting these organs during the time blood flow is stopped.

The supercold flush makes the brain tissues firm, and because there is no blood, surgeons do not have to clamp off delicate blood vessels. When the operation is completed, the heart is restarted electrically.

Such hypothermia has been used with some promise in patients terminally ill with brain cancer. It may help patients with less far-advanced brain tumors and may aid the surgical repair of brain blood vessels that have ballooned or burst.

Laser Surgery

Lasers—devices that can produce small, nondivergent, extremely intense light beams—have been finding increasing use as surgical tools.

Super-powerful laser beams have been used by eye surgeons to repair detached retinas. More recently, they have also been found useful in destroying some skin cancers.

Still more recently, there have been encouraging early results in a series of more than 100 patients for whom the carbon dioxide laser has been used to remove growths on vocal cords—polyps, cysts, and cancers.

The first step in the procedure is insertion of a tube to

provide line-of-sight access to the vocal cords. With the aid of a binocular microscope and a tiny beam of normal white light, the laser is aimed through the tube. By stepping on a foot pedal, the surgeon then can open a shutter on the laser and allow the beam to strike the diseased tissue for as little as one-tenth or as long as one-half of a second. With several such bursts, the beam vaporizes the tissue on which it is focused while simultaneously cauterizing nearby blood vessels so there is no bleeding. Because of the high accuracy, neighboring healthy tissue remains undamaged.

Laser operations have proven to be free of discomfort for patients. Most patients are able to eat, drink, and talk in a whisper shortly after the anesthetic wears off and to leave the hospital the following day.

Cryosurgery

Cryosurgery—the destruction of diseased tissue by extreme cold—has lent itself to a wide variety of uses, from removing tonsils to treating malignancies, and new uses for it are being reported often.

Cryosurgery is performed with an instrument called the cryoprobe—a hollow tube connected to a source of liquid nitrogen, which can be stored at temperatures far below zero. The probe is insulated throughout except at its tip. With a valve to control the flow of liquid nitrogen through the tube, the surgeon can cool the tip to any temperature down to $-196°$ C.

One advantage of the cryoprobe is that it freezes only the tissue of the specific target site, not the surrounding area. Tissue only about 1/25th of an inch away can remain unaffected. Another advantage is that the surgeon can produce temporary numbering only or can destroy the tissue simply by varying temperature and time of application. The technique is also bloodless and, if not entirely painless, produces less discomfort than other surgical methods.

Among the conditions for which cryosurgery has been reported to be promising are the following:

Vascular tumors. These growths filled with blood vessels may be difficult to treat with conventional surgery because of the possibility of profuse bleeding. Freezing tends to close the blood vessels.

Cervicitis. Women who suffer from this often-persistent infection that produces discomfort and annoying discharge often benefit from cryosurgery. They usually go home from the hospital the next day; there is no bleeding; and complete uncomplicated healing is usually experienced within three to five weeks.

Excessive menstrual bleeding. Freezing treatment of the uterine lining has been reported successful in women with menorrhagia (excessive menstrual bleeding) that had not responded to dilation and curettage (D & C)

Pituitary gland conditions. Cryosurgery may be used for reducing secretions of the pituitary gland when this may be helpful in controlling a vision-threatening complication of diabetes, diabetic retinopathy; in palliating advanced breast and prostate cancers; and in relieving the disfiguring condition *acromegaly* produced by runaway pituitary hormone production.

Involuntary movement disorders. Cryosurgery has been used with good results for Parkinson's disease, which produces uncontrollable tremors or muscular rigidity. Under local anesthesia, through a small opening made in the skull, with X-ray guidance the cryoprobe is moved toward the thalamus area of the brain. There the probe-tip temperature is lowered to slightly below 0° C. to numb but not destroy the target area in the thalamus. The patient is then asked to raise an arm and make other movements. If the probe is precisely on target, tremor will be gone. If not, the probe can be shifted slightly. Then the temperature is lowered to −70° C. and the trouble spot is quickly destroyed. Cryosurgery has also proved valuable in treating involuntary movement disorders in children, including dystonia, which produces writhing movements.

Eye conditions. The cryoprobe has been used to aid in the removal of cataractous lenses, to reattach detached retinas, and to treat dendritic keratitis, an ulceration of the cornea or window of the eye.

Cancer. There have been reports of promising results in some cases of cancer of the skin, tongue, mouth, bone, rectrum, and prostate. With freezing, malignant tissue may die and be sloughed off in a few days and there may be little or no disfigurement. Results of cryosurgical treatment of early cancer of the cervix are reported to be excellent.

Hemorrhoids. Developed some years ago, a rubber-band method of hemorrhoid treatment that could be used in a doctor's office involved slipping a special band over a hemorrhoid with a special instrument; with nothing further done, the band eventually caused the hemorrhoid to disintegrate and the band dropped off with it. More recently, a cryoprobe has been used to freeze the hemorrhoid after banding. The hemorrhoid then disintegrates faster and there is even less discomfort. With freezing, too, it is often possible to deal with more than a single hemorrhoid in a session.

Fetal Surgery

Surgery today is beginning to gain the ability to operate, when necessary, on an unborn child in the womb.

A few years ago, at a university medical center, a thirty-one-year-old woman who had previously suffered eight miscarriages and was seven months pregnant, again faced the loss of another baby. The only hope was an operation attempted only a few times before and never successfully.

The attending surgeon made a 6-inch incision from the woman's navel to an area over the urinary bladder, exposing a large area of the uterus. He then made a 1½-inch opening in the uterine wall and through this small aperture looked down into the amniotic sac, the thin capsule surrounding the baby. Opening the capsule, he dipped forceps into the waters within the capsule and brought up a fetal leg only a few inches long. Near the baby's groin he inserted a tiny tube into a vein and through this removed most of the baby's blood. Because of Rh disease, produced when an Rh-negative woman bears an Rh positive baby as the result of mating with an Rh-positive husband, vital red cells in the baby's blood had been attacked by antibodies from the mother's bloodstream. As a result of the attack, the baby was so anemic that she would have died *in utero*.

After withdrawing the baby's blood, the surgeon trans-fused, through the same tube, new blood rich in red cells. After that, the tube was removed, the incision in the baby's groin closed, the leg gently replaced in the amniotic fluid. Three weeks later a live baby girl was born, one month premature, still slightly anemic but not nearly as much so as three weeks before. Now, four years later, the little girl is healthy and normal in every respect.

Today the Rh problem can be treated in other ways. A special serum can be given to an Rh-negative mother to help prevent antibody formation.

But the procedure developed to combat the Rh problem surgically, along with other new procedures, may permit help for other problems of still-unborn babies. It is expected that fetal surgery can be applied to repairing heart and blood vessel defects, diaphragmatic hernias that may lead to lung malformation, fetal tumors, hearing defects, and hydroceph-alus, a disorder in which fluid concentrates in the head and may damage the brain.

One of many tools recently developed, for example, is a fiberoptic amnioscope, a viewing device that looks inside the womb and channels light to a particular site. The fetus swallows amniotic fluid, and surgeons have been able recent-ly to inject an X-ray contrast material into the fluid which then allows visualization of the fetus's tiny gastrointestinal tract on a fluoroscopic screen.

Outpatient Surgery

In recent years, with the advances in surgery and anesthesiology, it has become increasingly apparent that for some patients undergoing some operations, extended hospital stay is not essential. Any shortening of hospital stay, if it is not damaging in any way to a surgical patient, has many potential benefits. There are, of course, monetary savings. There is less interruption of family life. Out of the hospital and home earlier, encouraged by this very fact to become more active more quickly, patients may even do better, recover faster, find themselves able to go back to work sooner. In the case of children especially, there is less emotional upset.

One pronounced trend is in the direction of outpatient or come-and-go surgery, in which the patient is admitted for only a few hours and does not stay in the hospital overnight.

The idea is not brand-new; some hospitals have performed such surgery in their outpatient departments for years. What is new, however, is the expansion in the number of hospitals offering it and the conditions for which it is being used. About half of all hospitals in the country now have provisions for outpatient surgery. In addition, outpatient units not physically attached to or operated by hospitals are being built.

The American Medical Association recently has endorsed outpatient surgery under general and local anesthesia as good medical practice for "selected procedures in selected patients." At Children's Hospital Medical Center, Boston, no serious complications occurred in the course of almost 5,000 outpatient operations over a three-year period. Reports from other in-and-out surgery units indicate that postoperative complications have been minor, such as nausea after general anesthesia; there is less chance for complications because only relatively minor operations are performed on outpatients. It is also a fact that the total resources of the hospital are available when needed and most independent surgical

THE PROGRESS OF SURGERY

units have arrangements with nearby hospitals for transfer of patients in cases of emergency.

Generally, procedures performed on an outpatient basis involve little loss of blood or postoperative pain. Among the operations that may be performed are abortions, removal of tonsils and adenoids, repair of simple hernias, biopsies of tissue from the breast or other body areas for cancer tests, removal of noncancerous cysts and tumors, dilation and curettage (D & C).

Usually, anemic patients or those with chronic heart or blood vessel disease, neurological or endocrine gland disorders or other complicating diseases that are not well controlled are not considered suitable for outpatient surgery. Many surgeons prefer that patients over sixty have surgery on an inpatient basis.

The surgeon who is to perform the operation makes the appointment for outpatient surgery. There are variations in details, but at one outpatient surgery facility, the patient arrives on the scheduled day about 1½ hours before he is to undergo surgery. The receptionist and an anesthesiologist start a medical record. A nurse takes a blood sample. The patient goes to a dressing room and dons a disposable gown and paper foot-covers. His temperature is taken, and heart and lungs are examined by an anesthesiologist. The patient is made comfortable pending arrival of the surgeon and is given reading material or may listen to music through earphones.

Upon arrival of the surgeon, the patient is taken to an operating room. The surgeon scrubs, enters the operating room, performs the operation. The patient is taken to the recovery room, where an anesthesiologist is present until the patient is ready for discharge, usually within 3½ hours of his having entered the facility.

Generally, the saving to the patient is the cost of room and board for an overnight hospital stay. More and more health insurance plans cover the costs for outpatient surgery but many still do not, and a check should be made with the insurance company to make certain.

INDEX

Index

A

Abdominal operations. *See* individual operations and organs

Acids, stomach, 17, 87
  and peptic ulcer, 17-21, 22-23, 25
  regurgitation in hernia, 32, 33
  See also Hydrochloric acid

Adenoidectomy, 198-201
  infection, 198
  surgery, 199-201
    anesthesia, 200-201
    children and, 199-201
    psychological preparation, 201
    recovery from, 200-201
    surgical fee, 376

Adrenal gland, 93-94, 430
  cancer of, 93-94
  hormones in, 93-94

Advisory Board for Medical Specialties, 351

Alcohol
  and leukoplakia, 214
  and liver, 85
  and pancreas, 87
  and peptic ulcer, 19, 25

American Association of Cosmetic Surgeons, 296

American Association of Nurse Anesthetists, 395

American Board of Radiology, 424

American Cancer Society, 193

American College of Surgeons (F.A.C.S.), 340, 344, 350, 352-53

American Dietetic Association, 20

American Heart Association, 19

American Hospital Association, 351, 361, 371

American Medical Association, 346, 351, 360, 444

American Society for Aesthetic Plastic Surgery, 296

American Society of Anesthesiologists, 395

American Society of Plastic and Reconstructive Surgeons, 296

Amputations, 261-63
  phantom pain, 262
  psychological repercussions, 263

Anal fissure, 68-69

449

Anemia
and artificial heart valve, 133
and hemorrhoids, 66
and intestinal cancer, 58, 61
lab tests for, 427
and pancreas, 88
and preoperative care, 388
and spleen, 91
Anesthesia, 336, 389-98
choice of anesthesia, 396-97
choice of anesthetist, 396
forms of, 390-91, 393-96
history of, 389-90, 434-35
improvements in, 336, 436
nitrous oxide, 389, 390, 393
procedures, 391-93, 402, 403-
404
recovery from, 396-97, 411-
15
risks of, 391, 397-98, 404
See also individual operations
Aneurysm, 148-49, 230
Antisepsis, 387, 401-2, 403
Anus. See Anal fissure; Fistula
in ano; Hemorrhoids;
Rectal polyps
Anxiety
and amputations, 263
and cancer, 58, 75-76
how to deal with, 2-7
of parents about children, 9-
10, 54-55
in tonsillectomy and adenoidectomy, 201
in ulcerative colitis, 43
Appendicitis, 28-32
appendectomy, 29-31
anesthesia, 30
fee for, 374-75, 376, 377,
379
postoperative care, 30-31,
364
success rate, 31
causes, 29
complications, 29-30, 31-32
death from, 31-32

diagnosis, 28-29, 31
diet for, 30
pain, 28, 29, 31
vermiform appendix, 28
Arteriosclerosis, 20, 145-47
Artery operations, 145-48
aneurysm, 148
bypass, 146-47
diagnosis of obstruction, 147
endarterectomy, 146
need for surgery, 145-46
See also Heart disease, coronary artery
Arthritis, 253-60
arthrodesis, 256
arthroplasty, 256-57
osteoarthritis, 254, 257
osteotomy, 255
rheumatoid, 254, 255, 257
synovectomy, 254-55
total joint replacement, 257-
60
Arthritis Foundation, 258
Association of American Medical Colleges, 351
Association for Voluntary Sterilization, 320

B

Baldness, 310-12
Barclay, William R., 346
Bile, 16, 77-78, 80, 81, 82, 90,
432
Birthmarks, 313-14
Blacher, Richard S., 5-6
Bladder
cystoscopy, 154, 155-56, 159,
161, 429
function of bladder, 154
stones, 157
tumors, 159-60
cancer, 159-60

eye surgery, 442
hemorrhoids, 442
Parkinson's disease, 441
pituitary gland, 441
Cystoscopy, 154, 155, 159, 161, 429

D

Deviated septum. *See* Nose, deviated septum
Diabetes, 339
laboratory tests for, 428, 430
and pancreas, 86, 89, 90
and peptic ulcer, 19
Diagnostic aids. *See* individual operations; Laboratory tests; Radiology
Diaphragm, 32, 34, 103, 104
Diet and
anal fissure, 68
appendicitis, 30
diverticulitis, 36, 38-39
gallstones, 77-78, 79, 80, 81
ileitis, 45, 46
kidney stones, 156
intestinal cancer, 60, 61
pancreas, 88, 89, 90
peptic ulcer, 19-20, 22, 24-25
preoperative care, 384
See also individual operations
rectal cancer, 73
rheumatic fever, 132
stomach cancer, 57, 58
ulcerative colitis, 42
Digestive tract, 15-17, 19-20, 77, 82, 86-87
See also Esophagus; Intestines; Stomach
Dilation and Curettage (D & C), 169-71
early discharge after, 364

indications of, 169-70
cancer, 169
hormonal disturbance, 169-70
polyps, 169
operation, 170-71
surgical fee, 376
Directory of Medical Specialists, 297
Dislocations, 245-47
elbow, 246
knee, 246
shoulder, 245-46
spine, 247
surgery, 245-47
symptoms, 245-46
Distention in,
abdominal operations, 413
cholecystitis, 79
ileitis, 44, 46
intestinal cancer, 62
intestinal obstruction, 47, 51
megacolon, 52
ulcerative colitis, 42
Diverticulitis, 35-39
and cancer, 37
cause of, 36
diagnosis of, 35-36
diet and, 36, 38-39
medical treatment, 36
need for surgery, 36-37
operation, 36-39
postoperative care, 38
success rate, 38
pain, 35, 36
Doctor's Hospital (Texas), 259
Drugs and medication
for abscessed lung, 111
anesthetic, 390-91, 392-93
for appendicitis, 29, 31
anticholinergic, 19, 24
for boils and carbuncles, 292
for bursitis, 248-49
for cancer, 56, 61, 63, 191
for diverticulitis, 36, 38
for gallstones, 79, 80, 81

H

Hair transplants, 310-12
Harelip. *See* Plastic surgery, cleft lip and palate
Heart defects, congenital
adult, 128
aortic stenosis, 122
atrial septal defect, 120
best time for surgery, 126-27
care for child, 125-28
coarctation of aorta, 119
combination of defects, 125
patent ductus arteriosus, 118-19
pulmonary stenosis, 121-22
surgery, 126-28
convalescence, 128
preparing child for, 127-28
risks, 127
Tetralogy of Fallot (blue baby), 122-24
diagnosis, 123-24
medication, 123
palliative operation, 124
transposition of great vessels, 124-25
ventricular septal defect, 120-21
Heart disease, 133-40, 431
coronary artery, 136-40
angina pectoris, 136-37
bypass, 138, 139-40
causes, 136
cholesterol, 137
medical treatment, 137-38
postoperative care, 139
success rate, 139-40
surgery, 137-40
symptoms, 136, 137
and diet, 19-20
pacemaker surgery, 133-35
effectiveness, 134-35
transthoracic, 134
transvenous, 134

See also Heart defects, congenital; Heart operations
Heart-lung machine, 407-10
and chest surgery, 116
limitations of, 409-10
need for, 409-10
origin, 407-9
use in heart operations, 120-24
Heart operations, 114-40
closed-heart, 115
surgical fee, 376-77
description of heart, 115, 116-17
reaching the heart, 115
open-heart, 116
hypothermia, 438-39
transplant, 321, 322, 326-29
X-ray of, 420
See also Artery operations; Blood vessel surgery; Heart defects, congenital; Heart disease; Heart-lung machine; Rheumatic fever
Hemorrhage
of esophagus, 85
in head injuries, 230-31
of hemorrhoids, 64, 65, 66
of liver, 83
in peptic ulcer, 21
in rectal cancer, 72
in rectal polyps, 70
in ruptured spleen, 91
in ulcerative colitis, 41
of women, 169, 170, 172, 174
Hemorrhoids, 64-68
bleeding of, 64, 65, 66
and cancer, 65
cause of, 64-65
cryosurgery, 442
description of, 64
diagnosis, 65, 428, 431
hemorrhoidectomy, 66-67
anesthesia, 66

bile, 77
biopsy, 82-83
cancer, 84-85, 419
    operation, 85
circulation in, 82, 84, 85-86
cirrhosis of, 85-86, 427, 431
cysts and tumors, 84-85
description of, 82
laboratory tests on, 427, 428, 431
injury of, 83
transplant, 321, 322, 326-29
See also Hepatitis
Lobotomy, 232
Long, Crawford W., 389
Lumpectomy, 191
Lungs, 19-20, 110-14
abscess, 110-11
    diagnosis, 111
    symptoms, 111
bronchiectases, 113
cancer, 113-14
    biopsy, scalene, 113
    bronchoscopy, 113
    fee for removal, 376-77
    surgery, 113-14
    survival rate, 114
    X-ray treatment, 114
chest surgery, 115-17
collapse, 104
cyst, 112
description of, 110, 117
transplant, 321-22, 326-27, 328-29
tuberculosis, 112
    drugs, 112
    thoracoplasty, 112
See also Heart operations; Heart-lung machine; Heart disease; Heart defects, congenital; Rheumatic fever
Lymph nodes, 216-17
breast cancer, 190-91
lung cancer, 113-14
neck surgery, 216-17

stomach cancer, 56
tongue cancer, 215, 216

M

McDowell, Ephraim, 433-34
Male breast, 196-97
    cancer, 197
    enlargement, 196-97
Mammography, 186-87, 190
Massachusetts General Hospital, 258, 259
Mastectomy, 192-94
Mastoidectomy, 281-82
Mayo Clinic, 258, 259
Medical Economics, 374
Medical schools, 360
Megacolon, 52-54
    cause, 53
    diagnosis, 53
    operation, 53-54
        postoperative care, 54
        psychological preparation, 54-55
        recovery, 54
Microsurgery, 278, 435-36
Mucous
    in anus and rectum, 64
    cervical, 180
    in nose, 217-18, 219, 220
    in stomach, 15-16, 19
    in stools, 40
Myringoplasty. *See* Ear surgery, eardrum repair

N

National Board of Medical Examiners, 351
Neck surgery, 216-17

cancer, 216
lymph nodes, 216-17
Nephrectomy, 156, 158-59
Nervous system, 151-52
  See also Brain and nerve surgery
Nose, 217-20
  broken, 220
  deviated septum, 219-20
  surgical fee, 376, 378
  nasal polyps, 219
  sinus operation, 217-19
  sinusitis, 218
  sinus procedure, 218-19
  See also Plastic surgery, nose
Nuclear medicine, 423-24
Nurses, 368-69, 370
  as anesthetists, 395, 396, 398
  in operating room, 402
  private, 414

O

Organs
  hierarchy of importance, 5-6
  removal of, 335
  See also individual organs
  transplants, 321-30
  X-ray study, 418-22
Orthopedic surgery. *See* individual problem
Osteomyelitis, 250-51
Otoplasty, 302
Outpatient treatment, 380, 444-45
Ovary operations, 177-80
  cancer, 178, 179
  cysts, 177-78, 179
  oophrectomy, 179
    postoperative care, 179
    success rate, 179
    limitations, 179
  tumors, benign, 178

P

Pacemakers, 133-35
Pain
  anesthesia and, 389-97, 403
  of aneurysm, 148
  of angina pectoris, 136, 137, 138, 140
  of appendicitis, 28, 29, 31
  of arthritis, 254, 259
  of bladder stone, 157
  of breast surgery, 193
  of bursitis, 248, 249
  of cancer, 89, 109, 164
  children's, 9
  of diverticulitis, 35, 36
  of eardrum, 279
  of frozen shoulder, 249-50
  of gallstones, 78, 80, 81
  of glaucoma, 267
  of hemorrhoids, 64, 65, 68
  of hiatus hernia, 32
  of ileitis, 44
  of intestinal obstruction, 47, 48, 52
  of kidney stones, 155, 156
  in mastoidectomy, 281
  of osteomyelitis, 250
  of ovarian cyst, 178
  of pancreatitis, 87, 88
  of peptic ulcer, 18, 20, 21, 23
  in phantom limb, 262-63
  of rheumatic fever, 129
  of slipped disk, 236, 237
  of spinal column, 235
  of stomach cancer, 55
  of varicose veins, 141
Pancreas, 86-91
  acute pancreatitis, 87-88
  benign tumors, 89-91
  cancer, 89-91
  chronic pancreatitis, 88-89
  diabetes, 86, 89, 90
  laboratory tests on, 427, 428
  pancreatomy, 89
  role in digestion, 16, 86-87

diet, 132
medical treatment, 131-32
mitral valve damage, 129-30, 131, 132
surgery, 132-33
Rhinoplasty. *See* Plastic surgery, nose
Riley Hospital for Children, 9
Roentgen, Wilhelm Conrad, 418

S

St. Luke's Medical Center (Chicago), 325
Salivary glands, 207-8
cancer, 208
stones, 207-8
tumors, 208
Saphenous vein
artery operations, 146
in coronary bypass, 138
in varicose vein surgery, 142-44
Scars
appendectomy, 32
burns, 299
hernia, 34
peptic ulcer, 23-24
plastic surgery, 302, 304, 305, 307, 309, 310
pyloric stenosis, 27
sinus surgery, 218
skin grafting, 297-99
varicose vein, 145
Shoulder, frozen, 249-50
Sigmoidoscope, 59, 60
Sinus operations, 217-19
Skin and superficial tissue surgery, 288-94
boils and carbuncles, 291-92
cancer, 294
description of skin, 288-89
excessive perspiration, 293

lipomas, 292
moles, 290-91
pinched fat, 292-93
sebaceous cysts, 291
warts, 289-90
treatment, 289-90
types, 288
See also Plastic surgery
Slipped disk, 236-38, 345, **376**
Sphincters
cardiac, 16
pyloric, 16, 25, 26-27
rectal, 64, 69, 70, 73
Spinal cord surgery. *See* **Brain** and nerve surgery, **spinal** cord
Spleen
and blood cells, 91
description of, 91-93
removal of, 91, 93
surgical fee, 376, 378
Sterilization, 315-20
vasectomy, 316-17
operation, 316-18
psychological effects **of,** 318
voluntary, 315-16
women's, 318-20
effects, 320
laparoscopy, 318-19
tubal ligation, 318
Stomach, 429, 432
digestion in, 15-16
and hernia, 32, 33, 34
obstruction in infants, **25-27**
and peptic ulcer, 17-24
removal of, 21-22, 24, **25**
subtotal gastrectomy, **fee,** 375, 376
Stomach cancer, 55-58
diagnosis, 55
medical treatment, 56
need for surgery, 55-56
operation, 56-58
limitations after, 58
postoperative care, 57

psychological preparation, 58
removal of stomach, 56-57
success rate, 57-58
Stomach juices. *See* Acid, stomach
Strabismus, 270-72
Stroke, 149-52
cause of, 149
and diet, 19-20
developments in, 149-50
symptoms, 149-50
surgery, 150-51
bypass, 151
sympathectomy, 151-52
Surgeon
checks on, 344, 361-62
choice of, 348-56
connection with hospital, 353, 357
discharging patients, 415-16
ethics of, 341, 343, 345, 378-79
fame of, 353-54
fee of, 373-79, 382-83
general practitioner as, 355-56
getting information from, 3-8
male chauvinism of, 354-55
number of, 342
pediatric, 437-38
plastic, 295-97
and preoperative care, 384-88
qualifications of, 346-47, 348, 352-53
rapport with, 44, 354
training of, 336, 344, 349-51
the Boards, 350-51
See also Surgery
Surgery
advances in, 435-45
cryosurgery, 440-42
fetal surgery, 442-43
hypothermia, 438-39
laser surgery, 339-40
microsurgery, 435-36

power instuments, 436-37
alternatives to, 345, 346
See also individual problems
blood transfusions, 405-7
hepatitis, 406-7
matching, 406
on children, 8-11, 333, 437-39
elective, 338, 340-41
emergency, 338-39, 340
function of, 335
by general practitioners, 355-56
history of, 433-35
anesthesia, 434-35
margin of safety, 337
mortality rates, 335-36
necessity of, 340-47, 362
number of operations in U.S., 333
operating room, 399-410
antisepsis, 401-2, 403
equipment, 399-400
heart-lung machine, 408-10
operating team, 402-3
preoperative care, 384-88
procedure, 402-4
risk, 335-36, 345-46, 362
second opinions on, 340, 345, 346-47
surgical scrubbing, 387, 400-402
tissue review, 344, 361-62
total care, 348-49
types of, 351-52
See also Anesthesia; Costs; Hospital, individual operations; Postoperative care; Preoperative care; Surgeon

T

Testicle, undescended, 100-101